Health Education

Creating Strategies for School and Community Health

THIRD EDITION

Glen G. Gilbert, PhD
East Carolina University

Robin G. Sawyer, PhD
University of Maryland, College Park

Elisa Beth McNeill, MS
Texas A&M University

JONES AND BARTLETT PUBLISHERS

Sudbury, Massachusetts

BOSTON   TORONTO   LONDON   SINGAPORE

World Headquarters
Jones and Bartlett Publishers
40 Tall Pine Drive
Sudbury, MA 01776
978-443-5000
info@jbpub.com
www.jbpub.com

Jones and Bartlett Publishers
Canada
6339 Ormindale Way
Mississauga, Ontario L5V 1J2
Canada

Jones and Bartlett Publishers
International
Barb House, Barb Mews
London W6 7PA
United Kingdom

Jones and Bartlett's books and products are available through most bookstores and online booksellers. To contact Jones and Bartlett Publishers directly, call 800-832-0034, fax 978-443-8000, or visit our website, www.jbpub.com.

Substantial discounts on bulk quantities of Jones and Bartlett's publications are available to corporations, professional associations, and other qualified organizations. For details and specific discount information, contact the special sales department at Jones and Bartlett via the above contact information or send an email to specialsales@jbpub.com.

Production Credits
Acquisitions Editor: Shoshanna Goldberg
Senior Associate Editor: Amy L. Bloom
Editorial Assistant: Kyle Hoover
Production Manager: Julie Champagne Bolduc
Associate Production Editor: Jessica Steele Newfell
Associate Marketing Manager: Jody Sullivan
V.P., Manufacturing and Inventory Control: Therese Connell
Composition: Auburn Associates, Inc.
Cover Design: Scott Moden
Senior Photo Researcher and Photographer: Christine Myaskovsky
Cover Images: (top) © Monkey Business Images/Dreamstime.com; (middle) © Monkey Business Images/ShutterStock, Inc.; (bottom) © Monkey Business Images/ShutterStock, Inc.
Printing and Binding: Malloy, Inc.
Cover Printing: Malloy, Inc.

Library of Congress Cataloging-in-Publication Data
Gilbert, Glen G. (Glen Gordon), 1946–
  Health education : creating strategies for school and community / Glen G. Gilbert, Robin G. Sawyer, Elisa Beth McNeill. — 3rd ed.
      p. cm.
  Includes bibliographical references and index.
  ISBN 978-0-7637-5929-2 (pbk. : alk. paper)
  1. Health education—United States. I. Sawyer, Robin G. II. McNeill, Elisa Beth. III. Title.
  RA440.5.G48 2010
  613—dc22

                                                    2009031529

6048
Printed in the United States of America
13 12 11 10 09   10 9 8 7 6 5 4 3 2 1

We dedicate this book to
Rosemarie, Jessica Rose, Jennifer Evelyn, and Jeffrey Daniel Gilbert;
Anne Anderson-Sawyer and Katherine, Emily, Meg, and Gillian Sawyer;
and Cal, Molly, Jace, and Micah McNeill and Eugenia Williams.

Brief Contents

Contents

Chapter 3   **CONTEXTUAL CONSIDERATIONS FOR BEHAVIOR
CHANGE: INTERVENTION/METHOD SELECTION   47**

| **Chapter 4** | **METHODS OF INSTRUCTION/INTERVENTION** | **97** |

Chapter 5   **PRESENTATION AND UNIT PLAN DEVELOPMENT**   **185**

Chapter 6   PERSONAL COMPUTERS AND THE INTERNET   221

**Chapter 7   USE OF MEDIA IN HEALTH EDUCATION:
LITERACY, SELECTION, MARKETING,
DEVELOPMENT, AND EQUIPMENT   251**

Chapter 8   MINORITY HEALTH   287

Foreword

If a second edition of a college textbook signals its survival and utility in the classroom, a third edition marks the true measure of its success. Textbook authors often receive a second chance from their publishers on the grounds that they may have missed the mark with a first edition, but, if the second edition's revisions fail to capture or maintain a defensible share of the "market" (as measured by professors' decisions to adopt the book), it is toast. In the case of a book on health education methods and strategies, authors have the added burden of convincing the most critical audience of adopters: professors whose main expertise lies in the very subject of the book, both in content knowledge and professional preparation and practice.

With *Health Education: Creating Strategies for School and Community Health*, Glen Gilbert, Robin Sawyer, and Beth McNeill have not only survived these rigors of natural selection, but they have proved to be among the fittest chroniclers of the growing science and technological sophistication of health education methods and strategies for school and community health. I am impressed with their commitment to the concept that *best practices* in health education are *best processes*. They inherently apply the diagnostic approach that recognizes no inherent superiority in specific methods but recognizes the need to match the features of methods and strategies with the audience, purpose, and conditions of the educational application. They take this a step further in their position that a good strategy—created with good methods arrayed in a good plan—is only as good, ultimately, as its effective delivery. It is the "doing" of education, they argue, that makes a good educational diagnosis and a good educational plan good health education. They seek not only to inform students who take a course in this subject area but to inspire them by example from the pages of this book.

Lawrence W. Green, DrPH
Professor, Department of Epidemiology and Biostatistics
School of Medicine
University of California at San Francisco
Former Director, Office of Health Information and Health Promotion
U.S. Department of Health and Human Services

Preface

The philosophy presented in *Health Education: Creating Strategies for School and Community Health, Third Edition*, is based in the premise that the core of health education is the process of health education. There are many tools for health educators, such as epidemiology, statistics, and program planning, but what is truly unique about a health educator is the focus on "doing." To be an effective health educator, you must be skilled in conducting health education. As educators we may have access to the best knowledge available, but unless we are skilled and effective deliverers of this information, the usefulness of our work is clearly compromised.

This text is dedicated to the proposition that we must be good at the doing. Further, it is our belief that health educators need a more systematic approach to the selection of methods of intervention. This text assists health educators in reducing the possibility of a poor performance by encouraging the systematic development of sound, effective, and appropriate presentation methods.

Health Education: Creating Strategies for School and Community Health, Third Edition, is designed for any health educator or would-be health educator who wishes to become proficient in conducting health education programs. We strongly believe that the skills necessary to successfully plan for and deliver effective health education programs are fundamentally the same regardless of where they are practiced—in classroom, workplace, hospital, or community settings. The principles of sound methodology remain constant; therefore, this text is designed for multiple settings. It addresses the needs of the so-called "generic" health educator and provides the tools necessary for making appropriate programming decisions based on the needs of the clients and the educational settings.

A variety of learning aids are incorporated into this text. Each chapter contains health educator competencies, learning objectives, case studies (with new objectives and questions to consider), exercises, and a summary. Also included in this text are a glossary, a professional resource list, and up-to-date references.

This *Third Edition* demonstrates the evolving state of health education. Additions have been made to develop the reader's skills in writing measurable performance indicators. The unique qualities of adult learners are discussed, and tips to enhance the implementation of the various methods are offered. Included are updates on the use of technology in health education classrooms as well as an expansion of the content on health literacy. All chapters have been updated and include Internet references, allowing instructors and students to easily access current information.

Using the Jones and Bartlett website (http://healtheducation.jbpub.com/strategies) will increase the rewards for using this text. On the website, instructors will find PowerPoint presentations, test questions, teaching tips, and worksheets.

Responding to user requests, Objectives and Questions to Consider have been added to the case studies. Responses to each case study are located at the end of each chapter, appearing under "Case Studies Revisited." This affords the reader the opportunity to critically consider the case at hand before reading the authors' responses. This edition continues to feature the "Noteworthy" section, which includes relevant stories related to the chapter content.

We know that a good text must fulfill the user's needs. We constantly seek to improve *Health Education: Creating Strategies for School and Community Health*, and we look forward to hearing from students, instructors, and professionals who may have a comment, an idea, or a suggestion.

Acknowledgments

The authors wish to give special thanks to the reviewers of this edition: Debra L. Bakker, Calvin College; Lillian Cook Carter, Towson University; Retta Evans, University of Alabama at Birmingham; Ying Li, Western Washington University; Laura Miller, Edinboro University of Pennsylvania; Katherine Sharp, University of Maryland; and Christine Unson, Southern Connecticut State University.

We also would like to acknowledge the reviewers of past editions: Jill Black, Springfield College; Loren Bensley, Central Michigan University; Lynn Bloomberg, Worcester State College; Michael Cleary, Slippery Rock University; Lyndall Ellingson, California State University at Chico; Gerald S. Fain and Karen Liller, University of South Florida; Onie Grosshans, University of Utah; John Janowiak, Appalachian State University; Barbara J. Richards and B.E. Pruitt, Texas A&M University; and Katina Sayers, West Virginia University.

A special thank you goes to Eugenia Williams, a dear friend and the mother-in law of Beth McNeill, for the hours of text review and the non-sparing use of her red pen.

We would like to thank Carol Jackson, Sandy Walter, Robert Gold, Lawrence Green, Gail Jacobs, Fran Gover, Bev Monis, Rosemarie Taylor, Jennifer Morrone-Joseph, Susan Karchmer, and Judy Patek.

We thank our many students over the years at the University of Maryland, East Carolina University, University of Virginia, Portland State University, University of North Carolina at Greensboro, Texas A&M University, South Eugene High School, Colin Kelly Junior High School, Penge High School, London and Calverton School, Bryan High School, and the many other schools where we have conducted workshops and classes.

The authors also would like to thank Judy Patek, education administrator, Susan Karchmer, and Jennifer Morrone-Joseph formerly with Gallaudet University for their advice and expertise in writing Chapter 9. Their collective suggestions proved invaluable.

Thank you also to Starr Eaddy of St. Francis College for updating the ancillary materials for the *Third Edition*.

And finally, thanks to the staff at Jones and Bartlett, including Shoshanna Goldberg, Acquisitions Editor; Amy Bloom, Senior Associate Editor; Jessica Newfell, Associate Production Editor; and Jody Sullivan, Marketing Manager.

About the Authors

Glen G. Gilbert

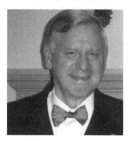

Glen is currently Professor and Dean of the College of Health and Human Performance at East Carolina University. He has taught university-level methods and strategies courses for over 15 years and has conducted in-service and consulting programs throughout the United States. He went on leave from his university post for two years to serve as Director of the School Health Initiative for the U.S. Public Health Service and worked with many state and federal agencies in seeking to plan and achieve the Health Objectives for the Nation. As a former secondary teacher, school teacher, and community health educator, Glen can relate to the real-world needs of health educators. He has authored over 70 professional publications and has taught at East Carolina University, the University of Maryland, Portland State University, the University of North Carolina at Greensboro, and the Ohio State University. He has been a department chair at three universities and served as interim Vice Chancellor of Research and Graduate Studies at ECU. He has been a health educator for over thirty years.

Robin G. Sawyer

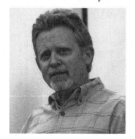

Robin is currently an Associate Professor and Associate Chairperson in the Department of Public and Community Health at the University of Maryland, teaching courses in human sexuality and adolescent health. A native of Great Britain, Robin earned his bachelor's degrees from the University of London and George Mason University, a master's degree from the University of Virginia, and a doctoral degree from the University of Maryland. His areas of research interest include college student contraceptive compliance, sexually transmitted infections, AIDS education, and date rape. He has received 13 national and international film awards for developing sexuality-related media and received numerous university teaching awards. Robin has published extensively and is a nationally known speaker, having made over 450 presentations at schools, colleges, and universities throughout the United States. His teaching gained national attention in the *Washington Post* and, most recently, he has appeared on the *Today Show* and the *Tyra Banks Show* and acted as a consultant for MTV.

Elisa Beth McNeill

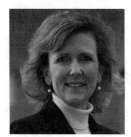

Beth is an Associate Instructional Professor of Pedagogy with the Department of Health and Kinesiology at Texas A&M University. She serves as the coordinator of the Health Education Teacher Certification Program. Beth is a 20-year teaching veteran of public schools, working with middle school, high school, and at-risk pregnant and parenting adolescents. She earned her master's degree and principals certification in Educational Administration. Beth is known for her innovative instruction; she teaches courses in human sexuality, elementary and secondary school health, secondary teaching, community and school health methodology, and first aid. Beth has presented at state, regional, and national conferences with multiple publications. She is currently in the final phase of completing her doctoral degree at Texas A&M University.

Introduction

- Pat is conducting a mandatory inservice on HIV prevention for new correction personnel at the local jail.
- Michael is conducting a five-part workshop on health and safety for 45 physical plant employees at a local factory.
- Maria is performing a one-time presentation on the pap and pelvic examination for a group of 15 Hispanic women in a local community center.
- Natalie is conducting an individual birth control session for a sophomore student at a university health center.
- William is teaching a 10-part unit on family life to a class of 25 ninth-grade high school students.
- Tanya is performing a patient education session for two hypertensive middle-aged males at a local hospital.
- Peter is working with the residents of an assisted living community to implement an intervention designed to keep seniors physically active.
- Dwayne is lecturing to 500 college students about sexually transmitted infections and safer sex, as part of a series on contemporary sexual issues.
- James is podcasting a presentation on breast self-examination that can be downloaded directly via the Internet.
- Delores is speaking to a congressional panel on the importance of comprehensive health education.

Although these **health educators** are dealing with very different audiences—from very large groups to individuals, from high school students to elected national officials, from young to old, from the workplace to the school, from the community to the House of Representatives—they all share one crucial factor that will invariably determine success or failure . . . how well they actually educate. The philosophy presented in this text is based on the premise that the core of **health education** is the **health education process**, composed of factual information, effective delivery, and motivational impact. This means that what is most important is how well and effectively we perform the function of educating people and motivating them to make good health decisions.

There are many tools available to health educators, such as epidemiology, statistics, and program planning, but the essence of being a health educator is the actual "doing" of health education—that is, the conveyance of clear, appropriate **health information**. As educators we may have access to the best knowledge available, but unless we are skilled and effective deliverers of this information, the usefulness of our work is clearly compromised. Anyone who has sat through a poorly prepared, often boring and uninspired presentation or class should question the thought processes that resulted in such a negative experience. Health educators, therefore, need a systematic approach to the selection of educational interventions.

Our goal is to favorably influence the voluntary health decision making of our clients.

This text is intended to assist the health educator or would-be health educator in developing sound, effective, and appropriate presentation methods to create learning experiences that facilitate voluntary changes leading to health-enhancing behaviors. It is founded on the proposition that we must be good at the doing . . . the health education. Our goal is to favorably influence the health decision making of our clients. Further, it is our belief that health educators need a systematic approach to the selection of methods of intervention.

The authors of this text strongly believe that the skills necessary to plan for, and deliver, effective health education programs are fundamentally the same, regardless of where they are practiced—in a classroom, workplace, Internet/online, hospital, or community setting, as shown in Figure 1-1. The fundamental duties of health educators, regardless of setting include:

- Assessment of target population needs
- Planning for intervention strategies
- Implementation of interventions
- Evaluation of success

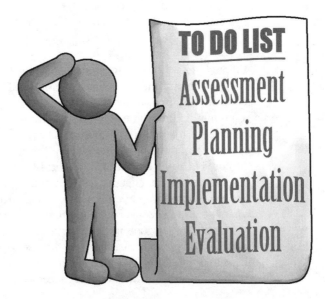

Figure 1-1
Health Educator Duties

These are basic components that can be used in any setting. Consequently, this text is designed for multiple settings and will address the needs of the so-called "generic" health educator.

This *generic health educator* concept has important ramifications for the training of health educators because it puts more emphasis on the acquisition of skills than on health content. Health educators practice in a variety of settings, including school health education, community health education, worksite health education, and patient health education, and it is clear that some skills would be used more in some settings than in others; yet the basic tools are generic to all settings. Health educators need to acquire these basic skills. It is ludicrous, for example, for an individual to believe he or she can function well as a health educator without training in educational principles. This text is organized and presented to facilitate the acquisition of many of these basic skills.

Process of Health Education

Remember always to be grateful for the millions of people everywhere whose despicable habits make health education necessary.
—Mohan Singh

It is important to remember that health education is, as the name implies, education about health. Health education has its roots in education and public health. It draws on many disciplines including psychology, sociology, education, public health, and epidemiology. It is a unique discipline in many ways. One of the challenges for the health educator is that although the principal tool is education, the sought after outcomes are often behavioral adaptations. Other disciplines in education focus almost exclusively on knowledge, which is a critical component of health education. Knowledge alone is unlikely to be robust enough to cause behavior change. The complexity of human behavior requires that approaches to health education target three key influences for behavior change:

- *Knowledge* about the behavior
- *Attitudes* associated with the behavior
- *Skills* necessary to enable behavioral adaptation

Health education strives to provide knowledge as well as the requisite skills necessary to apply that knowledge—while developing appropriate attitudes—to result in healthy behavior choices or behavior changes as needed (see Figure 1-2). Failure to address these three components will likely result in marginal outcomes. Health education is called upon to lower cholesterol, alter drug-taking behavior, and improve fitness—to name a few of the many complicated expectations. The dissemination of knowledge alone, clearly, would not be sufficient to accomplish such lofty goals.

To effectively accomplish the process of health education, health educators must learn to set meaningful, appropriate, and achievable goals and objectives. After setting clear, high-quality objectives, the health educator must seek to meet those objectives through appropriate ethical methods.

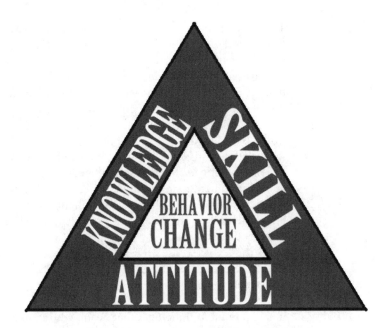

Figure 1-2
Triangle of Influences
on Behavior Change

History of Health Education

Health education has been offered in some form since the beginning of time. Humanity has always sought to lead a longer and healthier life. Means's classic text *A History of Health Education in the United States* reviews early health education activities in the United States. It is interesting to note Harvard College required hygiene in 1818 of all seniors (Means, 1962, p. 36). The American Public Health Association was formed in 1872, and the National Education Association started a Department of Child Safety in 1894 (Means, pp. 46–48). The American School Health Association was formed in 1927 as the American Association of School Physicians. The American Association for Health Education began as the American Association for Health and Physical Education in 1937, which is now part of the American Alliance for Health, Physical Education, Recreation and Dance (AAHPERD).

Education about health became more common in the 1800s and early 1900s with numerous reports and advocates. Some noted advocates included Horace Mann, Thomas Denison Wood, the American Academy of Medicine, the Metropolitan Life Insurance Company, the U.S. Public Health Service, and the U.S. Office of Education. The first reported academic department of health education was located at Georgia State College for Women around 1917. The first known recipient of a health education degree was Cecile Oertel Humphrey, who, after additional course work at Harvard during the summers of his program at Georgia State College, received a bachelor of science in health education. A thesis was required, and his was entitled "The Inferiority Complex—Its Relation to Mental Hygiene." No report is available on what has become of Mr. Humphrey (Means, 1962, p. 144). Teachers College, Columbia University, began an undergraduate degree in 1920 and was one of the early granters of graduate degrees in health education.

Health education has functioned as a separate discipline for approximately the last 30 to 60 years. As a relatively new discipline, it has always struggled for a strong sense of identity. One illustration of this is the large number of health education professional organizations, each with overlapping goals. Another is the odd fact that health education degrees are sometimes offered at higher-education institutions with few or, in some extreme cases, no health educators on the faculty. Despite these problems, health education continues to evolve into an important discipline with a unique orientation to addressing the health education needs of the world.

The demand for health educators is presently on the rise. The U.S. Department of Labor Statistics predicts an employment market growth of 26% over the next decade (Bureau of Labor Statistics, 2008). This is considered to be much faster than the average for all other occupations (Bureau of Labor Statistics). According to the National Employment Matrix, in the year 2006 there were approximately 62,000 health educators employed in the United States. The Bureau of Labor Statistics predicts that that number will increase to 78,000 by the year 2016. Much of this growth is attributed to the rising cost of health care. Insurance companies and governmental agencies are recognizing the cost-effectiveness of preventive health measures. Thus, these agencies are embracing the important contributions of the health educator in prevention efforts.

Throughout the history of health education, numerous agencies have recognized its potential to address health problems. Federal agencies have supported many studies and projects designed to improve the quality and impact of health education. An important effort was the Role Delineation Project begun in 1978 (funded by the then U.S. Bureau of Health Manpower and carried out by the National Center for Health Education), which examined the role of the entry-level health educator and generated a defined role. This defined role was based on surveys of practicing health educators in 1978. The end product was a defined role for the entry-level health educator. Although obviously in need of continual updating, the definition of the role was a significant step in the evolution of health education as a discipline. An important finding suggested that the health educator's role was essentially the same regardless of the health education setting. The result was the definition of the generic health educator, a concept very important for the training of health educators. It states that health educators should all possess certain common skills. These skills were later more fully defined as *competencies for entry-level health educators* by a panel of experts meeting at Ball State University. Still later these competencies became the basis for a test by the National Commission for Health Education Credentialing (NCHEC) to certify health education specialists. The competencies are also used by the National Council for the Accreditation of Teacher Education (NCATE) as part of the teacher-training accreditation review process.

Advancements in computers and telecommunications have significantly accelerated the evolution of the health education profession. Searching for health information is one of the most common reasons consumers use the Internet (Greenberg, D'Andrea, & Lorence, 2003). Not long ago, searching for information about any subject usually involved a trip to a local library and a walk through the dusty stacks of books, hoping that the volume in question had not already been borrowed by another inquisitive patron. Although libraries today still fulfill an important role as providers of the printed word, these institutions have altered their services to include direct access to data via the Internet. Today, most librarians are Internet experts.

Today, health educators have immediate access to data. National databases such as the Youth Risk Behavior Surveillance System (YRBSS) and the *Morbidity and Mortality Weekly Report* (MMWR) are just a click of the mouse away. Professionals, as well as lay persons, have instant access to the most current information available at the Centers for Disease Control and Prevention (CDC) or the National Institutes of Health (NIH). Additionally, the ability to collaborate and share information with others has been enhanced via the use of podcasting, video streaming, blogs, and bulletin boards. The information age has assisted in the evolution of the health education process.

Goals of the Text

After reading and synthesizing this text, the health educator will be able to:

- Plan properly for health education instruction.
- Develop quality lesson/presentation plans and unit plans.
- Plan for the special needs of target populations.
- Select appropriate methods through a systematic approach.
- Use methods of intervention properly.
- Utilize methods to promote health literacy.
- Identify appropriate strategies for the marketing of health promotion.

Format of the Text

Competencies   Each chapter begins with a listing of the generic entry-level and/or Advanced 1 or 2 competencies developed for the National Task Force on the Preparation and Practice of Health Educators, Inc. A complete listing of the competencies can be found in the appendix.

The entry-level health education competencies were first developed during the early 1980s and were published in 1985. Over the last few years, health education professionals have worked to reverify them through the Competencies Update Project (CUP), initiated in 1998 by the National Commission for Health Education Credentialing (NCHEC). This project examined how other professions distinguished themselves among levels of practice and attempted to identify current specifications of entry-level competencies.

The CUP model outlines distinct sets of competencies and subcompetencies for each of the three levels of practice (National Commission for Health Education Credentialing [NCHEC], Society for Public Health Education [SOPHE], & American Association fo Health Education [AAHE], 2006). The levels of practice are designated as:

- Entry: Baccalaureate/master's, less than 5 years' experience
- Advanced 1: Baccalaureate/master's, more than 5 years' experience
- Advanced 2: Doctorate and 5+ years' experience

The competencies and subcompetencies are aligned with the major categories of performance expectations of a proficient health education practitioner (SOPHE & AAHE, 1997).

Use of Competencies in the Text   Each chapter begins with the relevant entry-level competencies and subcompetencies and any appropriate new Advanced 1, 2 competencies. In some instances the entry-level and Advanced 1, 2 competencies are the same, and in these cases this similarity is noted.

A complete listing of the entry-level competencies and subcompetencies and Advanced 1 and 2 competencies can be found in the appendix.

Methodologies   Each chapter also begins with a graphic (Figure 1-3) that illustrates the components of proper method selection addressed in the chapter. As the caption explains, the heavy-bordered boxes identify the components addressed in this text. One or more of these boxes will be shaded to indicate the subject or subjects of a chapter.

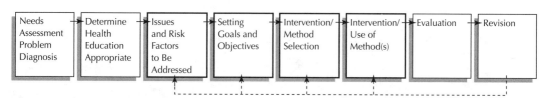

Figure 1-3 Method Selection in Health Education

Method Selection Components

Many public health and health education texts deal with program planning and evaluation. This text focuses on the *conducting* of health education—the pedagogy. **Pedagogy** is the art or profession of teaching. Pedagogy is what health education practice is about and is best accomplished by ensuring that the seven following components are applied.

1. **Needs assessment and problem diagnosis.** This text begins with the assumption that some type of needs assessment has been done, and it has been determined that health education is a viable alternative.

2. **Determination of whether health education is the appropriate intervention.** This text also begins with the assumption that it has been determined that health education is the appropriate intervention. Health education can be very complicated, expensive, and difficult, so this is an important assumption. Often other methods of health promotion may be more appropriate. Altering the environment, for example, might make better use of resources. If students are eating unhealthy lunches, it may be easier to ensure that they eat lunch at school where they will be offered only healthy choices. Such tactics can lead to much better behavior at relatively low cost. However, the long-term behavior may not be altered with only a change in the physical environment.

3. **Issues and risk factors to be addressed.** This text will consider some of the issues and risk factors to be taken into account when making decisions. See Chapters 2, 3, 9, and 10.

4. **Setting goals and objectives.** Goals and objectives are an important component of pedagogy and are addressed in Chapters 2 and 3.

5. **Intervention/method selection.** Selection of the appropriate intervention or method for health education is the major issue addressed in this text. See Chapters 4 through 10 and the appendix.

6. **Evaluation.** *The issue of evaluation is so major that it cannot be sufficiently addressed in this text.* The importance of this area cannot be overestimated. Entire books and courses are dedicated to evaluation, as is fitting for such important and lengthy material. Therefore, although there are many references to evaluation here, no chapter is dedicated to the issue. Instead, the reader is referred to books that can treat the subject in detail.

7. **Revision.** Good, practical evaluation will lead to revision of any intervention. Revision is an important tool that should be part of any program. However, because it should be based on evaluation, revision is not addressed in this text.

Objectives   Each chapter states the objectives to be achieved by the reader.

Case Studies   Case studies are used throughout the text and are revisited at the end of each chapter.

Case studies will provide opportunities to apply the principles found in each chapter to specific situations. A discussion of each case study can be found at the end of each chapter (under "Case Studies Revisited"). Following is an example of such a case study and its evaluation.

Example of Case Study

Objective: While reviewing the case study, the reader will identify multiple factors that contributed to the results of the intervention described.

The government authorizes $6 million to evaluate a large clinical trial aimed at influencing the health behaviors of Americans. A group of volunteers provides pamphlets and educational counseling at a large shopping mall, and each volunteer spends about an hour with over 5,000 people. The research design for evaluating the program is solid. Proper comparison groups are in place, and the instrumentation for assessing change is of high quality. We know what the behaviors, attitudes, and knowledge were before, during, and after the intervention (treatment), and we are certain threats to internal and external validity of the study have been controlled. The outcome measures are well matched with the objectives of the health education program. According to all measures, however, the intervention does not change anything.

Example of Case Study Revisited

There are, of course, many possibilities for the no-change results, but here are three questions that we want you to consider in particular:

1. Were the methods selected for the intervention appropriate and properly implemented?
2. Was adequate time provided for the intervention to achieve the objectives?
3. Were the people conducting the intervention properly trained? Were they in fact health educators?

Also note the following points:

- Although we do not have the objectives before us, it seems clear that few behavioral objectives could be reached by an intervention consisting solely of pamphlets and educational counseling by volunteers.
- An hour is not enough time to change most behaviors unless you have a very highly motivated clientele.
- Volunteers can play important and sometimes powerful roles but do not qualify as health educators.

This only moderately exaggerated example shows why health educators must work to improve the art and science of health education. Becoming a high-quality health educator requires hard work and dedication. A top-quality health educator is always working to develop communication skills, increase current knowledge of the subject matter, and remain a motivator. It is hoped that this text will provide some of the tools needed to accomplish the goals and objectives of health educators.

Summary, Practice Exercises, and References	Each chapter ends with a summary, a series of exercises, and a list of references and resources.
Glossary	A glossary can be found at the end of the text.
Proverbs	Scattered throughout the text are health education proverbs from "Mohan Singh," the pseudonym of Horace G. "Hod" Ogden. Before his death in 1998, Mohan Singh directed many programs for the institution now known as the Centers for Disease Control and Prevention (CDC) during his more than 20 years with the U.S. Public Health Service. He always felt it was important to keep life in perspective and that having a good laugh was one way to do that. We are certain he must be laughing about the continuing life of his sayings, often constructed on napkins in Atlanta and D.C. beverage houses. We are pleased to continue spreading these timeless messages for health educators willing to listen.

SUMMARY

1. A major goal of the text is a systematic approach to the selection of methods of intervention.

2. Education about health has been part of general education since antiquity. Health education as a formal discipline, however, is relatively new.

3. Successful health education interventions and presentations require the development of realistic and meaningful goals and objectives.

4. The basic skills required for effective health education, be it community, worksite, health care, governmental agency, or school, are essentially the same.

EXERCISES

1. Health educators perform an array of tasks in several diverse settings. Examine the following job descriptions. In which setting (community, worksite, health care facility, governmental agency, or school) do you believe these activities are most likely to be performed?

   a. The health educator asks a high-risk patient about medical procedures, operations, services, and therapeutic regimens to create activities and incentives that will encourage him or her to take advantage of available services.

   b. The health educator helps identify needs, mobilize resources, and build coalitions to improve the health status of a target area.

   c. The health educator provides employee counseling, education services, risk appraisals, and health screenings in order to comply with occupational health and safety regulations.

   d. The health educator teaches health as a subject while promoting and implementing the coordinated school health programs.

e. The health educator ensures that state and federal mandated programs are implemented while working closely with nonprofit organizations to secure resources, such as grants.

2. Prioritize the three key influences for behavior change (knowledge, attitude, and skills)

according to your opinion of their impact and importance.

3. Justify why the term *generic health educator* is an appropriate descriptor of a professional health educator.

REFERENCES AND RESOURCES

Bureau of Labor Statistics, U.S. Department of Labor. *Occupational Outlook Handbook, 2008–2009 Edition.* Retrieved January 11, 2008, from http://www.bls.gov/oco/cos063.htm

Greenberg, L., D'Andrea, G., & Lorence, D. (2003). *Setting the Public Agenda for Online Health Search: A White Paper and Action Agenda.* Retrieved February 9, 2008, from http://www.consumerwebwatch.org/pdfs/URAC.pdf

Means, R. K. (1962). *A History of Health Education in the United States.* Philadelphia: Lea and Febiger.

National Commission for Health Education Credentialing, Society for Public Health Education, & American Association for Health Education. (2006). *A Competency-Based Framework for Health Educators.* New York: Authors.

National Task Force on the Preparation and Practice of Health Educators. (1983). *A Guide for the Development of Competency-Based Curricula for Entry Level Health Educators.* New York: Author.

National Task Force on the Preparation and Practice of Health Educators. (1985). *A Framework for the Development of Competency-Based Curricula for Entry Level Health Educators.* New York: Author.

Society for Public Health Education & American Association for Health Education. (1997). *Standards for the Preparation of Graduate-Level Health Educators.* Washington, DC: Authors.

U.S. Department of Health and Human Services. (1981). *National Conference for Institutions Preparing Health Educators: Proceedings, Birmingham, AL, 1981.* DHHS Publication 81-50171.

2

CHAPTER

Planning for Instruction

Entry-Level and Advanced 1 Health Educator Competencies Addressed in This Chapter

Responsibility I: Assess Individual and Community Needs for Health Education
Competency A: Assess existing health-related data.
Competency B: Collect health-related data.
Competency F: Infer needs for health education on the basis of obtained data.

Responsibility II: Plan Health Education Strategies, Interventions, and Programs
Competency B: Incorporate data analysis and principles of community organizations.
Competency C: Formulate appropriate and measurable program objectives.
Competency D: Develop a logical scope and sequence plan for health education practice.
Competency E: Design strategies, interventions, and programs consistent with specified objectives.

Responsibility III: Implement Health Education Strategies, Interventions, and Programs
Competency A: Initiate a plan of action.
Competency B: Demonstrate a variety of skills in delivering strategies, interventions, and programs.

> Note: The competencies listed above, which are addressed in this chapter, are considered to be both entry-level and Advanced 1 competencies by the National Commission for Health Education Credentialing, Inc. They are taken from *A Framework for the Development of Competency Based Curricula for Entry Level Health Educators* by the National Task Force for the Preparation and Practice of Health Education, 1985; *A Competency-Based Framework for Graduate Level Health Educators* by the National Task Force for the Preparation and Practice of Health Education, 1999; and *A Competency-Based Framework for Health Educators—The Competencies Update Project (CUP)*, 2006.

Method Selection in Health Education

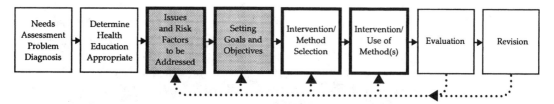

Heavy-bordered boxes indicate subjects addressed in this text; shaded boxes indicate subject(s) of current chapter.

After studying the chapter, the reader should be able to:

- Identify methods for analyzing needs of populations.
- Conduct an appropriate needs assessment for a given community setting.
- List the major considerations that should be made before selecting an educational objective.
- Assess the role of goals and objectives in program planning and evaluation.
- Write behavioral objectives in the cognitive, affective, and psychomotor domains for a given concept or contact area.
- List the most common mistakes in objective selection.
- Discuss ethical considerations in planning.

KEY ISSUES

Program planning
Conducting a needs
    assessment
Relationship of objectives and
    evaluation
Selecting objectives
Objective domains
Process objectives

Performance indicators
ABCD&E objectives
Outcome objectives
Writing goals and objectives
Selecting verbs
Common mistakes
Ethics as part of planning

Program Planning

Program planning begins with the identification of a "problem" that impacts quality of life. A variety of planning models exist to help health educators systematically develop programs. Effective program development will classically include the following tasks:

1. Assessment of needs
2. Diagnosis of the problem(s)
3. Development of appropriate goals and objectives
4. Selection of methods to create an intervention
5. Implementation of the intervention
6. Evaluation of program effectiveness
7. Revision of program as needed

Method selection is only one element of program planning. Program planning has issues that are beyond the scope of, and therefore not addressed by, this text. Many other books are devoted to those issues. We begin with the assumption that the "problem" has been identified and health education has been determined to be part of the needed solution. This is, of course, a major assumption. It is usually valid for school settings, where the **curriculum** framework for health education is already in place, and for health educators

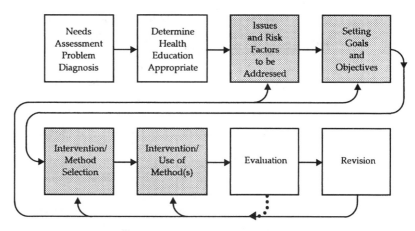

Figure 2-1
Method Selection in
Health Education

Shaded boxes indicate subjects included in this text.

working for a categorical agency that has decided to focus on one or two elements of health education. If the decision for health education has not been made, then the reader should turn to planning models and conduct a thorough diagnosis of the problem before turning to health education and this text. Figure 2-1 shows the full range of method selection, with shaded boxes indicating the subjects that are the focus of this text.

Needs Assessment

Although program goals and objectives are often set for the health educator by some other group, a **needs assessment** (step one of Figure 2-1) is always appropriate. The needs assessment may be informal or formal. An informal needs assessment may occur through frequent conversations and personal interactions with colleagues and clients. Formal approaches systematically assess the quality of life in an effort to identify differences between what currently exists and what may be a more desirable state (Bartholomew, Parcel, Kok, & Gottlieb, 2001).

Outside agencies will often develop excellent objectives, but may still fail to account for special characteristics found at the local level. The needs assessment, as the term implies, seeks to determine the needs of the targeted population. Before health educators set out to do something, it is important for them to know how this **target population** perceives its needs.[1] When assessing needs, the literature is always a good place to start. Conducting a *literature review* of current periodicals helps to establish a sound foundation for the proposed intervention while identifying common themes to be addressed as part of the **goals** and **objectives** of the program. When goals and

---

[1]Green and Kreuter use the term *diagnosis* to describe this phase of health promotion planning. They describe this phase in detail in their classic text *Health Promotion and Planning: An Educational and Environmental Approach*. It is also sometimes referred to as *reconnaissance*.

objectives are established for health educators, it reduces the complexity of their needs assessment, but they should still play a significant role in objective establishment, by interpretation if not by setting the objectives directly.

Generally, the better we know the target population, the more we should be able to accomplish. The amount of time and resources we devote to the needs assessment will depend on issues such as the duration, priority, and prior work experience with the group. If we have worked with the group recently, we may need to spend little time, but if this is a new group, it may require considerable time and effort.

Obtaining information about a target population's perceived need can come from multiple sources. *Social indicators*, found in public records like census or welfare reports, are useful for providing descriptive statistics that help to estimate population needs (Langmeyer, 1993). *Surveys and questionnaires* allow the health educator to collect information for a large sample of the target population. Additionally, selected community leader and agency representatives are often considered a valuable source of information. These *key informants* are often surveyed to help identify specific needs that might go undetected when attempting to correlate statistical data. A simple needs assessment survey is depicted in Figure 2-2. *Community forums*, similar

---

WORKSHOP NEEDS ASSESSMENT

Please answer the following questions as completely and honestly as you can. The information collected will be used in determining the content of the health education workshop.

1. What do you hope to get from this workshop/class?

2. Why are you here?

3. What is one thing you hope will be covered?

4. What is one issue that has been covered too much and would be a waste of time for this wokshop?

Other comments:

Figure 2-2
Simple Needs
Assessment Survey

to open town meetings, seek input from community members, allowing the health educator to gain perspective on whether the community will support a given program (Langmeyer, 1993). *Focus groups* aid the health educator by providing opinions of the potential recipients of the intended intervention. Each of these techniques empowers the health educator to develop tailored interventions that meet the needs of the target population.

Objective: While reviewing the case study, the reader will evaluate the feasibility of the drug education program described in relationship to its ability to achieve the desired outcome.

Case Study: Pat Pat has set the elimination of drug use by all adolescents in her community as her objective for a community-wide drug education program. She plans to work cooperatively with several local agencies including the schools and later to apply for federal funding to support the program. Following two years of this approach, she gets a small local grant to evaluate her program. Preliminary reports show that drugs are used by about 15% of adolescents in the community. (See Case Studies Revisited page 44.)

Questions to consider:

1. What are potential problems related to Pat's objective?
2. How might a needs assessment have better facilitated the plan for Pat's program?

Target Population

To develop an accurate picture of the target population, two types of information should be obtained by the health educator: demographics and statistics.

Demographics **Demographics** include information about age, ethnicity, gender, and other characteristics that describe a population. Discovering the target audience's developmental characteristics, knowledge levels, attitudes, health skills, and interests will likely impact the program objectives and method selection. If we are working with young people, we may turn to information on the developmental characteristics of this age group. Surveys may exist that will tell us something about the knowledge or interests of this age group. If such surveys do not exist, we may be able to conduct such surveys. This data collection, sometimes referred to as baseline data, provides information that helps us determine how to conduct our program and serves as a basis of comparison. Any major program must include such baseline data, because there will always be interest in what benefits have been accrued for the dollars invested.

Statistics   Statistics, obtained from both qualitative and quantitative methods of data collection, render useful information. Qualitative methods allow the target population an opportunity to express their thoughts, feelings, ideals, and beliefs (U.S. Department of Health and Human Services, 2000). These methods aid the health educator in identifying problems, barriers, or gaps that may not be recognized by an outsider. Quantitative methods render numerical representations of statistical information and provide a general perspective of an identified phenomenon. Table 2-1 categorizes a few of the methods commonly used to conduct an assessment of needs.

We should consider what statistical information may be available. International, national, regional, or local reports can provide vital information on needs. Such reports can also be used to demonstrate the importance of a topic. When they do not, it may be important to conduct our own needs assessment specific to our target population. Collecting such information also demonstrates an interest in tailoring the program to the needs of the local target group and may serve as part of the intervention program by pointing out individual needs. Identification of personal needs often leads to some attempt at behavior change. People who know they are at higher than average risk for some loss of health will sometimes try to reduce that risk. How serious they perceive the risk to be will often determine how they respond. Such information is often very important in selling the program to funding agencies, gathering local support, and encouraging participants to cooperate in the program.

It is important that health educators assess this demographic and statistical information to minimize unneeded work while taking into account the desires of the target group. Conducting a needs assessment puts a group on notice that you recognize its importance and value its opinions. These are necessary ingredients for success.

Table 2-1 Assessment Tools by Category

Statistics	
Qualitative Methods	**Quantitative Methods**
• Public forums	• National or regional vital statistics
• Key informants	• National or regional health surveys
• Informal interviews	• Questionnaires
• Focus groups	• State reports on health status
	• School- or community-based surveys
	• Self-constructed surveys

Focus Groups

He who lives by bread alone needs sex education.
—Mohan Singh

There are a number of ways to design and use focus groups as a needs assessment and planning tool. Basically a representative group of the target population (5 to 10 people) or a very similar group is assembled for a focused discussion. Sometimes incentives may be necessary to secure participation and meetings are often taped for later transcription. Prior to the meeting, questions are developed to gather the sought after information, typically including the demographics, beliefs, and health practices of the community, as well as the names of respected leaders. The focus group leader is responsible for ensuring that useful information is collected through both preassembled questions and careful follow-up of cues from the comments of the group. Often unanticipated information is collected that can alter the methods selected for the intervention.

A professional focus group facilitator can be employed, or a member of the planning team may become a good facilitator with practice.

The following are questions that encourage participants to respond by providing an opinion:

- What do you think about . . . ?
- How do you feel when . . . ?
- Think back to a time when you . . .
- What might influence you to . . . ?

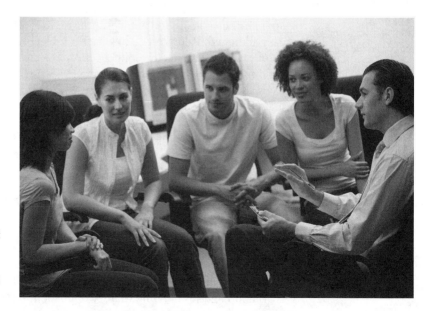

Focus groups are a useful needs assessment and planning tool. The organizer should concentrate on creating the right mix of people.

Focus group sessions last about an hour and address only five to six pre-assembled questions. Participants are seated in a manner to easily facilitate discussion, allowing the health educator to fade away from the group as participants share their thoughts (Krueger, 2003). The health educator should act as a neutral guide, posing questions and prodding to get a full response. Most good community health educators do at least a very brief version of a focus group before starting any program in a community.

The Goal–Objectives–Performance Indicators Link for Evaluation

Alice asked, "Would you tell me please, which way I ought to walk from here?"

"That depends a good deal on where you want to get to," said the Cat.

"I don't much care where," said Alice.

"Then it doesn't matter which way you walk," said the Cat.

"—so long as I get somewhere," Alice added as an explanation.

"Oh, you're sure to do that," said the Cat, "if you only walk long enough!"
—Lewis Carroll,
Alice in Wonderland and Through the Looking Glass

You may have heard the statement, "If you do not know where you want to go it is usually impossible to get there." These words of wisdom apply well to all health education endeavors. We often see health educators trying to get somewhere without being clear about where that somewhere might be. Even more interesting, we often see them trying to evaluate what they have done while trying to get there. Obviously, this is not a prudent practice. Health educators must know clearly where they want to go.

Goals, objectives, and performance indicators function very much like the elements of an archer and his or her target in that they clarify the purpose of the health education intervention. Goals, like the target, are broad statements of direction used to specify the overall intent of a program. Goals reflect the desired outcome but do not clarify indicators to measure success. Objectives are derived from goals. Like the rings of the archer's target, the objectives define areas to address in the accomplishment of the goal. An objective is a precise statement of intended outcome declared in measurable terms. Objectives are more accurate assessment tools because they tell what needs are specifically addressed (Palomba & Banta, 1999). Objectives have the inherent quality of exercising a directive influence. An objective, taken together with its performance indicator, is outcome-oriented, stated in measurable terms, and focused on a single outcome (Palomba & Banta). A **performance indicator** describes activities that provide information about acceptable progress toward the stated objective. A performance indicator acts as a quantifiable or qualitative measure of the accomplishment of the objective (Palomba & Banta). The performance indicators, like the archer's arrows, are used to "hit" the objectives, and the precision of their landing is an indication of success. Figure 2-3 graphically depicts this relationship. Taken together, an objective and its performance indicator should allow all to evaluate what is being changed, by whom, and by how much. Table 2-2 provides a simplified sample of a medical facility's goal, objectives, and performance indicators. These examples are part of a larger strategic plan to improve hospital services.

Clearly, the performance indicators support the objectives, which promote accomplishment of the hospital's stated goal. Establishing measurable goals and targets is not only vital for evaluation, but also essential for good planning in selecting an intervention.

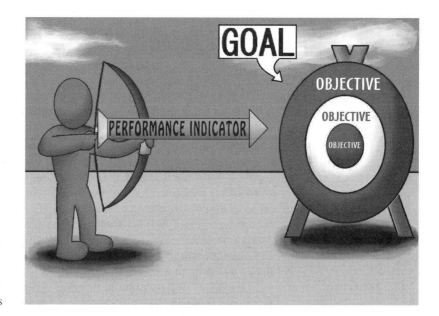

Figure 2-3
Relationships Among
Goals, Objectives, and
Performance Indicators

Table 2-2 Examples of Goals, Objectives, and Performance Indicators

Goal
Enhance Patient Education and Staff Training

Objective 1:	**Objective 2:**
Provide ongoing staff development across all disciplines that respond to staff-identified training needs and requirements.	Develop and implement an ongoing patient education program by 2010 according to identified opportunities for education, health promotion, and disease prevention.
Performance Indicators:	**Performance Indicators:**
a. Plan and conduct continuous medical education (CME) sessions, offering at least 9 credit hours/year.	a. Monitor the use of the website with the appropriate information targeting a 20% increase in use.
b. Plan and conduct skills training seminars in basic life support (BLS), cardiopulmonary resuscitation (CPR), and advanced cardiac life support (ACLS) at least twice a year.	b. Increase the use of mass media (TV, newspaper) by 10% to promote hospital programs/services.
c. Enhance staff development either by providing it onsite or by sending candidates to outside training facilities.	c. Host monthly public health care lectures or seminars.

There are clear links among goals, objectives, performance indicators, method/intervention selection, and evaluation.

Let us examine some examples (with discussion) of how inappropriate conclusions can be reached when we have no clear-cut targets.

1. "My program went well because we distributed 750 pamphlets on drug abuse."

   If the program objective was to distribute pamphlets, then the objective was met, but it was a very poor objective. Distribution numbers or numbers of people that visit a booth in a shopping mall are examples of very limited measures that tell us nothing about changes in knowledge, attitudes, or behaviors.

2. "My program went well because the 40 people attending the lecture on drug abuse seemed very interested and asked many questions."

   Looking interested tells us nothing about what is being learned. It does tell us something about the methods employed (process evaluation). It may indicate that people find the topic or method of presentation interesting, but it tells us nothing about what has been learned.

3. "My program went well because, after the five antidrug television spots were aired, the state drug use numbers went down."

   Although this is a positive trend, it does not tell us if that trend is related to our program. It may have nothing to do with our activities, and it would be inappropriate for us to assume so without further information.

4. "My program went poorly because, after our intensive intervention with all county high school students, the state drug use numbers went up."

   Again, we do not know if this trend had any connection to our program. The number for our students might be much better due to our program, but without clear objectives we cannot adequately measure our outcomes.

5. "My STI prevention program went poorly because, after our intensive intervention throughout the county, our STI statistics showed an increase."

   Again, we do not know if this trend had any connection to our program. The statistics for STIs commonly go up for a period of time following an intensive campaign because people seek treatment. If we set objectives to lower incidence rates in a short period of time, we would be setting up our program for failure.

It is difficult to evaluate these statements without knowing the objectives, but all suggest that the evaluation measures have not been well thought out.

Establishing well-planned targets allows the evaluation process to occur as a natural by-product of the implementation process. If the performance indicators are met, this should naturally meet the objectives and in turn help to meet the goal. Poorly defined targets will result in the inability to appropriately evaluate program effectiveness.

Objective: While reviewing the case study, the reader will identify two fundamental errors Jerry committed in planning and will describe the impact of these errors on his ability to justify the program.

Case Study: Jerry   Jerry was extremely enthusiastic about beginning a sex education program in his high school. The principal had been skeptical about the potential controversy and had put Jerry off for 2 years. Finally, the principal gave Jerry the administrative and financial support to begin a program, provided he furnish the principal with a course outline and specific objectives. In his haste to consummate the agreement, Jerry quickly prepared an outline, including objectives that promised a substantial decrease in unintended pregnancy and sexually transmitted infection rates. One year later, with budget reductions looming, Jerry is asked to justify the continued support of his sex education program. Much to Jerry's chagrin, the principal points to a higher number of pregnancies than last year, and no available data whatsoever of any sexually transmitted infection rates. What fundamental errors did Jerry make? (See Case Studies Revisited page 45.)

Questions to consider:

1. What fundamental errors did Jerry make?
2. How might his poor selection of objectives do irreparable damage to a program that is already under a watchful eye?

Writing General Goals

Goal: A broad statement of direction used to present the overall intent of a program or course.

Different authors and authorities use a variety of terms and definitions regarding goals and objectives. We will use the term *goal* to mean a broad statement of direction used to present the overall intent of a program or course. As shown in Figure 2-4, a goal functions to direct the focus of the health intervention. A goal does not need to be stated in measurable terms, since it is a broad statement. *Objectives* should always be stated in measurable terms and should complement and more fully explain the intent of a goal. A goal gives us a general sense of the intent of the program or class.

Some goals might include the following:

1. Participants will be able to recognize healthy meals.
2. Promote awareness of nonprescription drug use.
3. Participants will develop good parenting skills.
4. Know risk factors associated with unwanted pregnancy.
5. Students will understand the digestion process.
6. Participants will show appreciation for the environment.

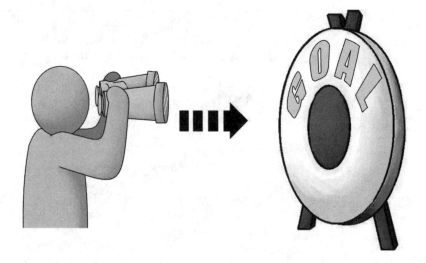

Figure 2-4
Targeting the Goal

Goals for Healthy People

Healthy People 2010 defines two overarching goals for the nation:

Goal 1: Increase quality of years of healthy life
Goal 2: Eliminate health disparities

These two goals are targeted by 28 focus areas each containing more precise goals and objectives to support the goals. A few examples are provided in Table 2-3.

Since these are national goals they have been written so that they are measurable. As explained earlier, this is not always the case with goals. Most are written as broad statements and are not measurable.

Narrowing Goals to Measurable Objectives

Goals provide a sense of where we want to go, but they usually do not provide clear, precise statements of our destination. We must break these broad statements into measurable objectives. One method for doing this is to use a worksheet to guide us to our objectives. After examining our problem, we set general goals. Next we break the problem down as far as we can go. We state our objectives as clearly and precisely as we can. See Figure 2-5 for a sample program planning worksheet.

Table 2-3 Samples of Healthy People 2010 Goals

Overarching Goals of Healthy People 2010
Goal 1: Increase Quality of Years of Healthy Life
Goal 2: Eliminate Health Disparities

Focus Area: Maternal, Infant and Child Health

Goal	Objectives
16-1 Reduce fetal and infant deaths	16-1a To reduce the number of fetal deaths at 20 or more weeks of gestation from 6.8 to 4.1 per 1000 live births plus fetal deaths by 2010. 16-1b To reduce fetal and infant deaths during prenatal period (28 weeks of gestation to 7 days or more after birth) from 7.5 to 4.5 per 1000 live births plus fetal deaths by 2010.
16-6 Increase the proportion of pregnant women who receive early and adequate prenatal care.	16-6a To increase maternal care beginning in first trimester of pregnancy from 83% to 90% of live births by 2010. 16-6b To increase early and adequate prenatal care from 74% to 90% of live births by 2010.

Focus Area: Immunization and Infectious Diseases

Goal	Objectives
14-25 Increase the proportion of providers who have measured the vaccination coverage levels among children in their practice population within the past 2 years.	14-25a To increase the number of public health providers measuring vaccination levels from 66% to 90% by 2010. 14-25b To increase the number of private health providers measuring vaccination levels from 6% to 90% by 2010.
14-27 Increase routine vaccination coverage levels for adolescents.	14-27a To increase vaccination coverage levels for adolescents aged 13 to 15 years having 3 or more doses of hepatitis B from 48% to 90% by 2010. 14-27b To increase vaccination coverage levels for adolescents aged 13 to 15 years having 2 or more doses of measles, mumps, rubella (MMR) from 89% to 90% by 2010. 14-27c To decrease vaccination coverage levels for adolescents aged 13 to 15 years having 1 or more doses of tetanus-diphtheria booster from 93% to 90% by 2010.

Source: Partners in Information Access for the Public Workforce, 2007.

SAMPLE PROGRAM PLANNING WORKSHEET

1. What needs to be done? List issue(s) or program(s):

   _____
   _____
   _____
   _____

2. State the general goal:

   _____
   _____

3. State the objective(s) to be evaluated as clearly as you can:

   _____
   _____
   _____
   _____
   _____

4. Can these objectives be broken down further? Break them down to the smallest unit. It must be clear what specifically you hope to see documented or changed: knowledge, attitudes, or a behavior.

   _____
   _____
   _____
   _____

5. Can each objective be evaluated? If not, restate it.

   _____

Figure 2-5
Program Planning
Worksheet for Narrow-
ing Goals to Objectives

Why Use Objectives?

Objectives serve many useful functions. They provide the health educator with a clear notion of what is to be accomplished. Consequently, it becomes much easier to select methods and to focus all efforts. This focus is vital if we are to develop comprehensive, coordinated approaches to influencing health behaviors. As mentioned in Chapter 1, behavior change is a function of the knowledge, skills, and attitudes of a target audience. Therefore, when writing objectives, it is important to begin with the question: What is the target? (See Figure 2-6.) Then we must define the target as specifically as we can.

Objectives make evaluation efforts possible. Without objectives, it is impossible to measure the achievement of change in knowledge, attitudes, or behavior. You cannot evaluate any type of change unless you first clearly and precisely state exactly what you intend to change.

Objectives, moreover, make it easier to convey our instructional intent to others. Learners in any setting do better when it is clear what is to be learned. This is true of participants in workshops as well as students in more formal educational settings. Plus, reviewing well-stated objectives allows learners to assess if a program is the correct program for them.

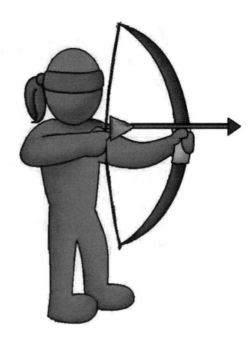

Figure 2-6
Finding the Target

Issues in Setting Objectives and Selecting Interventions/Methods

Some issues to be considered in setting objectives and selecting interventions or methods are as follows:

1. Maturity level of the learner
2. Content to be covered
3. Environment
4. Materials and equipment available
5. Time allotment
6. Group size
7. Time of day

When we set our objectives it is important to make them as realistic as possible given our resources. Of course, our objectives are often set by someone else, but the principles are the same. What can we accomplish in the time available with the resources at our disposal?

We must take into account the *maturity level of the learner*. Is the information pitched at the correct level for the learner? If it is too high, comprehension will be a problem; if it is too low, boredom and distraction

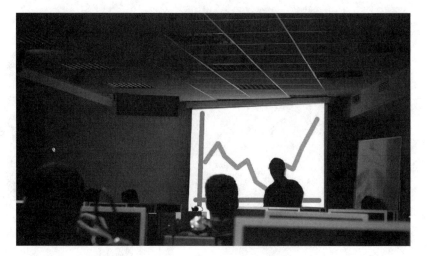

The success of your presentation depends on the correct environment and access to appropriate presentation tools.

will occur. Are the selected activities sufficiently varied to stimulate audience attention? This is an important concern when working with young people.

What type of *content* do you intend to cover? Large amounts of complex, didactic information may need to be broken down into smaller more understandable units, again depending on the level of the learner. Varying strategies might also alleviate the boredom factor and result in more effective learning.

What is the physical *environment* like? Can you, for example, lay out four "Annie" CPR mannequins on the floor of a very confined space to conduct important certification classes? Can you successfully perform group facilitation that might include sensitive issues in a space with little privacy? The available environment cannot be underestimated when considering objectives.

Can you obtain the *materials and equipment* you would like to include in a program? For example, is a certain video you would like to use available or affordable? Do you have access to a projector or DVD player? Before you include activities in program outlines and strategy selection, check to make sure that the resources are available. How much *time* do you have with specific groups, and how often will you meet? Is it worth spending 20 minutes incorporating an icebreaker exercise with a group that will only meet one time for 2 hours? The answer to this question depends on the specific objectives that you construct. Should you construct objectives that include behavior change when you will only meet with a group for a total of 2 hours? You must be realistic about which activities can be utilized and what objectives can be achieved within certain time constraints.

Group size will certainly drive your method selection. Presenting to a large group of 250 individuals will definitely require a different strategy than group process for a small number of people. Consider what might be the most effective ways to communicate with individuals and groups when considering group size.

Anyone who has had early morning classes or dozed during an after-lunch or dinner speech will appreciate the importance of *time of day*. Will you need to wake up the group, quiet them down, struggle to keep their interest, or what? Early morning or post-lunch groups might require a wake-up activity, so always consider this issue when developing strategy selection.

Often we must also determine if we can hope to achieve and perhaps measure outcome/impact objectives, or if we should focus on process objectives. Time and resources permitting, we should consider both.

Process Objectives

A **process objective** is concerned with what we hope to do along the path to our outcome objectives. This includes a look at how well we are implementing our methods. Are we maintaining interest, and are we providing high-quality information? Most curriculum packages are not implemented as designed. Often when programs are evaluated, the outcome of the evaluation is based on the faulty assumption that all users implement the program in the same way. Whether we are totally successful, partially successful, or unsuccessful, we must have a clear picture of what was done and not just what we hoped would be done in order to evaluate our results. Often programs are deemed ineffective when in fact the program was not implemented or only a few activities or methods from that program were actually used. This refers to program **fidelity**. How faithful to the planned program were the health educators? A lack of fidelity points to the need for training and marketing the total program to the intended user.

Some process objectives might address the following areas of concern:

- Getting people to participate
- Recognition of need
- Quality of workshop presentations
- Needs assessment
- Peer review
- Fidelity
- Self-assessment
- Changes in policy statements
- Quality control standards
- Participant satisfaction

Writing Outcome/Impact Objectives

Beware, lest the fragile lotus of health education be trampled by the elephants of reality.
—Mohan Singh

Outcome/impact objectives are concerned with what we are seeking to change in knowledge, attitudes, skills, and, consequently, behaviors. How will the participants be different as a result of our educational intervention? These outcomes can be assessed after a short-duration program or long-term program. Obviously, what we can expect must be based on the contact time, motivation, and intensity of our program. For a short-term program it may be realistic to expect gains in knowledge or skills but not attitude or behavior change.

Some outcome/impact objectives might address the following areas of concern:

- Changes in knowledge
- Changes in attitudes
- Changes in skills
- Changes in behavior
- Cost effectiveness

Writing Self-Contained Outcome/Impact Objectives

Objectives must be much more specific than goals. They must be measurable and clearly indicate what will be different after implementation of the health education program. There are many educational experts knowledgeable in the writing of educational objectives. Most health agencies and organizations will have their own method for stating objectives. Most such methods will be far less specific than what is recommended here and therefore easier to write. We have taken the components from other systems and have constructed a system called *self-contained objectives*. That means, of course, that all the elements are contained within the objective statement. The objective can "stand on its own" and make sense. Each objective makes clear what is expected, according to what source of information, and is stated in such a way that the achievement is measurable. The authors present this method first because it is a format that forces the user to examine important issues in the object process. Most agencies use some abbreviated version of this format. Objectives need not always be measured, but they must be measurable. In the real world there are not always sufficient funds, time, personnel, or the need to measure all objectives, but if measurement is not possible, then the objective is not clearly stated.

Correcting Errors   **Self-contained** or behavioral objectives designate the specific behaviors the target audience must demonstrate to indicate learning has occurred. Poorly written and, consequently, immeasurable objectives frequently suffer from a few basic errors. These common mistakes are listed here. Additionally, the authors have included an example that demonstrates the concept followed by clarifying commentary and a corrected alternative.

Error One

The objective is too vast or complex, representing multiple objectives (Smaldino, Lowther, & Russell, 2007).

Example 1: The participant will summarize each of the seven topics covered in the weekend workshop, evaluate the effectiveness of each session, and offer recommendations for improvement for next year's session.

There are three very complex ideas being represented in example one. If the participants are able to summarize the seven topics but cannot then offer recommendations for improvement, has the objective been met? This objective is attempting to measure too many complex behaviors at one time.

Example 1 Corrected: Following session two of the weekend workshop, the participant will list his or her top three concerns of the seven provided about environmental pollutants on the evaluation form.

Error Two

The behavior of concern in the objective is not measurable (Smaldino et al., 2007). This often occurs when the verb used to indicate behavior is not clearly defined; it is commonly referred to as a "fuzzy" verb.

Example 2: Following the demonstration, the learner will comprehend the sequence of events in developing a 10-step, decision-making model.

When measuring this objective, how will the health educator be certain that the learner "comprehends"? What does it mean to "comprehend" in this situation? Other examples of verbs that do not lend themselves to being measured include "appreciates," "understands," and "values." Although these verbs may be appropriate for setting goals, they lack the precision necessary to represent objectives.

Example 2 Corrected: Following the demonstration, the learner will list in order on the butcher paper provided the sequence of events to develop a 10-step, decision-making model.

Error Three

The objective describes instruction in place of what is to be learned (Smaldino et al., 2007).

Example 3: The patient will use the diabetic supplies to assess his or her glucose level after a fatty meal.

The preceding objective describes the method to be implemented but does not clarify what the learner should know, feel, or be able to do. Is the health educator attempting to measure if the patient knows how to use the supplies, how the patient feels about the glucose level, or if the patient is aware of what type of information the diabetic supplies can provide?

Example 3 Corrected: Using the diabetic supplies provided, the patient will accurately assess his or her blood glucose level by performing the finger-prick method described in the pamphlet.

It is evident the health educator's intent is to ensure the patient's ability to perform the skill being taught.

Error Four

The objective has vague performance parameters. It does not clarify what constitutes evidence of success (Smaldino et al., 2007).

Example 4: The student will record warning signs of cancer in his or her journal after viewing the cancer video.

If the video discussed the seven warning signs of cancer using the CAUTION model, it seems apparent that the objective intends to have the student list all seven. Without specifying the expectation, however, the student could list only two of the seven and, therefore, meet the requirements of the objective.

Example 4 Corrected: Using the CAUTION acronym described in the cancer video, the student will record the seven warning signs of cancer on a poster board.

The inability to measure the attainment of objectives, because of these common blunders, handicaps the health educator's ability to provide evidence of program success.

ABCD&E Formula for Writing Objectives

Avoiding the previously discussed errors is fairly simple by following the basic ABCD formula for writing objectives (Heinich, Molenda, Russell, & Smaldino, 1996). This method prescribes a step-by-step procedure for writing self-contained objectives, with each letter in the model representing an aspect of the objective that should be included. Take this a step further by using the ABCD&E formula.

A = Audience

Identifies who or what will perform the identified behavior:

- Learner
- Participant
- Parent
- Student
- Patient

B = Behavior

Uses an action verb describing what the audience is expected to do:

- The participant will be able to *list seven common depressant drugs.*
- The student will be able to *match drugs with the appropriate classification.*

- The participant *will show a willingness to take personal action* against drug use in the neighborhood by *volunteering*.
- The participant will be able to *demonstrate the mouth-to-mouth procedure*.

C = Condition

Describes the circumstances that enable the behavior to be performed. The condition indicates what the audience will need or how they have been enabled to perform the behavior:

- *Following the presentation*, the participant will be able to list seven common depressant drugs.
- The student will be able to match drugs with the appropriate classification *found in the course textbook*.
- *After participating in the discussion on community advocacy*, the participant will show a willingness to take personal action against drug use in the neighborhood by volunteering to be part.
- The participant will be able to demonstrate the mouth-to-mouth procedure for rescue breathing *on the mannequin provided*.

D = Degree

Indicates the criteria that must be met in order to constitute success:

- Following the presentation, the participant will be able to *list seven* common depressant drugs.
- The student will be able to match drugs with the appropriate classification found in the course textbook *with 80% accuracy*.
- After participating in the discussion on community advocacy, the participant will show a willingness to take personal action against drug use in the neighborhood by volunteering to be part of the neighborhood patrol *once a month*.
- The participant will be able to demonstrate the mouth-to-mouth procedure for rescue breathing on the mannequin provided *according to the American Red Cross guidelines with no errors*.

Many educators, including the authors of this text, propose the addition of the letter *E* to the model.

E = Evidence

Indicates the source of proof that the objective was met:

- Following the presentation, the participant will be able to list on the *butcher paper* seven common depressant drugs.
- The student will be able to match drugs with the appropriate classification, found in the course textbook, with 80% accuracy and *record them on the worksheet*.

- After participating in the discussion on community advocacy, the partici-pant will show a willingness to take personal action against drug use in the neighborhood by volunteering to be part of the neighborhood patrol *with a partner* once a month.
- The participant will be able to demonstrate, *to the instructor*, the mouth-to-mouth procedure for rescue breathing on the mannequin provided according to the American Red Cross guidelines with no errors.

In each of the preceding objectives there is a clear indicator of a source the health educator could assess to see if the objective has been satisfied. Although the addition of the "E" element is not always necessary to have measurability, its presence ensures a mechanism for evaluation.

The following are examples of self-contained objectives written using the ABCD&E method. Notice that, although all the components of the ABCD&E method are present, they are not necessarily written in sequential order. The order of the elements is not important, only that all the elements are represented.

Sample Objectives

1. Participants will be able to list and describe to their group members, the four local agencies available to provide child abuse prevention support as presented during the workshop.
2. In their post-workshop evaluations, participants will report improved self-efficacy in communication with family members according to the guidelines presented during the workshop.
3. Students will show a willingness to take personal action to improve the environment by voluntarily participating in one of three community-organized cleanups or by voluntarily taking personal action to reduce waste in their community.

Table 2-4 outlines the ABCD&E components of the sample objectives. The italicized words highlight the component represented.

Educational Domains

An important consideration is the characteristics of the objectives we are seeking to achieve. Most health education programs work in more than one "domain" as defined in the classic, *Taxonomy of Educational Objectives* (Krathwol et al., 1964). The three major domains are cognitive, affective, and psychomotor. Cognitive refers to the recall and synthesis of information, typically what is considered knowledge. Affective refers to the change of an attitude. Psychomotor refers to the performance of a physical skill. Sometimes skills are also included as a domain of their own. Examples include refusal skills or the ability to analyze the unscientific nature of appeals used in health advertising.

There is disagreement as to the relationship of these domains and health behavior. Knowledge, attitudes, physical performance, and skills all have important relationships, but they act in different ways at different times and

Table 2-4 Outline of Self-Contained Objectives Using the ABCD&E Method

Breaking down the parts of the objective using the ABCD&E method				
	Audience	**Behavior**	**Condition**	**Degree**	**Evidence**
1	*Participants*	will be able to *list* and *describe*	*as presented during the workshop*	the *four* local agencies available to provide child abuse prevention support	to their *group members*
2	*Parents*	will *report*	*according to the guidelines presented in the workshop*	*improved* self-efficacy in communication	in their post-workshop *evaluation*
3	*Students*	will *show* a willingness to take personal action to improve the environment by (1) *participating* in (2)	*community-organized clean-ups*	Note: two degrees 1. *voluntarily* 2. *one of three*	*Could be assessed by checking to see if student volunteers (evidence-implied)*

with different people. Knowledge can change behavior at times and at other times seems to have no relationship to behavior change. Most people, if they know their partner is HIV positive, will take extra precautions or avoid sexual contact altogether. However, although most of us know the relationship of diet to heart disease and cancer, we will still elect to eat high-fat, low-fiber foods on occasion. Several highly respected health educators, for example, are overweight. What motivates one person may not motivate another. A model or theory may never explain the behavior of some individuals. Therefore, it is probably wise to use a variety of methods addressing as many domains as practical.

Other Objective-Writing Formats

There are many styles of writing objectives, and the health educator may be forced to adapt to the style adopted by the agency or school. Self-contained objectives are suitable for most purposes, and we recommend their use. Further, once you can author self-contained objectives, it becomes relatively easy to master other methods (see Figure 2-7). However, there are advantages to other styles. Some formats make it easier to use objectives over and over again with little change and may be used for different content areas.

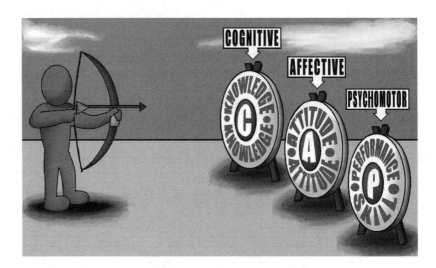

Figure 2-7
Targeting Educational
Domains

A general instructional objective will function much like a goal, as described previously in this chapter.

1. General instructional objectives (learning outcomes).
   a. Write each objective as an *intended learning outcome*.
   b. Use a verb that is general enough to encompass a domain of student performance. Omit the lead-in phrase, "The student will be able to. . . ." Use verbs such as *knows, understands, applies*.
   c. Include only one learning outcome for each general objective.
   d. Keep these objectives free of subject matter so that they can be used with various units.
   e. State each general objective so that it is definable by a set of specific learning outcomes. (For short units, two to four general objectives will usually suffice.)
2. Specific instructional objectives (learning outcomes).
   a. Place the specific instructional objectives under the general learning objectives. Be certain they are relevant to the general learning outcome under which they are placed.
   b. Use a verb to begin each specific learning outcome. This verb should specify definite, observable student performance. Avoid using verbs such as *sees* and *realizes*, which are vague and not observable.
   c. Under each general learning outcome, list a representative sample of specific learning outcomes to describe the performance of those students who have achieved the objective. (It is impossible to list all learning outcomes.)
3. When writing instructional objectives, the following outline may be used as a template.
   I. Content and population
      A. General instructional objective (learning outcome)

    (1) Specific instructional objective (learning outcome)
    (2) Specific instructional objective (learning outcome)
    (3) Specific instructional objective (learning outcome)

Examples

1. Drugs (high school/college level).
   A. Knows systems of classification.
      (1) Lists various systems of classification.
      (2) Explains the advantages and disadvantages of each system.
      (3) Designs an original system.
2. Stress control (high school/college level).
   A. Understands breathing techniques.
      (1) Discusses uses of these.
      (2) Demonstrates them.
      (3) Expresses willingness to use technique.
3. First aid—choking (junior high/elementary level).
   A. Knows correct procedures.
      (1) Explains when and when not to use the techniques.
      (2) Recites the steps.
      (3) Performs the procedures.

The outline format gives the health educator the ability to reuse objectives and provides a strong foundation for writing more specific self-contained objectives if needed.

Suggested Recipe for Writing Health Education Outcome/Impact Objectives

1. Make a rough outline of what you hope to accomplish in the educational setting. Jot down key elements of what you hope to achieve.
2. Try to state each specific item of information, feeling, and skill as a behavior objective.
3. Check your verb to see that it is specific (see Table 2-5).
4. Can you measure your objective? Remember that you do not have to follow through on measuring each objective, but it must be possible to do so, or it is not a true behavioral objective. Assessment of affective objectives is controversial because many people do not believe they can be measured. Generally, affective assessment is based on a measurable action that a "reasonable person" would assume represents a held attitude or feeling.
5. Ask yourself if each objective is something the targeted population has gained or could gain from your instruction. If the answer is no, it is not a good objective.
6. Ask yourself the following: When participants finish with the lesson, workshop, or unit, how will they feel or act? What new knowledge or

Table 2-5 Suggested Verbs for Health Education Goals and Objectives (by Domain)

Goals	
Analyze	Contemplate
Appreciate	Comprehend
Conceptualize	Know
Enjoy	Be aware of
Perceive	Understand
Consider	Commit
Apply	Plan

Objectives by Domain		
Cognitive	*Affective*	*Psychomotor*
Arrange	Show a willingness	Construct
Design	Choose	Conduct
Itemize	Agree to	Demonstrate
Categorize	Promote	Act out
Classify	Accept responsibility for	Clean
Compute	Volunteer	Operate
Match	Initiate	Perform
Report	Share	Sort
Discuss	Defend	Disassemble
Identify	Justify	Install
List	Express	Repair

skills will they possess that were not present before this event? Have you selected objectives appropriate to the needs and domains? For example:

A. Cognitive domain: What do I want the audience to *know*?
- Cognitive/know . . . recall of information
- Cognitive/know . . . synthesis of information

B. Affective domain: What do I want the audience to *feel or believe*?
- Objective . . . seeking willingness to take action
- Objective . . . reporting attitude change

C. Psychomotor domain: What do I want the audience to be able *to do*?
- Perform a physical skill
- Perform an analytical skill, which requires physical action

7. When psychomotor objectives represent physical skills that can be performed (e.g., mouth-to-mouth resuscitation), the focus of evaluation must be the physical performance. Mouth-to-mouth resuscitation requires cognition, but focus is on the performance of the skill. It is possible to have psychomotor skill as part of the objective even though it is not the focus of learning. A participant may be asked to visit an agency to discover the services provided; however, merely visiting the agency is not the focus. Visiting the agency is a condition required to help achieve the objective. Conditional requirements are not truly classified as psychomotor skills because they function to describe what is necessary to achieve the objective.

After writing your objectives, double-check each one with the following questions:

1. Have you avoided "fuzzy" verbs? (See Table 2-5 for suggested verbs.)
2. Can you measure the outcome of your objective?
3. Is the standard by which achievement will be measured clearly stated?
4. Is each objective something that is really worth achieving?
5. Is there a sufficient number of objectives to cover your true intention of instruction?
6. Are the three educational domains appropriately represented in respect to achieving the desired outcomes?
7. Are you guilty of not stating your true intentions just because you find it difficult?

Objective-Writing Exercises

Read the following scenarios, take a few moments to consider appropriate outcomes for each situation, and then write down what you would consider to be appropriate behavioral objectives. What are the most needed skills, beliefs, or knowledge? Obviously, you will have to give some consideration to the actual content you would potentially cover in each situation and how you would divide your time. Remember that you need to consider such basic principles as size of group, setting, time, number of objectives, domain of objectives, and so on.

1. You are a middle school health education teacher. You are about to teach your *first* lesson on heart health to a class of 20 seventh-grade students of mixed academic ability. This particular unit consists of five class periods, and each period is 50 minutes long.
2. You are a community health educator facilitating a program on smoking cessation for 10 middle-aged adults. The program consists of 10 two-hour weekly workshops, and you are planning to conduct the *first* workshop.
3. You have been invited to a local high school to deliver a 1-hour informational presentation on AIDS to a special assembly consisting of 400 ninth-grade students.
4. You are teaching a 2-hour workshop on CPR to 15 grocery store employees in the employee lounge. Your goal is CPR certification of the group.
5. You are a middle school health education teacher beginning the third of five 50-minute class periods on the topic of alcohol. For this period you have decided that the goals should focus on attitudes about the negative aspects of alcohol use. One strategy you have selected is the development of posters by the students depicting alcohol messages. There are 30 students in the class.

6. You are a community health educator who has been asked to facilitate a 90-minute workshop for approximately 25 Hispanic women on the importance of pelvic examinations. Levels of fluency in English are poor.

7. You are a college health educator who has been asked to conduct a 1-hour workshop on safer sex for approximately 20 students in a co-ed residence hall.

8. Two students in a campus residence hall have recently experienced date rape. As the campus health educator you have been requested by that residence hall's resident assistant (RA) to conduct a 1-hour presentation on date rape. The RA expects about 50 students to attend the presentation scheduled to be held in the first-floor lounge.

9. You have been facilitating a weekly 6-week course on childbirth. The class meets for 90 minutes and consists of six couples in various stages of pregnancy, from 36 to 41 weeks. This is the last of the six sessions, and you are planning objectives that will allow you to wrap up the course.

10. You are a high school health educator teaching in a very progressive and enlightened school district. You are teaching human sexuality and are about to begin a 2-day, 50-minute-period unit on homosexuality. You are planning objectives for this first class.

Common Mistakes in Objective Selection

Beware of the following common mistakes in setting objectives:

1. Selecting an objective that is not achievable.
2. Using verbs that are not specific.
3. Selecting objectives that do not truly represent what you wish to achieve.
4. Selecting objectives that are not realistic given the resources available.
5. Stating an activity and not an objective.

The National Health Objectives

When the 1990 Health Objectives were released, they received little attention outside the Public Health Service. They soon became an important force driving agendas and setting funding priorities for all sectors of government. Having clear, specific objectives has forever changed the U.S. Public Health Service. The process in setting the Year 2000 Objectives became much more politicized because public and private groups were aware of their influence. The objectives have become powerful tools in setting government and private policy. The 2010 objectives have grown in number and complexity and have been the subject of much debate. The U.S. Department of Health and Human Services released its framework for Healthy People 2020 in 2009 and plans to launch the Healthy People 2020 goals, objectives, and action plans in January 2010 (U.S. Department of Health and Human Services, 2008).

The U.S. Public Health Service Office of Disease Prevention and Health Promotion was established as a coordinating and policy development unit of the Office of the Assistant Secretary of Health. The unit was charged with coordinating the development of the Surgeon General's reports and the health objectives for the nation. In 1979 the first Surgeon General's report on health promotion was released ("Healthy People: The Surgeon General's Report on Health Promotion and Disease Prevention"), which reviewed the gains made in health promotion. In addition, the report established broad national goals according to life stages and focused on reduction of mortality.

During the same period a process was put in place to develop national health objectives. This took over a year, with first drafts developed by 167 invited experts serving on panels centered around 15 subject areas held and sponsored by the Centers for Disease Control and Prevention (CDC) in Atlanta. Members were drawn from a variety of backgrounds. The purpose was to develop national, not federal, objectives. It was felt that by establishing clear targets, agencies would focus on meeting those objectives—a common practice for business for many years but a new concept for much of government. Available research was used to determine appropriate targets, and the compilation of information pointed to the need for additional data (needs assessment). A major effort was made, but the task became even more complicated when the process was repeated for the year 2000 objectives. By this time people knew that influential people, including virtually all federal funding sources, were paying careful attention to the objectives. As a result, major lobbying efforts became part of the process of setting the objectives.

Some of the original drafts of the years 2000 and 2010 objectives differ significantly from the final product. The Office of Disease Prevention and Health Promotion and the CDC are to be commended for pulling together the various factions and completing the target objectives. This is an important example of what needs to be done for any health education program. Clear objectives must be established at the outset if the project is to be successful and to make measurement possible. The national health objectives have resulted in significant changes in the way the U.S. government, and especially the U.S. Public Health Service, does business.

Ethics as Part of Planning

Many ethical issues are involved in health education intervention. We are attempting to change people in some way. Will these changes and methods of change be ethical? To ensure that the answer is yes, certain steps should be taken to protect people's rights. Until recently, the most widely adopted code of ethics was the Society for Public Health Education (SOPHE) code. A brief version of the SOPHE code is given in Figure 2-8. This code stated that a health educator should influence people without coercion and that changes of behavior should be voluntary. A more recent code of ethics has been developed by the Coalition of National Health Education Organizations and has superseded the SOPHE code (see appendix).

To guide professional behaviors of its members toward highest standards, SOPHE adopted a Code of Ethics in 1976 and acknowledged the need for periodic review and improvement of the Code.

- I will accurately represent my capability, education, training, and experience, and will act within the boundaries of my professional competence.

- I will maintain my competence at the highest level through continuing study, training, and research.

- I will report research findings and practice activities honestly and without distortion.

- I will not discriminate because of race, color, national origin, religion, age, or socioeconomic status in rendering service, employing, training, or promoting others.

- I value the privacy, dignity, and worth of the individual, and will use skills consistent with these values.

- I will observe the principle of informed consent with respect to individuals and groups served.

- I will support change by choice, not by coercion.

- I will foster an educational environment that nurtures individual growth and development.

- If I become aware of unethical practices, I am accountable for taking appropriate action concerning these practices.

Figure 2-8
SOPHE's Code of
Ethics (Brief Edition)

Human Subjects Review

When we design programs and select intervention methods, it is important we keep ethical considerations in mind. For example, if we are conducting any data collection, we must go through a formal review process to protect the rights of human subjects in research. These *institutional review boards* (IRBs) are a requirement for any programs that receive federal funding. They are established by government, colleges, universities, and other agencies to review ongoing research projects. They have formal guidelines to protect the rights of subjects, including the right to know what will happen, the right to privacy, and the right to be free from harm.

Ethical Obligations to Employer

Quality health education is not easy, and it is not accidental.

We are responsible to our employer, which means we are obligated to give full effort to our job. If we have been hired to work a 40-hour week, we must ethically devote 40 hours to the work as defined by our employer. It is not ethical for us to define what our work is unless we are self-employed. If we believe our employer is asking us to do something that is unethical, it is our obligation to discuss it with him or her. If it is then clear we are being asked to do something improper, we should report it to the next-higher authority, resign, or do both. If we are asked to teach something we do not believe in due to religious or other conflicts, we are obligated to discuss this with our

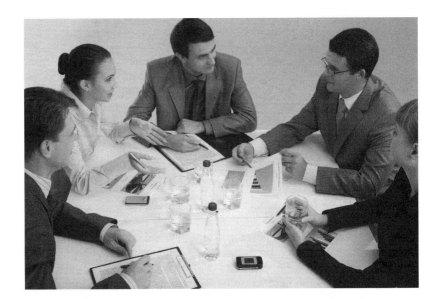

Institutional review boards use formal guidelines to monitor ongoing research projects that involve human subjects.

employer. Perhaps someone else can teach that topic or other accommodation can be made, but it is not ethical for us unilaterally to change the curriculum or lesson to fit our personal beliefs. We must work through channels to either get it changed, teach it, or allow someone else to teach it.

We also have the obligation to keep up to date and to employ the best methods. We often hear of the shortcomings of health education programs. After reading this text, you will probably recognize that we do have the tools to be successful, but many practitioners are not applying what we know. This is an ethical issue. Quality health education is not easy, and it is not accidental—it takes hard, dedicated work.

Objective: While reviewing the case study, the reader will identify two or more examples of ethical compromises committed by Nathaniel.

Case Study: Nathaniel

Nathaniel has been assigned to teach a personal health course at a local community college. The outline calls for 2 days of coverage of HIV/AIDS issues. Nathaniel is not very conversant in these issues, so he substitutes 2 additional days in the nutrition area, which he enjoys. Several students and student reporters go to the dean to urge the dean to be certain AIDS is covered in personal health courses. The dean says that it is part of all personal health courses. Several students have just completed Nathaniel's course and state emphatically that it is not. The dean is very angry when she discovers that Nathaniel has not covered the prescribed material. Can Nathaniel defend his position? (See Case Studies Revisited page 45.)

Questions to consider:

1. What alternative methods could Nathaniel have selected to ensure the requirements of the syllabus were fulfilled?
2. Do you believe his actions are defendable? Explain.

For more information and tools related to this chapter visit http://healtheducation.jbpub.com/strategies.

EXERCISES

1. You have been asked to develop a sexuality unit for ninth grade high school students. What do you think would be appropriate goals for such a unit? Also, write three sample objectives you feel would be reasonable, being sure to include at least one from the *affective* domain.

2. Select a health topic and target population. Now, in thinking of how to justify the development of your program, list specific resources or agencies from which you could obtain supportive data. (These must be *real* sources.) You will need to conduct some research and then cite addresses or Internet information related to the agencies or other sources you would use to support your proposal.

3. What are the three major reasons for developing objectives?

4. Describe four important factors to consider when developing objectives or selecting methods.

5. What are the major differences between goals and objectives?

6. Describe how you could utilize national health objectives like Healthy People 2010 or 2020 to develop your own local program objectives. Illustrate your answer by selecting any specific health topic.

7. Identify the ABCD&E components of the following objective samples.

a. Following session two of the weekend workshop, the participant will list his or her top three concerns about environmental pollutants on the evaluation form.

b. Following the demonstration, the learner will list in order on the butcher paper provided the sequence of events to develop a 10-step decision-making model.

c. Using the diabetic supplies provided, the patient will acccurately assess his or her blood glucose level by performing the finger-prick method described in the pamphlet.

d. Using the CAUTION acronym described in the cancer video, the student will record the seven warning signs of cancer on a poster board.

CASE STUDIES REVISITED

Case Study Revisited: Pat   Since Pat's only stated objective was to end drug use, she has failed by her own standards. Pat has not set realistic objectives in measurable terms for her program, and because of this mistake the program was virtually certain to fail. Further, Pat has not determined through a needs assessment what the current status of the community is in terms of its needs and interests and the prevalence of drug use. If, for example, Pat had discovered that drugs were being used by 35% of adolescents in the community, she could structure her objectives to reflect a modest but realistic behavior or attitude change. Pat has failed to plan carefully for instruction. (See page 17.)

Case Study Revisited: Jerry   Through his haste and poorly conceived, unrealistic objectives, Jerry has placed the entire sexuality program in jeopardy. He made the same two fundamental errors in planning as Pat did in the earlier case study. First, Jerry did not conduct a thorough needs assessment before designing program goals and objectives. If Jerry promises a reduction in sexually transmitted infections, he will need to obtain data as to their existing prevalence in order to make a subsequent comparison. The likelihood of even being allowed to collect such sensitive data in a public school is at best marginal. Second, in constructing his objectives Jerry was extremely unrealistic as to what any single program could accomplish. Constructing program *goals* related to reducing rates of unintended pregnancy and sexually transmitted infections would be appropriate, but specific behavioral *objectives* that need to be measurable should be much more modest and reasonable in scope. As discussed in Chapter 10, setting such unattainable objectives in a controversial area such as human sexuality can do irreparable and sometimes fatal damage to a program that may be constantly under scrutiny. (See page 23.)

Case Study Revisited: Nathaniel   Nathaniel's actions were poorly thought out and based on selfish motives. If Nathaniel was supposed to teach to an already existing syllabus, then he should have prepared sufficiently to be able to cover all topics. Alternately, Nathaniel could have used a more knowledgeable guest speaker or colleague to cover a particular topic. Nathaniel has certainly not helped himself professionally by angering his dean, and his actions would be difficult to defend. (See page 43.)

SUMMARY

Selecting or writing the appropriate educational goals and objectives is important for any health education program.

1. The selection of an objective should always consider the resources available to achieve that objective.

2. A needs assessment is an important step before selecting or writing objectives or selecting methods.

3. Goals may be general, but objectives must be specific and measurable.

4. In writing objectives, the educational purposes (process or outcome) must be considered.

5. All domains should be considered if adequate time and resources are available.

6. Methods should be selected with proper ethics in mind.

REFERENCES AND RESOURCES

Bartholomew, L. K., Parcel, G. S., Kok, G., & Gottlieb, N. H. (2001). *Intervention Mapping: Designing Theory- and Evidence-Based Health Promotion Programs*. Boston: McGraw-Hill.

Bloom, B. (1956). *Taxonomy of Educational Objectives: The Classification of Educational Goals Handbook I: Cognitive Domain*. New York: David McKay.

Gilmore, G. D. (1977). Needs assessment process for community health education. *International Journal of Health Education, 20,* 164–173.

Green, L. W., & Kreuter, M. W. (1991). *Health Promotion and Planning: An Educational and Environmental Approach*. Mountain View, CA: Mayfield.

Green, L. W., Levine, D. M., & Deeds, S. G. (1975). Clinical trials of health education for hypertensive outpatients: Design and baseline data. *Preventive Medicine, 4,* 417–425.

Green, L. W., Levine, D. M., Wolle, J., & Deeds, S. G. (1979). Development of randomized patient education experiments with urban poor hypertensives. *Patient Counseling and Health Education, 1,* 106–111.

Heinrich, R., Molenda, M., Russell, J. D., & Smaldino, S. E. (1996). *Instructional Media and Technologies for Learning*. Englewood Cliffs, NJ: Merrill.

Krathwohl, D., Krathwol, D. R., Bloom, B. S., & Masia, B. (1964). *Taxonomy of Educational Objectives: The Classification of Educational Goals Handbook II: Affective Domain*. New York: David McKay.

Krueger, R. A. (December 2003). Designing and conducting focus group interviews. Summary and proceedings from the State Health Access Data Assistance Center's (SHADAC) conference call on conducting data collection using focus groups. Retrieved June 6, 2009, from http://www.shadac.org/files/FocGrp_KruegerCall Summ_Dec03.pdf

Langmeyer, D. B. (September 1993). ARCH factsheet number 27. *ARCH National Resource Center*. Retrieved March 13, 2008, from http://www.arch respite.org/archfs27.htm

Morisky, D. E., DeMuth, N. E., Field-Fass, M., et al. (1985). Evaluation of family health education to build social support for long-term control of high blood pressure. *Health Education Quarterly, 12,* 35–50.

Morisky, D. E., Levine, L., Green, L. W., et al. (1983). Five-year blood pressure control and mortality following health education for hypertensive patients. *American Journal of Public Health, 73,* 153–162.

Palomba, C. A., & Banta, T. (1999). *Assessment Essentials: Planning, Implementing, and Improving Assessment in Higher Education*. San Francisco: Jossey-Bass. Retrieved March 15, 2008, from http://neasc.umf.maine.edu/data/developing_goals_and_objectives.htm

Partners in Information Access for the Public Health Workforce. (2007). Healthy People 2010 Information Access Project. Retrieved March 28, 2008, from http://phpartners.org/hp

Popham, J., & Baber, E. (1970). *Establishing Instructional Goals*. Englewood Cliffs, NJ: Prentice-Hall.

Ross, H., & Mico, P. (1980). *Theory and Practice in Health Education*. Palo Alto, CA: Mayfield.

Smaldino, S., Lowther, D., & Russell, J. (2007). *Instructional Media and Technologies for Learning* (9th ed.). Englewood Cliffs, NJ: Prentice Hall.

Taba, H. (1962). *Curriculum Development*. New York: Harcourt, Brace and World.

Toohey, J. V., & Shireffs, J. H. (1980). *Health Education, 11,* 15–17.

U.S. Department of Health and Human Services. (1980). *Promoting Health/Preventing Disease: Objectives for the Nation*. Washington, DC: Government Printing Office.

U.S. Department of Health and Human Services. (1992a). *Healthy Communities 2000: Model Standards*. Washington, DC: Government Printing Office.

U.S. Department of Health and Human Services. (1992b). *Healthy People 2000: National Health Promotion Objectives: Full Report, with Commentary*. Boston: Jones and Bartlett.

U.S. Department of Health and Human Services (USDHHS). (2000). *Healthy People 2010* (2nd ed.). Washington, DC: U.S. Government Printing Office.

U.S. Department of Health and Human Services (USDHHS), Centers for Disease Control and Prevention. (2007). General considerations regarding health education and risk reduction activities. Retrieved March 13, 2008, from http://www.cdc.gov/hiv/resources/guidelines/herrg/gen-con_community.htm

U.S. Department of Health and Human Services (USDHHS), Office of Disease Prevention and Health Promotion. (2008). Healthy People 2020: The road ahead. Retrieved March 29, 2008, from http://www.healthypeople.gov/hp2020/

Contextual Considerations for Behavior Change: Intervention/Method Selection

Contributions by
Dr. Pam Doughty
Texas A&M University

Entry-Level and Advanced 1 Health Educator Competencies Addressed in This Chapter

Responsibility I: Assess Individual and Community Needs for Health Education
Competency A: Assess existing health-related data.
Competency C: Distinguish between behaviors that foster or hinder well-being.
Competency D: Determine factors that influence learning.
Competency F: Infer needs for health education from obtained data.

Responsibility II: Plan Health Education Strategies, Interventions, and Programs
Competency D: Develop a logical scope and sequence plan for health education practice.

Responsibility III: Implement Health Education Strategies, Interventions, and Programs
Competency C: Use a variety of methods to implement strategies, interventions, and programs.

Responsibility IV: Conduct Evaluation and Research Related to Health Education
Competency A: Develop plans for evaluation and research.

Method Selection in Health Education

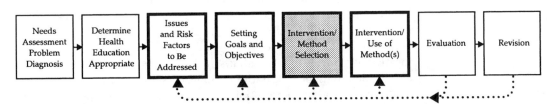

Heavy-bordered boxes indicate subjects addressed in this text; shaded boxes indicate subject(s) of current chapter.

Responsibility VII: Communicate and Advocate for Health and Health Education
Competency A: Analyze and respond to current and future needs in health education.

Note: The competencies listed on pages 47–48, which are addressed in this chapter, are considered to be both entry-level and Advanced 1 competencies by the National Commission for Health Education Credentialing, Inc. They are taken from *A Framework for the Development of Competency Based Curricula for Entry Level Health Educators* by the National Task Force for the Preparation and Practice of Health Education, 1985; *A Competency-based Framework for Graduate Level Health Educators* by the National Task Force for the Preparation and Practice of Health Education, 1999; and *A Competency-Based Framework for Health Educators—The Competencies Update Project* (CUP), 2006.

OBJECTIVES

After studying the chapter, the reader should be able to orally:

- List the major considerations in selecting an educational intervention/method.
- Employ appropriate theories and models in method selection.
- Present a rationale for proper selection of a method.
- List the most common mistakes in method selection.
- Describe effective learning environments.

KEY ISSUES

Objectives
Theories and models
Educational principles
Adult learners
Learning preferences
Characteristics of the learner
   and the community
Group size
Contact time
Budget

Resources/site/environment
Characteristics of the
   educational provider
Cultural appropriateness
Using a variety of methods
Learning environments
Seating arrangements
Packaging the total
   intervention strategy

Objectives as Drivers of Selection

Selecting the appropriate educational intervention is vital to achieving your objectives. Therefore, the objectives should drive the selection of all educational interventions and methods. In other words, the methods selected must be appropriate for the objectives sought. The previous chapter described the components of setting goals and objectives. This chapter emphasizes the importance of systematically identifying and reviewing objectives before selecting methods. Such a review is always the first step in selection. Interventions and methods must be linked with the objectives they are likely to achieve.

We use the term **intervention** to describe the total overall strategy to achieve our objectives. A **method** refers to one component of the intervention, such as an educational game or a health fair. Each is only one of perhaps many methods we could employ to achieve our objectives. All educators have the selection process in common, but the health educator must also consider how the chosen strategies might influence clients' attitudes that influence health and directly influence health behaviors. Further, the health educator must often work with very modest amounts of time and limited resources. Given that health educators may be asked to help clients modify complex and deeply rooted practices, selecting the correct methods is indeed a challenge. Nevertheless, we do have an arsenal of methods and a knowledge base to help us with these decisions. This chapter will review the contextual issues to be considered when selecting an intervention strategy (method) and explore environments that best facilitate their delivery.

Health Education Theories and Models

In theory there is no difference between theory and practice. In practice there is.
—Yogi Berra

In most health interventions, changing behavior is the goal; however, altering human behavior is extremely difficult, as anyone who has ever tried to quit smoking or stop eating sweets can tell you. So, how does one go about fostering behavior change? First, one must understand what types of things help to start the behavior; why people continue with a behavior, even if they know it is bad for them; and how unhealthy behaviors can be stopped or replaced with healthy ones. **Theories** have been developed to answer just such questions. These behavior change theories link objectives and methods to provide strategies for interventions. A theory serves to help explain why behavior occurs, what the determinants are that facilitate or hinder behavior, and how the health educator might most effectively design an intervention to promote what is desired (Glanz, Rimer, & Lewis, 2002). A theory attempts to make sense of interrelated concepts, definitions, and propositions to analytically explain or even predict a phenomenon (Kerlinger, 1986). Planning interventions from a theoretical perspective allows the health educator to focus on what has been identified as aspects that foster or hinder healthy choices. Theory provides a systematic approach to tailor, target, implement, and evaluate health promotion programs that will enhance the likelihood of success.

Constructs, Theories, and Models

Theories are built upon a set of identified **constructs**. Much like bricks function as base units that are built on to create buildings, constructs work in a similar way to serve as the base units of unique theories. As the health educator begins to analyze the dynamics facilitating or hindering a behavior, guiding general principles or constructs begin to emerge. A construct is a representation of such a concept within a theoretical framework (Green & Kreuter, 2005). These general guiding principles are called **concepts**, and they make up constructs. Constructs and concepts are the same except concepts are called constructs when used within a theoretical model. For example, one concept, **self-efficacy** (which is prominent in many health behavior theories), is a person's perception of self-control over his or her environment and behavior. This fundamental concept was first identified in the Health Belief Model created in the 1950s by a group of Public Health Service social psychologists (Glanz et al., 2002). The self-efficacy concept is represented by different construct titles in various theories, but it is essentially the same idea. Whereas Albert Bandura names the construct "self-efficacy" in his Social Cognitive Theory, Icek Ajzen refers to the same concept as "perceived behavior control" in his Theory of Planned Behavior.

Just as constructs form the foundation for the development of a theory, theories are used in the same manner as building blocks of a model. Models combine theories (often in a sophisticated manner) to produce an educational framework for the development of appropriate health education interventions. Figure 3-1 presents a graphic explanation of the relationships between constructs, theories, and a model.

Figure 3-2, the Transtheoretical Model (TTM), is built on the combination of three separate theories or hypothetical truths—Decisional Balance, Stages of Change, and Self-Efficacy. Benefits and costs are constructs for Decisional Balance Theory; pre-contemplation, contemplation, preparation, action, and maintenance are concepts of Stages of Change; and confidence and temptation influence the concept of Self-Efficacy. Altering human behavior is not only extremely difficult, but it also requires complex strategies for successful implementation. Understanding constructs, theories, and models will be essential in effective intervention.

PRECEDE-PROCEED Model

A variety of models exist to supply structure and to support program planners in the development of health promotion interventions. One of the most widely used models in health education is Green and Kreuter's PRECEDE-PROCEED planning model. "The PRECEDE-PROCEED model provides a comprehensive structure for assessing health and quality-of-life needs

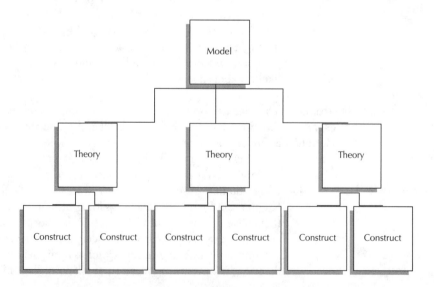

Figure 3-1
Constructs, Theories, and a Model

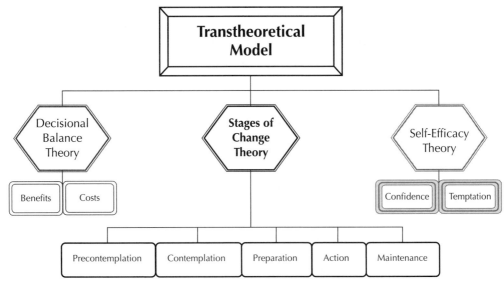

Figure 3-2
Transtheoretical Model

and for designing, implementing, and evaluating health promotion and other public health programs to meet those needs" (Green & Kreuter, 2006, p. 1). The model has been used to design interventions for diverse health issues including weight control, nutrition education, tobacco cessation, alcohol and drug abuse prevention, cancer prevention, and injury prevention.

The PRECEDE-PROCEED model is divided into two sections, each containing multiple phases. Understanding the constructs of the PRECEDE-PROCEED model will assist health educators in determining possible interventions as they investigate behaviors that are contributing to the health concern. The first half of the model, PRECEDE, includes the following concepts:

> **P**redisposing
> **R**einforcing
> **E**nabling
> **C**onstructs in
> **E**ducational
> **D**iagnosis and
> **E**valuation

PRECEDE is designed to aid in the diagnosis of health concerns and in the planning process for the development of interventions. There are four phases in the PRECEDE part of the model. Phases one (social assessment) and two (epidemiological behavior and environmental assessment) are steps for the needs assessment where the overall magnitude of the problem is outlined. Factors that predispose, reinforce, and enable the targeted behavior are examined in phase three (educational and ecological assessment). This phase assesses the existing knowledge, skills, and attitudes regarding behavior and gives insight into possible theories for intervention development. Phase three identifies the determinants of change, objectives for change, and priorities that can be converted into a program plan (Green & Kreuter, 2005). Prior to the actual development of a program, phase four is assessed to evaluate existing health education efforts and current policies. Phase four of the model (administrative and policy assessment and intervention alignment) serves to identify potential gaps in the educational efforts while preventing duplication of existing health promotion efforts.

The second half of the model, PROCEED, includes the following:

Policy
Regulatory and
Organizational
Constructs in
Educational and
Environmental
Development

This half of the model is composed of phases five through eight (not addressed in this text) that act as a guide for the implementation and evaluation of the developed intervention. Figures 3-3 and 3-4 show a graphic representation of the two halves of the model.

The ultimate goal of any health intervention is to develop healthy behaviors. If we want people to wear helmets when biking, we must consider what factors might be encouraging or discouraging them to do so. To influence behavior, it is important to consider the existing knowledge, skills, and attitudes of the person or group in order to understand the factors that predispose, reinforce, and enable the behavior. Predisposing factors provide the rationale or motivation for behavior and include elements such as the person's or group's knowledge level, beliefs, values, attitudes, confidence, perceptions, and personal preferences (Glanz et al., 2002; Green & Kreuter, 2005). Could it be that children do not wear bike helmets because they do not believe that they will have an accident? If this is true, it is likely they see no value in wearing the helmet. In order to effectively promote the use of a helmet, the health educator would need to address and change these children's predisposed values.

Reinforcing factors are the positive and negative consequences of action that provide motivation for the continuance or cessation of behavior. Reinforcing factors are positive and negative rewards that come from an outside source. Some reinforcing factors included social support, peer influence, advice, and physical consequences of behavior (Green & Kreuter, 2005). Many children do not wear bike helmets because their friends tease them if they wear them. The teasing from peers is a negative reward that decreases the likelihood that the helmet will be worn.

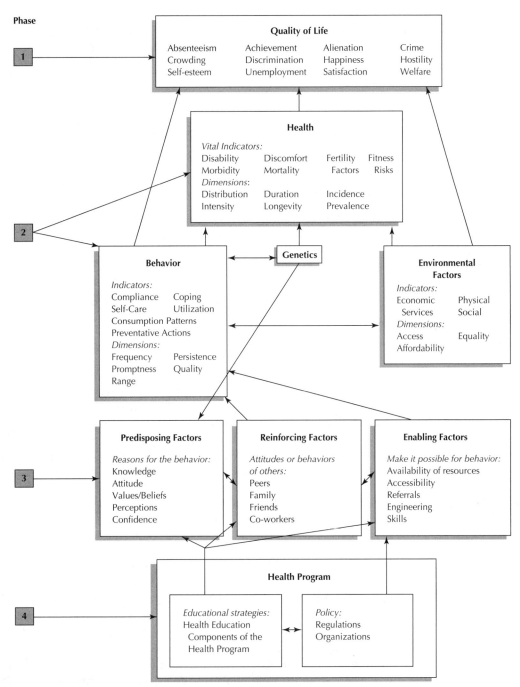

Figure 3-3
Representations of PRECEDE: Diagnosis and Planning Tasks
Source: Adapted from Green & Kreuter, 2005.

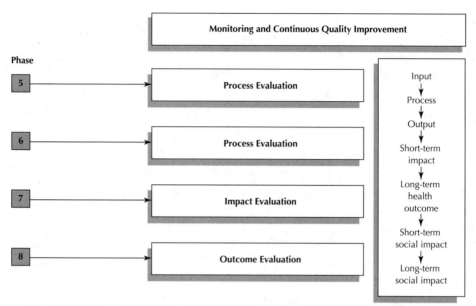

Figure 3-4
Representations of PROCEED: Evaluation Tasks
Source: Adapted from Green & Kreuter, 2005.

Enabling factors facilitate the performance of an action, and the absence of these factors prevents action (Green & Kreuter, 2005). Enabling factors include new skill sets and resources such as programs, services, and adequate finances to facilitate the behavior. Children without the financial resources cannot purchase a bike helmet and are clearly not going to be enabled to wear them. Providing helmets as an incentive for program participants, however, will enable them to wear their helmets.

Theory/Model Selection

If we think in terms of predisposing, reinforcing, and enabling factors as capacities to encourage healthy choices, then it makes sense to identify the most appropriate theory or model to strengthen these capacities. The selection of the most effective theoretical constructs for the model will be determined by what has been identified as encouraging and discouraging aspects of a behavior. Ideally, if a barrier to the performance of the behavior is tied to deficiencies in skills, then a theory containing constructs that emphasize skill improvement should be selected. This same line of thought would also hold true for barriers related to inappropriate attitudes or inadequate knowledge. It is not uncommon for a health educator to select constructs from a mixture of theories to create one that is tailor-made for the target population. The Individual Behavior Change Framework (IBCF) shown in Figure 3-5 shows the relationships among predisposing, reinforcing, and enabling factors to the constructs of knowledge, skills, and attitudes for behavioral change.

This IBCF is not a linear scaffold, but each of the factors is influenced by the other constructs. For example, to promote the wearing of bike helmets,

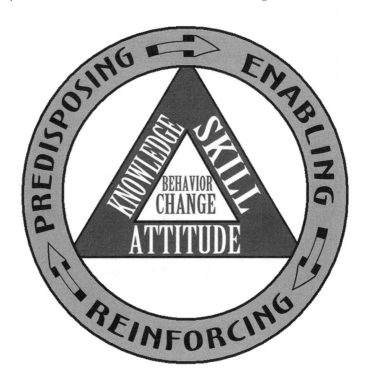

Figure 3-5
The Individual Behavior
Change Framework
Source: Co-contributed by
Dr. Pam Doughty

it is important to discover the knowledge, skills, and attitudes of the population regarding the wearing of helmets. Most people know they should wear a helmet, but they do not for a variety of reasons. Attitude may be a more significant predisposing factor than a lack of knowledge about its importance. If children think they look silly in the bike helmet, they are less likely to wear one. If their friends are all wearing helmets, however, it could reinforce their willingness to wear one as well. Providing helmets and teaching children the necessary skills to properly fit the helmet will promote and enable the children to perform the behavior.

Objective: After reviewing the case study, the reader will identify the concepts of the IBCF and the effectiveness of their use in Molly's program.

Case Study: Molly   Molly, a local health educator, was asked to design an intervention to increase fruit and vegetable consumption in adolescents. The high school agreed to pilot her program. As part of her intervention she provided lessons to increase the knowledge of the students and included multiple methods to develop positive attitudes about fruit and vegetable consumption. Following the intervention, the students were surveyed to measure their willingness to eat fruits and vegetables. Her analysis of the data indicated the students showed a favorable intention. She decided to test their intentions by replacing all snack machines with refrigerated vending machines containing healthy alternatives, such as fresh fruits and vegetables (see Figure 3-6). To adjust for the increase in cost, the price for each item was slightly higher. After 2 weeks, 95% of the fruits and vegetables had not been purchased. Her supervisor asked her to figure out what went wrong with her intervention. (See Case Studies Revisited, page 90.)

Question to consider:

What strategies would you consider adding or eliminating to increase the likelihood of students selecting the healthy foods from the snack machine?

Theoretical   A theory is often selected to serve as a guide for the development of inter-
Perspectives   ventions based on the specific concepts identified as influencing factors of
the behavior. The health educator ponders the question, "Which theory is best for this situation?" Theories serve to explain health behaviors and suggest intervention strategies. Different theories emphasize different aspects of behavior. Some theories focus on the individual as the unit of change whereas others examine change within families, institutions, communities, or cultures (National Cancer Institute, 2005). Theories are often categorized

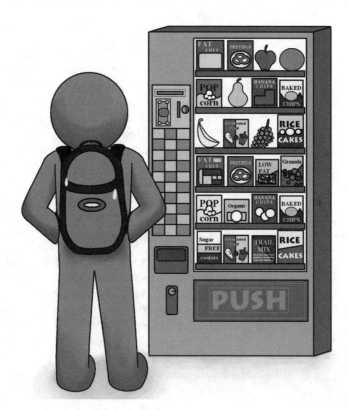

Figure 3-6
Healthy Vending
Machine Choices

according to two broad perspectives depending on the direction of the intervention. These viewpoints include the cognitive-behavioral perspective and the community-level perspective. Cognitive-behavioral theories highlight the importance of modifying behavior at the individual/intrapersonal and interpersonal levels. Health education efforts that target individual behavior choices include counseling, patient education, and other one-on-one approaches to behavior change. Cognitive-behavioral theories examine the actual behavior choices of the individual, as well as the dynamics of the individual's mindset or intrapersonal perspective. Intrapersonal factors might include the individual's motivation, beliefs, knowledge, attitudes, past experiences, and skills (National Cancer Institute). At the interpersonal level, theories of health behavior assume individuals exist within, and are influenced by, a social environment. In a cognitive-behavioral perspective, the theory would consider how the interpersonal factors of the social context (thoughts, opinions, and advice of other influential people) sway an individual's behavior. Cognitive-behavioral theories are built on the premise that changing the behavior of individuals will eventually result in changes in a group, which will spread to influence the whole community.

Community-level theories, on the other hand, support initiatives to serve communities and populations. They attempt to encourage behavior change from an indirect and more global approach that should trickle down to facilitate change at the individual level. For example, a health educator might design a campaign to reduce underage drinking by asking local businesses to display promotional posters in their window fronts. Community perspectives attempt to modify behavior by using community members, organizations, and social contexts as a vehicle for behavior change. An advantage of community-level approaches is that they expose the health education efforts to a greater number of individuals. Table 3-1 categorizes the more commonly used theories/models in health education by perspective.

"Effective practice depends on using theories and strategies that are appropriate to a situation" (National Cancer Institute, 2005, p. 6). Awareness of the available theories and their constructs will enable the health educator

Table 3-1 Categorized Theoretical Perspectives

Cognitive-Behavioral		Community-Level
Individual/Intrapersonal Level	*Interpersonal Level*	
Health Belief Model (HBM) Transtheoretical Model (TTM) • Decisional Balance • Stages of Change • Self-Efficacy Theory of Planned Behavior (TpB)	Social Cognitive Theory (SCT)	Social Ecological Model (SEM) Community organization models Diffusion/Innovation Model (DI)

to systematically approach intervention development. The following sections review a few of the more dominant theories/models.

Theories from a Cognitive-Behavioral Perspective

What people think and know affects how they will act. Although knowledge is necessary for behavior change, it is not sufficient to alter most behaviors. It is critical that the health educator consider the individual's perceptions, motivations, skills, and social environment as key influences of behavior (National Cancer Institute, 2005). We must also account for the individual's attitudes and skill level to enable behavior change. The following cognitive-behavioral theories/models attempt to address these key influences.

Health Belief Model

The Health Belief Model (HBM) stipulates that the willingness of people to take health-related action depends upon their attitudes and beliefs about the:

- Threat posed by a health problem (susceptibility, severity)
- Benefits of avoiding the threat (benefits)
- Factors influencing the decision to act (barriers, cues to action, and self-efficacy)

Motivation is a central focus of HBM; therefore, it is a good fit for addressing problem behaviors that evoke health concerns (e.g., cancer screenings, immunizations, or high-risk sexual behavior and the possibility of contracting HIV) (National Cancer Institute, 2005). The key concepts of HBM are as follows (Denison, 2002; Rosenstock, Strecher, & Becker, 1994):

- **Perceived susceptibility:** One's perception of the chances he or she will contract a health condition.
- **Perceived severity:** One's perception of how serious a condition might be and its medical, clinical, or social consequences.
- **Perceived benefits:** One's confidence in the effectiveness of the behavior to reduce the threat of the health condition.
- **Perceived barriers:** One's perception of the negative consequences (physical, emotional, financial, and social) for taking action.
- **Cues to action:** Factors that motivate or remind one to take action.
- **Self-efficacy:** One's confidence in the ability to take action and the perception that successfully executing the behavior will produce a desired outcome. Self-efficacy was added to the original model by Bandura in 1977 to account for more habitual behaviors such as management of diabetes.

The following is an example of the HBM in action. Individuals diagnosed with diabetes are encouraged to check their glucose (blood sugar) levels frequently to assess the effectiveness of their diabetes management plan. When glucose levels are in a normal range, the diabetic does not feel sick and may, therefore, elect to skip the recommended blood testing. In order to motivate the diabetic to follow the prescribed treatment regime, he must accept the fact that he has diabetes and that it requires management (perceived susceptibility). He must also understand that failure to control his glucose levels can result in serious medical complications such as stroke, heart disease, and nerve and kidney damage (perceived severity). By monitoring his glucose levels, the diabetic patient can reduce the likelihood of the aforementioned complications (perceived benefits) with the minimal effort of pricking his finger and reading the glucose meter (perceived barrier). The alarm on the cell phone of the diabetic could be set to serve as a reminder that it is time to check his glucose level (cue to action). The use of a daily log to record meter readings can serve as a confidence builder in the patient's ability to control his diabetes (self-efficacy).

Transtheoretical Model

The Transtheoretical Model (TTM) is composed of constructs from several theories that center on the Stages of Change Theory. As the name implies, it attempts to assess a person's readiness to change by identifying where he or she might fall along a continuum of behavior change. According to the theory, people are thought to move through five stages—precontemplation, contemplation, preparation, action, and maintenance—as they attempt to modify a problem behavior (Grizzell, 2007). At most stages the individual considers the constructs from the Decisional Balance Theory to evaluate the pros and cons of the behavior change while also incorporating the constructs related to self-efficacy. The individual must assess how confident he or she is to execute the behavior change and resist temptations that could result in noncompliance. This analysis serves as the motivation to move, either forward or backward, to another stage in the continuum. As the individual progresses through the five stages, the probability of sustained behavior change is more likely. This model has been applied to a wide variety of problem behaviors, including smoking cessation, exercise, low fat diet, radon testing, alcohol abuse, weight control, condom use for HIV protection, use of sunscreens to prevent skin cancer, drug abuse, medical compliance, mammography screening, and stress management (Velicer, Prochaska, Fava, Norman, & Redding, 1998).

Each of the five stages is summarized and a sample application is provided.

- **Precontemplation:** In this stage of the theory, the individual has no intention to take action in the foreseeable future, typically within the next 6 months (Velicer et al., 1998). Perhaps the individual is uninformed, underinformed, or has been unsuccessful with behavior change in the past; thus, she is not considering a change in behavior. A college student may not be aware of the potential health risks associated with drinking four to five alcoholic beverages within a 2-hour time span. The individual may not know that her binge drinking can lead to difficulty concentrating, memory lapses, and mood changes. To efficiently motivate self-change, individuals in precontemplation must first recognize a need for change.

- **Contemplation:** An individual in the contemplation stage recognizes a need and intends to change. As the binge-drinker begins to acknowledge negative consequences of heavy drinking—being hung-over or throwing up—she will compare these negative aspects to the benefits of appropriately regulating her drinking behavior to avoid embarrassing situations or to save money. Ideally the benefits will outweigh the costs, providing motivation to move into the next stage.
- **Preparation:** In this stage the individual attempts to make a plan for action to be implemented within the next month (Velicer et al., 1998). The binge-drinker may choose to take only enough cash in her wallet to purchase two drinks for the entire evening or may commit to having only one drink within an hour.
- **Action:** In the action stage the individual implements strategies that change her behavior. The binge-drinker has determined that if she only gets a new drink on the hour, she will be able to suitably regulate her alcohol consumption. While at the party, she sips slowly and waits until a full hour has passed before getting another alcoholic drink.
- **Maintenance:** In this stage the individual is striving to prevent relapse and is more confident in her ability to continue her behavior change for at least 6 months (Prochaska, 1994). The binge-drinker may discover additional strategies such as drinking water or other nonalcoholic fluids during the hour time frame, making it easier to adhere to her plan.

Ideally, an individual would arrive at the maintenance stage and stay there; however, the model is more spiral in nature, allowing for the individual to move back and forth along the continuum with successes and failures. Correctly identifying the target population's stage of change enables the health educator to tailor the health intervention to a group or an individual's readiness to change.

Theory of Planned Behavior (TpB)

The Theory of Planned Behavior (TpB), developed by Icek Ajzen (1991), suggests that behavior can be predicted because behavior can be planned. To date, behaviors explored using TpB include smoking, drinking, contraceptive use, dieting, wearing seat belts, exercising regularly, voting, and breastfeeding (Fishbein, Middlestadt, & Hitchcock, 1994). Ajzen theorizes that human actions are guided by three principles—behavioral beliefs, normative beliefs, and control beliefs.

- **Behavioral beliefs:** These beliefs include the person's thoughts or feelings about the likely outcome of the behavior and the evaluation of these outcomes. Behavioral beliefs create an attitude of importance about the behavior change. For example, if Tammy, an adolescent mother, determines that breastfeeding her newborn will provide additional immunity for her baby while helping her to lose her pregnancy weight, she may be more inclined to try breastfeeding.

- **Normative beliefs:** Beliefs about the expectations of others and the motivation to meet those expectations (what Ajzen [2006] calls normative beliefs) also play a role. Normative beliefs establish the foundation for the formation of the individual's subjective norm. A subjective norm is a conviction about whether most people approve or disapprove of a behavior (Glanz et al., 2002). As others acknowledge and encourage individuals to strive for the behavior change, they verify the subjective norm and increase the individual's motivation to be successful. Normative beliefs can facilitate or inhibit the performance of the behavior. When deciding whether or not to breastfeed, Tammy asks her friend Joanna what she thinks about it. Joanna replies, "Oh, that is so disgusting; I can't believe anyone would do that." The negative response from Tammy's peer could decrease her willingness to continue her breastfeeding behavior. Conversely, if Joanna said, "I heard that breastfed babies have higher IQs," the positive response could act as encouragement for Tammy.
- **Control beliefs:** Control beliefs, according to Ajzen (2006), represent ideas about the presence of factors that facilitate or impede performance of the behavior and the individual's perceived power over these factors. Control beliefs capture an individual's confidence in the ability to perform the behavior (Ajzen, 2006). When Tammy considers the cost and time necessary to use alternative methods of feeding, she might determine that it is easier and more cost effective to breastfeed.

Each of the belief constructs in Ajzen's theory is directly related to the attitudes of the individual. In combination, behavioral beliefs, subjective norms, and control beliefs lead to the formation of behavioral intention. Ajzen (2006) suggests a positive correlation exists between these three constructs and behavioral intention; as attitudes become more favorable, behavioral intention should become stronger. The three constructs collectively help Tammy to form a positive association with breastfeeding, thus increasing her willingness or intention to practice the behavior. Intention, according to TpB, is assumed to be an immediate antecedent of behavior.

Social Cognitive Theory

The Social Cognitive Theory (SCT) is unique from most of the cognitive-behavioral perspectives because its emphasis is on the interpersonal aspect of behavior. At the interpersonal level it is assumed that individuals are influenced by both physical environment, such as space or equipment, and social environment, such as family members, co-workers, friends, and health professionals (National Cancer Institute, 2005). Many theories examine the relationship between behaviors and the social context; however, the Social Cognitive Theory is considered to be the most robust and is a more frequently used interpersonal theory in health education.

SCT provides a framework for designing, implementing, and evaluating programs by considering the relationship among the environment, the people, and their behavior (Bandura, 1986a). The environment provides situations for the individual to learn new behaviors or have existing behaviors modified by others. As the individual evaluates his own thoughts and feelings about the impact of his behavior in relationship to the outcomes on his social environment, he is motivated to either maintain or alter his current actions. Behavior is not simply the result of the environment and the person, just as the environment is not simply the result of the person and behavior (Glanz et al., 2002).

According to SCT, changing health behavior is highly dependent upon a person's self-efficacy. A person—with confidence—has the ability to attain behavioral goals, even when faced with obstacles (National Cancer Institute, 2005). The ability to exercise control over one's own behavior motivates a person to act and be persistent through challenges (Institute of Medicine, 2002). As behavior in a person changes, it results in changes in the way one responds to one's own environment, thus setting up a reciprocal relationship where the environment and behavior influence one another. For example, Calvin, a new employee at the bank, notices that most of his colleagues bring their lunch to work and eat quickly so they can use the remainder of their lunch hour to work out in the on-site exercise room. Although this was not something he did at his previous place of employment, he is now considering altering his lunch routine to include exercise. The availability of the gym in the physical environment along with the positive examples set by his co-workers in his social environment provide motivation for Calvin to consider modifying his lunch behaviors.

The concepts represented in the SCT are founded on constructs from cognitive, behaviorist, and emotional models of behavior change (National Cancer Institute, 2005). A closer examination of the concepts provides insight into SCT's usefulness as an effective approach to behavior change. The concepts (Glanz et al., 2002, p. 169) include:

- **Environment:** This consists of factors physically external to the person. The physical environment might include the availability of space or resources such as equipment. The on-site gym and workout equipment make it easier for Calvin to exercise during the day, and their availability clearly communicates his employers' desire for employees to practice healthy behaviors at work. Calvin's physical setting facilitates the performance of the behavior. The social environment includes the interactions between the person and other influential people. While working out, Calvin has the opportunity to meet other employees who share a common interest, expanding his social network. Not only does the gym remove a physical barrier to exercise, but the commitment to exercising by Calvin's co-workers also provides a positive social interaction.
- **Situation:** Situation refers to the positive and negative thoughts about the behavior in relationship to one's environment. It includes a person's perception of the place, time, physical features, and the activity (Glanz et al.,

2002). For example, if Calvin perceives that there is enough time to get a workout in and if he believes that participating in the lunchtime workout will impress his employer, his motivation to comply could be greater.

- **Reciprocal determinism:** Reciprocal determinism is the idea that a dynamic interaction exists among the person, the behavior, and the environment where each influences the other. Behavior is shaped by our environment; our behavior also can affect the environment, which in turn can affect our thoughts, which in turn affect our behavior. While working on the bench press, Calvin realizes he needs a spotter to safely lift the bar. Although Sam is only an acquaintance, Calvin's environmental need motivates him to ask Sam for help. Not only is Sam willing to help, but he also offers Calvin some tips to improve his form. When it is time for Sam to work on the bench press, Calvin volunteers to spot him. Calvin's desire to return the favor fosters a positive experience for both men, thus reinforcing the likelihood that they will help each other out again. Before long Sam and Calvin begin to schedule regular workouts at the same time.

- **Self-efficacy:** Self-efficacy is often considered the most important prerequisite for behavior change, which explains why it is considered a ubiquitous construct in health behavior theories (National Cancer Institute, 2005). It represents a person's confidence in the ability to perform a particular behavior by taking action and overcoming barriers. At the gym Calvin notices the addition of a new electronic rowing machine. If Calvin believes the use of the rowing machine will enhance his workout and that he is capable of following the printed guidelines to use the equipment correctly, he is more willing to give it a try. Although he may feel uncomfortable about trying the unfamiliar equipment, he draws on his previous success with other pieces of equipment to build his confidence in his ability to successfully use the rowing machine. Self-efficacy is a critical concept in that it serves as the initial motivation to try. The Roman poet Virgil captured the concept of self-efficacy in his statement, "They are able who think they are able" (Pajares, 2002).

- **Behavioral capacity:** This concept represents the fundamental knowledge and skills necessary to perform the behavior. If a person is to perform a behavior, he or she must know what the behavior is and have the skills to perform it. In order to safely perform an exercise or utilize the gym equipment, Calvin needs to have an understanding of how it works.

- **Expectations:** These represent what a person believes will occur if the behavior is performed. Through trial and error a person discovers that certain outcomes occur when a situation is repeated. The individual then can perceive the cause and effect relationship. As Calvin continues to lift weights, he notices that his biceps are getting larger and that the amount of weight he can lift is increasing. He attributes the cause of this change to be the effect of his lifting behavior.

- **Expectancies:** These are a value assessment of the positive and negative results of the behavior. Individuals strive to minimize negative outcomes

They are able who think they are able.
—Virgil (about 40 B.C.)

and maximize positive ones. As Calvin considers his family history of cardiovascular disease, he comprehends the important role his exercise regime plays in the prevention of chronic disease.

- **Self-control:** Self-control is the ability to set and work toward achieving personal goals related to the behavior. In order for the goal to be reached, the behavior must be performed. Calvin has decided to compete in a marathon. His goal requires him to train hard to build up the endurance needed to compete. Without exercising, Calvin will be unable to successfully attain his goal.

If they can do it, so can I!

- **Observational learning:** Observing the successes and failures of others who have similar attributes contributes to a person's beliefs about his or her own capabilities (Pajares, 2002). Mentally the individual believes, "If they can do it, so can I!" While lifting, Calvin notices Peter, who is also in his early 30s, completing a 30-minute circuit training that combines the rowing machine with treadmill and exercise bike. Calvin thinks about his marathon training and decides that using a circuit method to train would be beneficial. Observations of Peter's behaviors motivate Calvin to change his exercise regime in order to meet his goal.

- **Reinforcements:** These are internal and external motivators that increase or decrease the likelihood of reoccurrence of the behavior. Reinforcements provide a reason for performing or ceasing a behavior. Reinforcements can be tangible, such as an award, or intangible, such as praise from others. As Calvin continues to work out, he begins to feel stronger. This good feeling is an intangible motivator that increases the likelihood that Calvin will continue to exercise. Even marking his workout days on the calendar serves as a tangible reward, representing his efforts to meet his exercise goals.

- **Emotional coping responses:** These are techniques used by a person to manage excessive emotional stimuli. Negative emotional stimuli, such as anxiety or nervousness, can act as a barrier to the performance of a behavior. The responses can include managing one's thoughts about a situation or using external devices to reduce or enhance the emotional level. Suppose Calvin has an important presentation scheduled for the afternoon. Although he does not want to miss his workout, he is fearful he will not have enough time to get showered and dressed before his presentation. To ease his emotions, he decides to set the alarm on his watch to remind him to stop in time. The use of the external device serves as a strategy to manage his concern.

The comprehensive nature of the theory, with its many constructs, allows for application to many health issues. Social Cognitive Theory has been used to study a wide range of health problems including childhood obesity, alcohol abuse, smoking, childhood bullying, and self-management of chronic diseases such as arthritis, hypertension, and diabetes. The inclusion of interpersonal factors in cognitive-based perspectives provides insight into the social nature of behavior.

Theories from a Community-Level Perspective

If we are to contribute significantly . . . we must broaden our perspective . . . beyond the individual level.
—Albert Bandura

Exploring health from an individual perspective has merit; however, it is limited in its ability to influence the masses. Not only did Bandura recognize the importance of considering the social context at the individual level, but he also touted the need to amplify our health education efforts by using community-level perspectives. Bandura stated, "If we are to contribute significantly to the betterment of human health, we must broaden our perspective on health promotion and disease prevention beyond the individual level. This calls for a more ambitious socially oriented agenda of research and practice" (Bandura, 2004, p. 162). Community-level models explore methods to mobilize community members and organizations to change the way social systems function from an ecological perspective (National Cancer Institute, 2005). The major premise of ecological models is that interventions that address behavior on multiple levels will lead to greater changes that sustain themselves for long-term health-promoting habits. Multilevel ecological models have been widely applied in several areas such as tobacco control and even used to guide public health and the science policy agendas of Healthy People (U.S. Department of Health and Human Services [USDHHS], 2000). The Social Ecological Model (SEM), one example of an ecological model, considers the intricate interaction among individual, relationship, community, and societal factors. Each level functions to examine the behavior in relationship to the other levels (Dahlberg & Krug, 2002).

- **Individual:** The first level is similar to cognitive-behavioral perspectives in that it considers factors about the individual such as age, education, income, substance use, or history of abuse. When considering the use of oral tobacco among adolescents in rural communities, one would need to think about the characteristics of adolescent development. It would be important to consider the educational immaturity and desire to explore risky behaviors among adolescents when developing intervention efforts.
- **Relationship:** The second level expands to examine how relationships with peers, intimate partners, and family members increase the risk for the behavior. If using oral tobacco is the norm of a teen's closest social circle, it is likely to influence the teen's acceptance of the behavior.
- **Community:** In the third level, characteristics of settings such as schools, workplaces, and neighborhoods are explored. These characteristics are examined to identify elements that contribute to the behavior. The use of oral tobacco is generally more accepted in rural communities. The "mom and pop" owners of the local grocery may not see any harm in selling tobacco to minors. This discovery would direct health education efforts to target community members as part of the educational regime.
- **Societal:** Level four strives to look at the big picture to determine societal factors and cultural norms that create a climate in which the behavior is encouraged or inhibited. Societal factors such as health, economic, educational, and social policies are reviewed to discover avenues to effectively intervene. A community may discover it lacks policies that regulate

the sale of tobacco to minors. Proposing regulatory legislation within a community could provide an opportunity to enlighten the public on the negative ramification of tobacco use among adolescents. This, in turn, could act to alter the cultural norm.

Health education efforts can begin at any level in the model; however, it is the inclusion of each level in health promotion strategies that increases the chances of having a successful intervention.

Multiple strategies exist for intervening at the community level, each involving different approaches to affect change. Most community organizing models contain key concepts that are necessary to consider if measurable change is to be achieved. These key concepts (National Cancer Institute, 2005) include:

- **Empowerment:** The use of techniques to build confidence in the ability of individuals, organizations, or communities to improve their own quality of life. Presenting concerns to influential members of the community, along with a charge for them to help solve the social problem, allows community members to assume greater power over their own circumstances. This, in turn, fosters the development of community leadership in their effort to create desired changes. Case in point: As a result of community growth, the landfill will no longer be able to accommodate the amount of refuse being created. Projections indicate that the landfill will be at maximum capacity in 5 years. The director of the waste management system provides information to the mayor's office indicating a need to identify solutions to the land space problem. The mayor decides to form a committee with representatives from the local clergy, school district, chamber of commerce, and the Lions Club to explore options for the community. Bringing together influential players allows the community members to assume greater power and to expand their power from within to create desired change.
- **Community capacity:** Considers the ability of a community to identify and address social problems. Capacity looks at the willingness of community members to trust and to work with others for the greater good of the whole. Do community members share responsibility for each other and bond together with common activities, such as neighborhood watch groups? If a community wants to reduce the amount of refuse created by the community, health promotion efforts might emphasize the need for all the members of the community to join the efforts to reduce, reuse, and recycle.
- **Participation:** Identifies ways for community members to act as equal partners in the problem-solving efforts. Participation could be built through the formation of a neighborhood recycling program. Homeowner associations could encourage recycling programs and even provide some supplies to achieve this goal.
- **Relevance:** Considers the importance of allowing community members to create their own agenda based on what they believe to be the pressing needs. One must consider the importance of the issue of concern from the community members' point of view. Perhaps the explosive community

growth has resulted in traffic complications due to an inadequate number of lanes. Although the landfill situation looks bleak and is an issue of distress, a more pressing dilemma of immediate concern to community members might be an inadequate transportation system.

- **Issue selection:** Involves the dissection of a problem into smaller solvable parts. This concept breaks the issue down to allow community members to see smaller changes that will impact the larger problem. Perhaps the creation of policies related to the amount of garbage each household would be allowed to contribute (without additional charge) would motivate community members to self-regulate the amount of garbage they produce, thus encouraging the practice of the reduce, reuse, recycle concept. The addition of the new policy, in conjunction with neighborhood recycling promotion, represents small changes that function collectively to make a significant impact toward solving the landfill problem.

- **Critical consciousness:** Includes strategies to help community members identify the root cause of its social concern. The community may choose to disclose the problematic landfill situation by using television, radio, and newspaper ads, and a waste management hotline could be created to provide additional information for community members who seek it.

The preceding community organization model places emphasis on building power and encourages community members to develop their skills as active citizens (Parachini & Covington, 2001). The model is a grassroots-based, conflict-oriented approach designed to mobilize disadvantaged people to act on their own behalf (Fisher, 1997). Other community-based models differ in that there is less emphasis on grassroots efforts and more focus on the use of policy and regulatory infrastructures to promote change.

Another popular theory that addresses social problems from a community-based perspective is the Diffusion of Innovation Theory. Diffusion of Innovation is an attempt to maximize the exposure of previously successful programs. The previously successful intervention is often considered a "new" and innovative approach to the health concern. This approach attempts to avoid the phenomenon of "reinventing the wheel" by increasing the number of people who are reached by successful interventions (National Cancer Institute, 2005). The concepts of Diffusion of Innovation explain the process by which innovation, such as an idea, product, or social practice, is communicated from one person to another over time among members of a social system (Rogers, 2003). The concepts central to the theory are summarized as follows (Rogers):

- **Innovation:** The "new" idea, object, or practice is discovered by an individual, organization, or other unit of adoption. Consider the promotion of family planning methods in third world countries. Although strategies to regulate reproduction are common in the United States, other nations, such as Indonesia, Thailand, and Colombia, struggle with multiple barriers that inhibit the adoption of family planning behaviors. One common barrier to family planning models is the limited number of health professionals

Neither contemplation of the navel nor the writing of pamphlets can be shown to be cost-effective.
—Mohan Singh

available to provide services. It is common to have one doctor for thousands of people in Indonesia, thus the "innovation" would be to build a clinic without walls where laypersons become part of the staff under the direction of the physician.

- **Communication channels:** Communication channels represent the means by which ideas are transmitted from one person to another. This can occur on an interpersonal or a mass media level. Laypersons working in the clinic work to educate clients on the various methods of birth control along with instruction on proper use. These laypersons might include religious leaders and other influential members of the village (Crossette, 1994).

- **Social system:** The joining of groups of individuals together to adopt the innovation represents the use of social systems. According to Rogers, social systems represent, ". . . a set of interrelated units that are engaged in joint problem solving to accomplish a common goal" (2003, p. 23). Uniting community organizations with governmental efforts also facilitates the adoption of an innovation. In Buddhist Thailand, for example, cutting fertility from more than 6.5 births to 2.1 per woman in a quarter of a century had much to do with government support and the efforts of the independent Population and Community Development Foundation (Crossette, 1994).

- **Time:** The amount of time it takes to adopt the innovation. How long it will take to institutionalize (be accepted as a normal procedure) the practice of using laypersons to provide family planning can have direct impact on the strength of the innovations. Innovations that have quick institutionalization are likely to sustain themselves and have a greater impact on public health.

Diffusion of Innovation Theory has been used to promote condom use, smoking cessation, and the use of new technologies by health practitioners. Like other community approaches it employs a multilevel approach to behavior change.

Change Strategies   Basically, health promotion strategies facilitate change from a continuum of two approaches: changes in people's behavior or changes in the environment (National Cancer Institute, 2005). These approaches can be subdivided into three ecological levels: individual, interpersonal, or community. Efforts that target the individual strive to alter a person's knowledge, skills, and attitude about behavior with the notion that changes in the individual behaviors might indirectly lead to changes in the environment. For example, when individuals adopt the practice of riding a bike to work, it results in an increased demand for bike lanes in the community. Innovations that emphasize community-level theory strive to make changes in the environment that indirectly influence the behaviors of the individual. As the number of bike lanes in the community increases more individuals ride their bike to work. Interpersonal-level theories tend to fall in the middle, investigating the relationship between individuals and their environments.

Figure 3-7 summarizes the continuum change strategies and the useful theories for each ecological level.

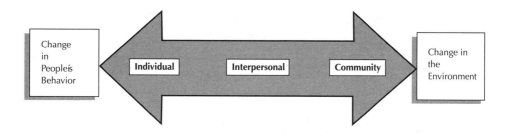

Ecological Level	Individual	Interpersonal	Community
Useful Theories	Health Belief Model Stages of Change Theory Decisional Balance Theory Self-Efficacy Theory Theory of Planned Behavior	Social Cognitive Theory	Social Ecological Model Community Organization Diffusion of Innovation Theory
Examples of Strategies	Individual counseling Health fairs Newsletters/flyers	Support groups Peer counseling	Bond elections Promoting change through policy

Figure 3-7
Change Strategies by Ecological Level
Source: Adapted from National Cancer Institute, 2005, p. 46.

Using Theories and Planning Models

Theories and planning models are tools available to practitioners to create solutions to health problems (National Cancer Institute, 2005). Like all tools, the ability to use them effectively comes with practice. Becoming comfortable with behavior change theories and planning models enhances a practitioner's ability to effectively plan innovations that maximize health promotion efforts. These tools provide a systematic approach to solving problems by looking at the health concern from a comprehensive perspective while narrowing the scope of the issue into manageable components.

Case Study: John

Objective: After reviewing the case study, the reader will discuss three or more obvious barriers to the success of this workshop.

John is offering a workshop for low-income expectant mothers as part of his work for the March of Dimes. He personally likes role-playing as a method, so he has written up several role-plays about life after the delivery. The site for the two-hour workshop is a nice upscale hotel, and he has mailed approximately 100 invitations. This is a very culturally diverse community with many Asians, Salvadorians, and Mexican Americans. John is surprised at the low participant turnout and very indignant when the few mothers-to-be in attendance walk out rather than participate in role-plays. (See Case Studies Revisited page 90.)

Questions to consider:

1. Based on the number of invitations sent, how many participants should John expect to attend?
2. What might be some barriers associated with the location John selected to host his workshop?
3. How might John's selected method (role-play) act as a barrier?
4. What suggestions would you make to help John improve his planning efforts?
5. How might the use of a planning model, such as PRECEDE-PROCEED have helped John identify these potential pitfalls?

Educational Principles

You should also review basic educational principles when determining which methods to employ. Have you applied as many educational principles as possible, such as reinforcement, repetition, and practice? Reviewing these principles will often trigger new ideas about which methods to use or not to use.

In order to address health issues through health education, it is important that we draw on the vast knowledge base that education has developed to tell us how to educate learners. The following principles, adapted from Gilbert's text (1981), are of enormous importance to health educators.

Principles Related to Motivation Teaching is effective only when clients are motivated to learn. Some principles of motivation follow:

- Learning is more effective when the learner is motivated by results intrinsic to the experience.
- Individuals tend to repeat behaviors that are rewarded (reinforced).
- Immediate reinforcement is more effective than delayed reinforcement.
- Fear and punishment have uncertain effects upon learning. They may facilitate or hinder it, depending on the learner's individual reaction at the time.
- An individual learns best when he or she believes the learning is important.
- Learners can be helped to understand a concept, principle, or generalization by being shown how varied experiences relate to it and how it can be applied to a new situation.

Principles Related to Needs and Abilities Clients can learn only to the extent of their abilities, and they are usually motivated to learn only that which they perceive as necessary. Therefore, educators must determine the needs and abilities of their client base. Principles related to this task follow:

- Behaviors sought should be within the range of possibility for the learner involved.
- Generally, the higher the educational level of any given group, the greater is the effectiveness of using the printed word.
- The lower the educational level, the greater is the need for oral or visual media.
- There are marked individual differences in any given group of learners.
- Individuals usually slant persuasive communications to fit their own biases. It is important to protect learners from your biases.
- Creative individuals show a preference for the complex and the novel.
- When problems or issues are a common concern, group thinking is an effective approach to learning.

Principles Related to the General Nature of Learning

Health educators, like any other educators, should be familiar with the following principles of the functions of learning:

- In order for learning to occur, repetition is usually required. Three exposures to the content are recommended.
- Learning should be an active process that involves the dynamic interaction of the learner with that which is to be learned.
- Other things being equal, recent experiences are more vivid than earlier ones.
- Learning generally proceeds from the general to the specific, and then to the general (whole–part–whole).
- Transfer learning is not automatic. The ability to apply prior knowledge or skills to a new context must be taught.
- Behaviors or skills sought must be practiced.
- Learning generally progresses from the known to the unknown, from the concrete to the abstract, and from the simple to the complex.
- Periods of practice interrupted by periods of rest result in more efficient learning than do longer periods of practice with few or no interruptions.
- Time spent recalling and discussing what has been read facilitates learning more than mere rereading.

Characteristics of Learner and Community

We must always consider the characteristics of the individuals and groups we are working with, namely, the following:

Age
Gender
Reading ability
Language skills/proficiency in English
Biases and beliefs held
Readiness to learn

Cultural and ethnic background
Motivation to learn
Learning preferences

Successful application of the previously mentioned theories and models depends on how these characteristics are addressed. For example, if this is a court-ordered alcohol education program, you may have good attendance in terms of the number of bodies, but it is usually a great challenge to get the minds in those bodies interested and attentive. Most community workshops mix ability groups, making it a further challenge to maintain a high interest level.

Principles Related to Adult Learners

Adult learners present a unique dynamic to the learning environment. The wide range of experiences and perspectives of adults dictate that they see a connection between learning objectives and application to their own lives (Edmunds, Lowe, Murray, & Seymour, 2002). Additionally, adults typically vary significantly in their preferences for how they learn as well as their aptitudes and abilities for learning. Edmunds, Lowe, Murray, and Seymour suggest several key differences between adult and child learners, including:

- Unlike children who rely on others to determine what is important to learn, adults are autonomous, preferring to decide for themselves.
- Adults are unwilling to accept information at face value and need to validate the information from their own perspective.
- Adults expect what they are learning to be immediately useful, unlike children who anticipate learning to be useful in the future.
- Adults use previous experiences as a canvas on which to add new information, unlike children who are often relatively inexperienced with limited viewpoints.
- Adults have the potential to be knowledgeable/creditable resources in the learning environment compared to the limited ability of children.

Robert W. Pike (2003), expert in human resource development and adult learning, has identified four fundamental principles related to adult learning. He refers to these as "Pike's Laws of Adult Learning." Although adults are the target of Pike's laws, his principles appear to be fairly universal for most learners.

His first law is related to experiential learning. Just as babies and children enjoy learning through experience, educational experts have discovered that adult learning is also enhanced by hands-on experiences. The ability to manipulate items or props in a hands-on situation enables the learner to "experience" the material and fit the new information into existing schemes.

Pike's second law is centered on the notion of self-directed learning. Learners are more apt to believe in and support their own ideas. Thus, the role of the educator is to design learning environments that allow participants to generate ideas, concepts, or techniques. The educator serves as guide, leading and clarifying, rather than as an all-knowing professor of information.

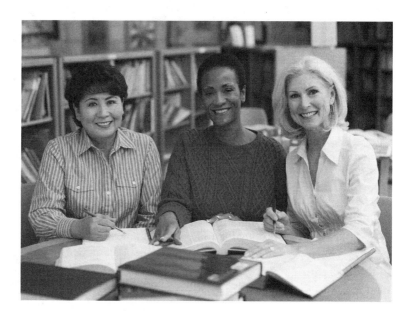

Adult learners need to see a connection between their personal lives and the learning objectives presented in the classroom.

The learning environment is often an overlooked aspect of learning. According to Pike's third law, there is a proportional relationship between the amount of learning and the amount of fun participants are having (Pike, 2003). Although having fun should never be the primary goal of an educational program, it is often a natural by-product of effective interventions. Creating a relaxed, comfortable environment where participants feel free to laugh, cry, and share personal experiences functions to tear down barriers to the learning process.

Pike's fourth law of learning sounds like the resounding gong of most health educators—behavior change equals learning. Actual changes in behavior are clear indicators that learning has occurred. The ultimate goal of all educational endeavors is to make a positive change in the participant's current knowledge, skill level, or attitude toward the behavior. The ability to apply the learning is what counts most; thus, providing ample opportunities to practice will increase the likelihood of retention (Edmunds et al., 2002).

Learning Preferences   It is common knowledge that individuals process information in different ways. A learning preference is a preferred method of taking in, organizing, and making sense of information. Learning preferences are often referred to as learning styles. Stewart and Felicetti (1992) define a preferred learning style as those educational situations under which a student is most likely to learn. "If students' learning styles are compatible with the teaching style of their instructors, they tend to retain more information, effectively apply it, and have a better attitude toward the subject" (Wirz, 2004). Learners can be classified according to their learning style/preference: visual, auditory, or tactile/kinesthetic.

Visual learners learn best by seeing. This type of student uses cues from the body language and facial expressions of others to fully understand the subject matter. Visual learners often think in pictures and learn best from visual displays such as diagrams, illustrations, videos, flip-charts, demonstrations, and handouts, and by eliciting memories (Wirz, 2004). If given the task of assembling a bicycle, the visual learner would rely heavily on his or her mental image of a completed bicycle and the graphic display in the directions as cues to complete the task.

Auditory learners learn best by listening. These learners interpret the meaning by listening to the tone, pitch, speed, and other nuances of speech. Ideal methods for auditory learners include lectures and small or large group discussions. When assembling the bike, the auditory learner would likely read the printed directions out loud, because written information has little meaning for him or her until it is heard (Figure 3-8).

Tactile/kinesthetic learners learn best by doing, moving, or touching. They prefer movement and concentrate best when do not have to sit still for long periods of time. Hands-on methods that allow the individual to explore and practice best facilitate learning for this group. The tactile/kinesthetic learner would likely toss the directions to the side when attempting to assemble a bike.

A health educator can easily accommodate varied learner preferences by selecting a mixture of methods within a program. Varying the strategies used for

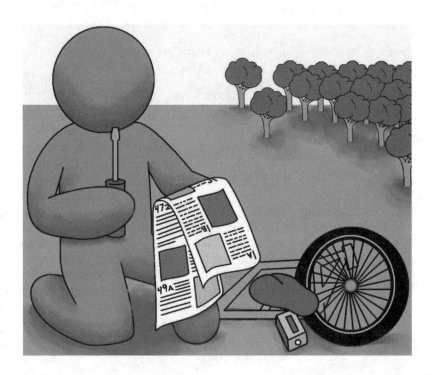

Figure 3-8
Learning Preferences

intervention decreases boredom while giving learners the opportunity to experience the content in a venue that optimizes their educational learning style.

Group Size   The size of the group will play an important role in method selection. Large groups, say over 100, make individual interaction difficult. Methods must be selected while keeping in mind the size of the group. Lecture is a way to share a considerable amount of cognitive information in a short time but usually is not effective for reaching affective or psychomotor objectives. Small groups offer flexibility in many ways but also put more pressure on the individual to participate. Ideally, small group size is from 4 to 6; however, groups can be as small as 3 or as large as 10 (Allen, Duch, & Groh, 2001). Groups with an odd number of members are recommended for greater success in working through conflicts. For projects involving research that culminates in a written report and/or an oral presentation, teams of three to five members can be quite effective (Howard, 1999).

Contact Time   The time you have to spend with a group will play a major role in the selection of appropriate methods. Certain methods simply cannot be used in a short period of time. Many activities require a certain amount of trust to be successful. Developing trust often involves icebreaking activities, which usually require time in order to create openness among the participants. Short workshops do not lend themselves to these activities. As the amount of contact time decreases the method selected must maximize the learning opportunity by ensuring that essential content is effectively delivered.

Objective: After reviewing the case study, the reader will identify two or more problems associated with the method James selected for his intervention.

Case Study: James   James is conducting a 2-hour workshop on alcohol abuse with 20 individuals who have been referred to this mandatory workshop for drinking and driving offenders. James has not worked with this type of group before and decides to use an icebreaker exercise designed to reveal personal details of the participants. The group members immediately become hostile and bombard poor James with comments like, "I don't want to be here anyway," "This information is no one's business but mine," "Just get on with the facts and let's all get out of here!" James cuts short the icebreaker and concludes the workshop as quickly as possible with a less than successful lecture on the dangers of alcohol abuse and driving. (See Case Studies Revisited page 90.)

Questions to consider:

1. What characteristics of the learners should James have considered when developing his intervention?
2. Why might the use of a personal icebreaker in this situation be an inappropriate method to select?

Budget Quality health education need not be expensive, but it does require an appropriate budget. To compete successfully with unhealthy media messages and long-held unhealthy habits, we need and deserve a reasonable budget. Do you have enough money to use the best methods for the health education program? If you have limited resources, can you still achieve your objectives, or would you be better off limiting the number of programs but improving the quality of the programs offered?

Quality health educators should receive quality salaries for their time, and that requires an appropriate budget. Photocopies, DVDs, computer software, and other tools of the health educator all cost money.

Resources/Site You must consider all the resources you have at your disposal. Do you have good facilities to break out into small groups? If you have access to a microcomputer lab, it opens up totally new possibilities. Will you have a quiet space for presentations? What about parking or transportation? If you have access to well-appointed teaching facilities, it opens up the use of many methods. This is especially true of those methods that include technology. Do the participants have Internet access? Of course, many quality health education programs have been offered without any facilities by reaching into homes or utilizing community settings. You work with what is available, and often the local setting is much better for achieving your objectives.

Characteristics of the Educational Provider If you are the primary provider, what are your strengths as a health educator? What methods are you uncomfortable using? Although you should be willing to take some chances if you are to be successful, it is important you not

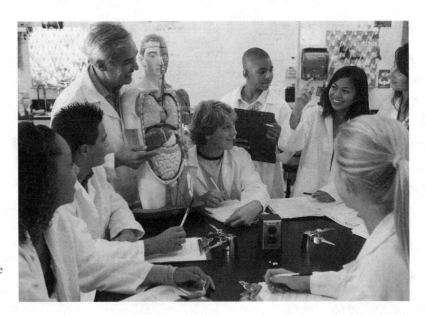

Be sure that the size of your group is appropriate for the type of program you are conducting.

set yourself up for disaster by selecting a method that will make you so uncomfortable that you cannot do a credible job. If certain methods seem central to achieving your objectives, it may be vital to employ them. Therefore, you may need to practice the method so you can be effective in using it, or perhaps you should bring in an outsider to conduct the method. Using such guests can often increase your comfort with a method while providing a needed activity for your target population. Again, the important principle is to use the correct method given your objectives.

The health educator must also be very cognizant of the influential role his or her personal attitude will have on the educational environment.

It is critical that you communicate a sense of excitement and support for the intervention. If you are not energized about the content being presented, why should your participants be? People are naturally drawn to optimistic individuals; thus, the health educator should strive to maintain a positive, supportive attitude that will in turn foster a positive learning climate.

Cultural Appropriateness

It is extremely important that you consider the cultural characteristics of the group you are targeting. Many programs have failed because of this issue. The best protection is to establish an advisory group from the group being targeted. This small group can preview your methods and give you some idea of what response to expect from the participants. Another, less formal way to get some idea is to sit down with a few participants prior to the event and ask them if they think the method would work and be appropriate. (See also Chapters 8 and 9.)

Using a Variety of Methods

Why use a variety of methods? Following are some reasons:

1. It makes it more likely you will achieve your objectives.
2. It may prevent disruptive behavior.
3. It may ensure participant interest.
4. It is more fun for the presenter and learner.
5. Not all learners respond positively to the same methods.

Remember, in health education we are often working with hard-to-reach groups, and anyone gets tired of the same presentation method. Always do what you can to make your presentation interesting, and you will have a better chance of achieving your objectives. By keeping people interested you will also minimize disruptive behavior, such as demonstrated lack of attention or even outright hostility. During community workshops some participants may actually walk out. The first time you have a large number of people walking out on your presentation, you will be very upset, but the problem may simply be a lack of variety or poor method selection. Variety is more fun for you too. You will lose interest if you do things the same way each time. Try new methods, and you will find your task much more enjoyable.

Some Comments on Method Choice

At the elementary and secondary levels, straight lecture or textbook methods are *considered nonfunctional* (Fodor & Dalis, 1974, p. 53).

Each instructor must develop his or her own technique of facilitating. Learning is greatly increased if students are motivated and interested in what they are doing. One of the major criticisms of health education programs is that they are dull. Developing a caring, humanistic approach toward participants should help health educators make their classes more exciting and challenging for the students. The learning process can and should be made enjoyable and interesting.

Any teaching technique or procedure must actively involve the learner if it is to be effective. According to Pike (1994), the average adult can "listen with understanding" for approximately 90 minutes, and "listen with retention" for approximately 20 minutes. As the level of intelligence decreases, the ability to retain information naturally decreases. Pike recommends the "90/20/8 rule," suggesting that no session we teach run more than 90 minutes, the method should be changed at least every 20 minutes, and participants should actively manipulate the content every 8 minutes (Booth, 2007). Active participation can be either direct or vicarious. In direct participation, the student is physically involved in the activity; in vicarious participation, he or she is a viewer of an activity that is going on in another place or another time. Either way, the goal is for the individual to be affected positively and provided perceptions and experiences contributing to the attainment of desirable long-range cognitive, affective, and action goals (Kime, Schlaadt, & Tritsch, 1977, p. 96).

Different learning opportunities should not be used for the sake of variety alone. True, a variety of learning techniques is of value in that variety tends to break the monotony for the teacher as well as for the student, but there are other important reasons for using different learning opportunities: (1) to meet a variety of objectives, (2) to meet a variety of student needs and interests, and (3) to stimulate a variety of senses (Oberteuffer, Pollock, & Harrelson, 1972, pp. 138–139).

One of the most important generalizations that emerges from systematic comparisons of programs and experiments with positive results and those with negative findings (no effect) is that the greater the variety in educational methods used, the more likely the program or experiment will show positive results. This generalization applies both with individuals and with populations. At the individual level, variety in education methods apparently helps to surround the learner with communications appealing to different senses and modes of learning that are mutually supportive (Green, 1976, p. iv).

Montambeau and Finch (2000) believe that learning is related to the method selected, as shown in Figure 3-9. The more active and involved the learner becomes, the more likely he or she will be to learn. Hence, the least effective strategy is simple lecture, with no learner activity, and the most effective occurs when the learner is teaching others and, thus, immediately applying what has been learned to the fullest extent.

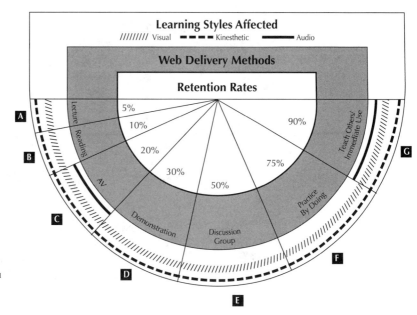

Figure 3-9
Learning Retention
Rates According to
Strategy
Source: From Montambeau
& Finch, 2008. Reprinted
with permission.

The Learning Environment

The mental/emotional environment can be influenced by the physical environment in which we conduct our classes or workshops. We must do what we can to make the total environment as pleasant as possible. If we have control over the space, we should strive to develop a cheerful, positive appearance that is conducive to learning. It is common sense that a room that is warm and pleasant is an enhancement for good learning. Select warm colors and organize the space to be inviting. Adding colorful paper and posters also sets a positive mood. Be certain to change the colors and posters on a regular basis. Like variety in method selection, variety in the environment stimulates learning. Often in community settings we have limited control over the physical setting.

Objective: After reviewing the case study, the reader will explain the relationship between the learning environment and learner performance.

Case Study: Susan Susan inherits a classroom that is run-down and gloomy in appearance. Many years ago it was painted a battleship gray, which has now faded. The bulletin boards are old and worn. She believes that this is contributing to a negative atmosphere and wants to do something about it. She has requested through her principal that it be refreshed. She discusses the problem with her students, who organize a fund-raising drive that results in $145 for paint and paper. Over the break students volunteer to help scrub

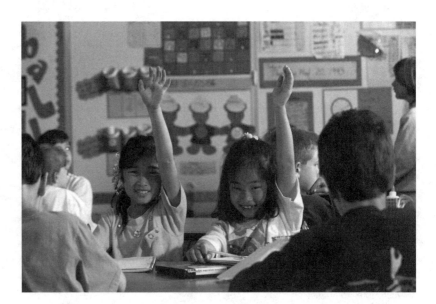

Rooms that are decorated cheerfully with warm colors offer an inviting learning environment.

and paint the room. The transformation is dramatic. The 3 days of vacation time spent painting result in a major change in the total environment. Susan notices a significant change in the classroom climate. (See Case Studies Revisited page 91.)

Questions to consider:

1. Do you believe Susan's outcomes in the classroom climate were worth her personal investment? Why or why not?
2. How might the inclusion of the students in the renovation project foster an effective learning environment?

Noise Levels   Noise can be a major distraction in the learning environment. Select a site free of distractions as much as possible. Soft background music can sometimes overcome some noise from the outside. Other noise can come from participants and can also be a distraction or could simply indicate a high degree of interest. Noise must be evaluated in terms of what helps achieve learning. Many classrooms are so quiet that learning is unlikely to be taking place. Noise, therefore, is not always bad. If we desire to increase learning retention, noise levels will likely increase if the methods used involve active learning. Participants need opportunities to show enthusiasm and ask questions. The reason for the noise is an important consideration. All participants should have an opportunity to hear and be heard.

Seating Arrangements

The way you organize your seating is very important. Most situations allow for some change. Determine what would be the best seating arrangement for the objectives you hope to achieve. If you want interaction, a circle might be best. If you feel you need most interaction to be between you and the group, a semi-circle might be best. If it is a large group, you might consider multiple rows with your position elevated. If you want small-group work, you might consider small clusters. Figures 3-10 through 3-15 depict various seating arrangements.

Cluster Seating (Figure 3-10): Arranging four or five desks in such a manner that the participants face one another.

Positives:

- Facilitates group work and activities.
- Facilitates learning from others and peer education.
- Allows for hands-on learning.

Negatives:

- Some participants will have their back to the instructor, requiring participants to turn during active instruction.
- The arrangement could distract from the ability to practice independently.

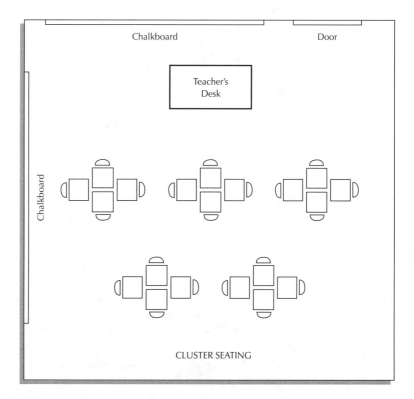

Figure 3-10
Interaction and Small-Group Work

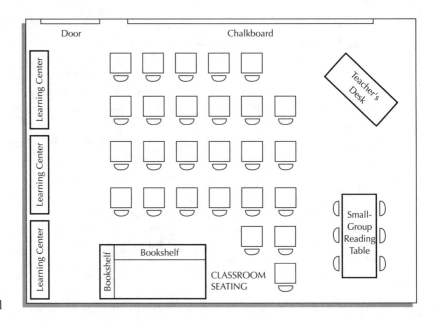

Figure 3-11
Flexibility with Control

- Group dynamics could inhibit learning (mismatched ability level or personality of the participants).
- Limits the instructor's ability to regulate activity.

Traditional Classroom Seating (Figure 3-11): Participants are all facing the front of the room in parallel rows and columns.

Positives:

- Emphasizes the role of the health educator as the instructional leader.
- Accommodates a maximum number of people.
- Ideal for independent activities.
- Allows focus of attention to be centralized on the instructor, screen, or board.
- Provides participants with a sense of personal space.

Negatives:

- Creates natural barriers to conversation, thus limiting discussion among participants.
- Limits the mobility of the presenter to the front of the room.
- The zone of teaching emphasis becomes the front and center of the arrangement. Participants seated on the sides, back, and corners might not participate equally with those seated in the middle or front.

Circular Seating (Figure 3-12): All seats are positioned fairly close, facing into the center of the room.

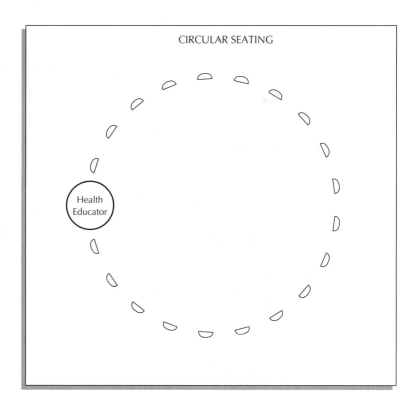

Figure 3-12
Guided Interaction

Positives:

- Promotes a sense of equality among participants.
- Facilitates equal interaction and participation.
- All participants are "exposed" to the health educator and other participants.
- Promotes the role of the health educator as "part of the group" in lieu of an authority figure.

Negatives:

- Loss of anonymity might make some participants feel uncomfortable.
- The proximity of desks promotes side conversation among neighboring participants.
- Limits the ability of the instructor to control off-task behavior.

U-Shaped Seating (Figure 3-13): Desks are arranged in parallel rows on one side of the room facing the parallel rows on the opposite side with an open space in the middle. The two rows are connected by an additional per-pendicular row of inward-facing desks. The health educator can be located in the open portion of the U shape or can minimize his or her presence by standing behind the perpendicular row.

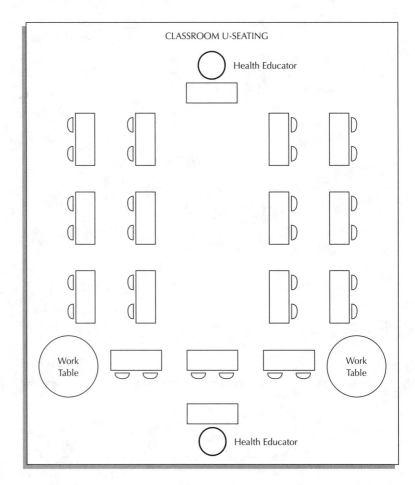

Figure 3-13
Flexibility with
Emphasis on Interaction

Positives:

- Useful for demonstration.
- Useful for debate.
- Encourages eye contact among participants.
- Health educator has greater freedom of movement.
- Promotes interaction among participants.
- Seating can be easily altered to create buzz groups.

Negatives:

- Creates a barrier among participants by dividing the room into sides.
- The zone of emphasis becomes the middle, potentially de-emphasizing students located at the ends and corners.
- The proximity of desks promotes side conversation among neighboring participants.
- The arrangement could distract from independent practice.

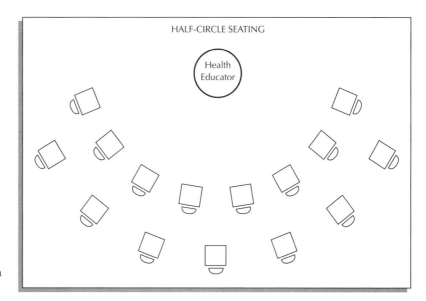

Figure 3-14
Controlled Interaction
with Health Educator in
Controlling Position

Half-Circle Seating (Figure 3-14): Seats are arranged in a semi-circle facing the health educator located in the middle.

Positives:

• Facilitates class discussions with an understanding that the health educator is the discussion leader.
• Allows the health educator greater freedom of movement among participants.
• More relaxed than parallel rows with minimal loss of control by instructor.

Negatives:

• Requires a large amount of space.
• The zone of emphasis becomes the middle, potentially de-emphasizing students located at the ends.

Board Room Seating (Figure 3-15): Design is similar to the U shape with parallel and perpendicular seating; however, the space between desks/tables is removed, creating a conference table.

Positives:

• Facilitates problem-solving activities by increasing the proximity of participants and reducing personal space.

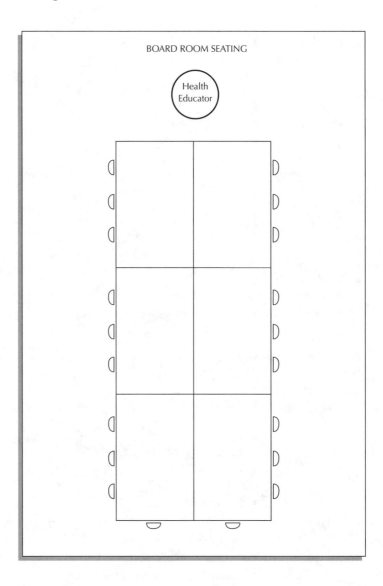

Figure 3-15
Controlled Interaction

- The instructional leader is clearly defined but easily shifted to other members in the group.
- Promotes a business-like environment and a sense of formality.

Negatives:

- The close proximity of participants could be uncomfortable for learners.
- Not conducive for larger groups.
- Eye contact is limited among participants seated on the same side.

It is important to plan ahead and not let seating happen simply by accident. Arrive early for workshops and plan your environment. Arrange the seating and let people know it is not okay to change it. If you do not want people sitting in the back, then do not place seats in the back. If you are in the classroom, do not let students pick where they sit until you know them well. Certain students or participants should never sit together. Be certain to also consider any special needs students have such as hearing or sight limitations. Putting someone in an incorrect seat can produce a behavioral problem. For example, a participant who cannot hear may become very disruptive simply because he or she cannot participate.

Using the Total Environment

In the past many health education programs have assumed that the few contact hours of the program could lead to major changes in the target population without giving consideration to the total environment in which individual members exist. It is important that we give consideration to the total physical and mental climate in which these people live.

Although we may not have the capability to significantly alter this environment, we can probably provide the knowledge or skills to alter perceptions of the environment. That is, we might help participants overcome feelings of lack of control or helplessness or we might provide information on where to get help to change the environment.

Case Study: Maria

Objective: After reviewing the case study, the reader will describe two or more environmental barriers ignored by Maria, which may have resulted in poor compliance.

Maria has conducted a prenatal care workshop for residents in the community who qualify for subsidized housing. The major objective was to increase knowledge regarding the reasons to seek prenatal care and increase compliance. Maria selected a variety of methods that emphasized the positive health outcomes among women who received prenatal care. The workshop was well attended, and the information seemed to be received with interest. Post-workshop assessment showed knowledge was significantly increased. A 6-month follow-up, however, shows no increase in seeking care compliance. (See Case Studies Revisited page 91.)

Questions to consider:

1. If Maria's goal was to increase prenatal care among her participants, how might her stated objective have led to inappropriate method selection?
2. What do you believe might be potential barriers to this target population that hinder prenatal care?

Packaging the Total Intervention Strategy

How your methods fit together to form your intervention package is important in achieving your objectives. Are the methods complementary and reinforcing? Do the methods break up the time together so that you can more easily hold the attention of your intended audience? Have you appealed to different styles of learning? Have you applied as many educational principles as possible, such as reinforcement, repetition, and practice?

Common Mistakes in Method Selection

Beware of the following common mistakes in method selection:

1. Selecting a method that you personally like but that is not the best method for achieving your stated objectives
2. Underestimating or overestimating the time required to conduct a method properly
3. Selecting an inappropriate method for the characteristics of the group
4. Not reinforcing key points

Principles of Engagement

The Centers for Disease Control and Prevention has developed a set of principles of engagement to promote quality community involvement in community health projects. These principles, presented in Table 3-2, can and should be applied to community health programs.

For more information and tools related to this chapter visit http://healtheducation.jbpub.com/strategies.

Table 3-2 Principles of Community Engagement

Before Starting a Community Engagement Effort . . .

1. Be clear about the purposes or goals of the engagement effort, and the populations and/or communities you want to engage.
2. Become knowledgeable about the community in terms of its economic conditions, political structures, norms and values, demographic trends, history, and experience with engagement efforts. Learn about the community's perceptions of those initiating the engagement activities.

For Engagement to Occur, It Is Necessary to . . .

3. Go into the community, establish relationships, build trust, work with the formal and informal leadership, and seek commitment from community organizations and leaders to create processes for mobilizing the community.
4. Remember and accept that community self-determination is the responsibility and right of all people who comprise a community. No external entity should assume it can bestow to a community the power to act in its own self-interest.

Table 3-2 Principles of Community Engagement (continued)

For Engagement to Succeed . . .
5. Partnering with the community is necessary to create change and improve health.
6. All aspects of community engagement must recognize and respect community diversity. Awareness of the various cultures of a community and other factors of diversity must be paramount in designing and implementing community engagement approaches.
7. Community engagement can only be sustained by identifying and mobilizing community assets, and by developing capacities and resources for community health decisions and action.
8. An engaging organization or individual change agent must be prepared to release control of actions or interventions to the community, and be flexible enough to meet the changing needs of the community.
9. Community collaboration requires long-term commitment by the engaging organization and its partners.

Source: U.S. Department of Health and Human Services, 1979.

EXERCISES

1. Select one of the theories/models or elements of a theory/model described in this chapter and apply it (them) to a specific health intervention. For example, consider HIV education for a community youth group. You could apply the Health Belief Model as a whole, elements of the Health Belief Model, or maybe you want to focus on the Theory of Planned Behavior of condom use. State the health issue on which you will focus, select the theory/model/element, and then briefly outline an intervention, describing the methods that will operationalize the theory.

2. One of the educational principles related to motivating the learner states: *Fear and punishment have uncertain effects upon learning. They may facilitate or hinder learning.* You are conducting a workshop for middle-aged women on preventing cervical cancer. Briefly describe how this educational principle could have an impact on your workshop.

3. One of the educational principles related to the needs and abilities of the learner states: *The lower the educational level, the greater the reliance on oral or picture media.* You are conducting a workshop for 10-year-old children on safety in the home. Briefly describe how this educational principle could have an impact on your presentation, and give concrete examples of how you would incorporate this principle.

4. You are planning to conduct a series of community workshops on weight control. List four *characteristics of the learner* that should be considered in planning, and briefly describe why each is important.

5. Interview a health educator regarding what models and theories he or she uses in the practice of health education.

CASE STUDIES REVISITED

Case Study Revisited: Molly   Molly addressed most of the concepts in the IBCF; unfortunately, her failure to account for predisposing and enabling factors has limited the effectiveness of the intervention. The program successfully provided the requisite knowledge about the importance of fruit and vegetable consumption, the necessary skills for evaluating healthy snack choices, and promoted a positive attitude about eating healthy. She failed to consider financial burden (enabling factor) associated with eating healthier foods. It is also possible, however, that the snacks in the vending machine were not the personal preferences of the students. Perhaps Molly should have included in her program a method that allowed students to determine what should be found in their healthy vending machine. The method would provide Molly with direction for the selection of fruits and vegetables while addressing predisposing factors related to personal preference. Reducing the cost of the items seems like an obvious solution; however, this may not be a viable option without additional funding to subsidize the cost of the healthier food. Molly might consider adding methods to promote the vending machine foods as "student choices" and tout the benefits of the healthier foods for just a few more cents, thus pointing out the positive aspects of the change and reinforcing the likelihood of snack purchase. (See page 55.)

Case Study Revisited: John   John has much to learn about workshop conduct and method selection. John sent out 100 invitations . . . how many people should he expect to attend? If health educators get a 50% attendance rate from invitations, they are usually thrilled! Is it likely that low-income individuals will be willing or even able to travel to an upscale hotel outside their community? John's attendance might have improved had he conducted the workshop at a site in the target community. Because of a personal interest in a strategy, John may have selected an inappropriate method for this population. Did he consult local community leaders about his presentation and discuss the most effective approaches he could utilize? Probably not. When health educators work with groups that they are unfamiliar with, it is essential that research or consultation of some type be performed in order to optimize effective strategy selection. (See page 69 and Chapters 8 and 9.)

Case Study Revisited: James   James obviously had not made a good match between his strategy selection and learner characteristics. In addition, using a revealing icebreaker exercise in a short, once-only workshop where trust could never be established was an error and not a good use of limited contact time. This example points to the necessity of thoroughly examining all the elements of learner characteristics and presentation conditions (group size, contact time) before proceeding with an intervention. Too many health educators have had to learn the hard way . . . through painful experience. (See page 75.)

Case Study Revisited: Susan   Susan has demonstrated an understanding of the effects that the environment can have on learning, and she has shown a great deal of initiative in enhancing her own particular environment. The atmosphere in Susan's classes may not change overnight, but she has optimized the possibility for change. Additionally, including the students as participants in the renovation project gives the students a sense of ownership and responsibility for learning in their classroom. Health educators should not underestimate the effects that the physical environment can have on learning, and in some cases how easily the environment can be improved. (See page 79.)

Case Study Revisited: Maria   Maria has conducted a useful workshop that obviously met her objective, providing some needed factual information. Unfortunately, her objective did not adequately support her goal of increasing compliance to seek prenatal care. Maria failed to consider the total environment (physical and mental) of her population and just what compliance would necessitate. Maria provided no information on the accessibility of the clinic or how to get there, and she failed to emphasize the very low costs involved. Including objectives, selecting methods to address skills related to accessing the clinic, and considering attitudes concerning barriers associated with cost might have produced more favorable compliance. She gave no real thought to the total environment of this group or the potential barriers to effecting a positive behavior change. (See page 87.)

SUMMARY

Selecting the appropriate educational intervention is vital to achieving your objectives.

1. The selection of a method should always take into account the objectives to be achieved.

2. Some other important considerations are
Educational principles
Theory and model application
Adult learners
Characteristics of the learner
Learning preferences
Group size
Contact time
Budget
Resources/site/environment
Characteristics of the educational provider
Cultural appropriateness
Using a variety of methods
Packaging the total intervention strategy

3. The total environment must be considered when planning for instruction.

4. Principles of community engagement can greatly enhance the likelihood of success.

REFERENCES AND RESOURCES

Ajzen, I. (1991). The theory of planned behavior. *Organizational Behavior and Human Decision Processes, 50*, 179–211.

Ajzen, I. (2006). Constructing a TpB questionnaire: Conceptual and methodological considerations. January 2006. Retrieved June 9, 2008, from http://www.people.umass.edu/aizen/pdf/tpb.measurement.pdf

Ajzen, I., & Fishbein, M. (1973). Attitudinal and normative variables as predictors of specific behaviors. *Journal of Personality and Social Psychology, 27,* 41–57.

Ajzen, I., & Fishbein, M. (1980). *Understanding Attitudes and Predicting Social Behavior.* Englewood Cliffs, NJ: Prentice-Hall.

Allen, D. E., Duch, B. J., & Groh, S. E. (2001). Strategies for using groups. In B. J. Duch, S. E. Groh, & D. E. Allen (Eds.), *The Power of Problem-Based Learning* (pp. 1–274). Sterling, VA: Stylus Press.

American Association for Health Education, National Commission for Health Education Credentialing, & Society for Public Health Education. (1999). *A Competency-Based Framework for Graduate-Level Health Educators.* Allentown, PA: The National Commission for Health Education Credentialing, Inc., American Association for Health Education, and the Society for Public Health Education.

Bandura, A. (1977). Self-efficacy: Toward a unifying theory of behavioral change. *Psychological Review, 84,* 191.

Bandura, A. (1977). *Social Learning Theory.* Englewood Cliffs, NJ: Prentice Hall.

Bandura, A. (1986). The explanatory and predictive scope of self-efficacy theory. *Journal of Social and Clinical Psychology, 4,* 359–373.

Bandura, A. (1986a). *Social Foundations of Thought and Action: A Social Cognitive Theory.* Englewood Cliffs, NJ: Prentice Hall.

Bandura, A. (2004). Health promotion by social cognitive means. *Health Education & Behavior, 31*(2), 143–164. Retrieved June 23, 2008, from http://www.sophe.org/ui/socialCognitive2.pdf

Bardsley, P., & Beckman, L. (1988). The health belief model and entry into alcoholism treatment. *International Journal of the Addictions, 23,* 19–28.

Becker, M. (Ed.). (1974). *The Health Belief Model and Personal Health Behavior.* Thoroughfare, NJ: Slack.

Becker, M., & Janz, N. (1985). The health belief model applied to understanding diabetes regimen compliance. *Diabetes Educator, 11,* 41–47.

Berra, Y. (n.d.). Yogi Berra quotes. Retrieved April 7, 2009, from http://www.brainyquote.com/quotes/quotes/y/yogiberra141506.html

Booth, A. (2007). In search of the information literacy training "half-life." *Health Information & Libraries Journal, 24*(2), 145–149.

Casey, T. A., Kingery, P. M., Bowden, R. G., & Corbett, B. S. (1993). An investigation of the factor structure of the Multidimensional Health Locus of Control scales in a health promotion program. *Educational and Psychological Measurement, 53,* 491–498.

Champion, V. (1985). Use of the health belief model in determining frequency of breast self-examination. *Research in Nursing and Health, 8,* 373–379.

Clark, N. M., & Dodge, J. A. (1999). Exploring self-efficacy as a predictor of disease management. *Health Education & Behavior, 26*(1), 72–89.

Cornish, E. (1980). Toward a philosophy of futurism. *Health Education, 11,* 10–12.

Creswell, W. H. (1984). Health education issues. In L. Rubinson & W. F. Alles (Eds.), *Health Education: Foundations for the Future.* St. Louis: Times Mirror/Mosby.

Crossette, B. (1994, September 7). A third-world effort on family planning. *The New York Times,* A8. Retrieved July 7, 2008, from http://query.nytimes.com/gst/fullpage.html?res=9D01E2D81038F934A3575AC0A962958260

Cummings, K. M., Becker, M. H., & Maile, M. C. (1980). Bringing the models together: An empirical approach to combining variables used to explain health outcomes. *Journal of Behavioral Medicine, 3,* 123–145.

Dahlberg, L. L., & Krug, E. G. (2002). Violence—a global public health problem. In E. Krug, L. L. Dahlberg, J. A. Mercy, A. B. Zwi, & R. Lozano (Eds.), *World Report on Violence and Health* (pp. 1–56). Geneva, Switzerland: World Health Organization.

Dalkey, N., & Helmer, O. (1963). An experimental application of the Delphi method to the use of experts. *Management Science, 9,* 458.

Dennison, D. (1977). Activated health education. *Health Education, 8,* 24–25.

Dennison, D. (1984). Activated health education: The development and refinement of an intervention model. *Health Values*, 8, 18–24.

Dennison, D., Frauenheim, K. A., & Isu, L. (1983). The DINE microcomputer program: An innovative curricular approach. *Health Education, 14*, 44–47.

Dennison, D., Prevet, T., & Affleck, M. (1980). *Alcohol and Behavior: An Activated Health Education Approach*. St. Louis: C.V. Mosby.

Denison, J. (2002). Behavior change—a summary of four major theories. Family Health International. AIDSCAP Behavioral Research Unit. Retrieved June 23, 2009, from http://fhi.org/nr/rdonlyres/ei26 vbslpsidmahhxc332vwo3g233xsqw22er3vofqvrfjuvb wyzc1vqjcbdexyz13m5u4mn6xv5j/bccsummaryf&o urmajortheories.pdf

DiBlasio, F. A. (1986). Drinking adolescents on the roads. *Journal of Youth and Adolescence, 15*, 173–189.

DiClemente, C., Prochaska, J. O., Fairhurst, C., Velicer, W., Velasques, M., & Rossi, J. (1991). The process of smoking cessation: An analysis of precontemplation, contemplation, and preparation stages of change. *Journal of Consulting Clinical Psychology, 59*, 295–304.

Donnermeyer, J. F., & Davis, R. R. (1998). Cumulative effects of prevention education on substance use among 11th grade students in Ohio. *Journal of School Health, 68*(4), 151–157.

Edmunds, C., Lowe, K., Murray, M., & Seymour, A. (2002). Ultimate adult learning. The ultimate educator: Achieving maximum adult learning through training and instruction; Chapter 3. Retrieved July 11, 2008, from http://www.ojp.usdoj.gov/ovc/assist/educator/files/chapter3.pdf

Eiser, J. R. (1985). Smoking: The social learning of addiction. *Journal of Social and Clinical Psychology, 3*, 357–446.

Fishbein, M. (Ed.). (1967). *Readings in Attitude Theory and Measurement*. New York: Wiley.

Fishbein, M., Middlestadt, S. E., & Hitchcock, P. J. (1994). Using information to change sexually transmitted disease–related behaviors. In R. J. DiCemente & J. L. Peterson (Eds.), *Preventing AIDS: Theories and Methods of Behavior Interventions* (pp. 61–78). New York: Plenum Press.

Fisher, R. (1997). Social action community organization: Proliferation, persistence, roots, and prospects. In M. Minkler (Ed.), *Community Organizing and Community Building for Health*. Rutgers, NJ: Rutgers University Press.

Fodor, J., & Dalis, G. (1974). *Health Instruction*. Philadelphia: Lea and Febiger.

Frazer, G. H., Kukulka, G. G., & Richardson, C. E. (1988). An assessment of professional opinion concerning critical research issues in health education. In J. H. Humphrey (Ed.), *Advances in Health Education: Current Research* (Vol. 1). New York: AMS Press.

Gilbert, G. G. (1981). *Teaching First Aid and Emergency Care*. Dubuque, IA: Kendall/Hunt.

Glanz, K., Lew, R. A., Song, V., & Cook, W. A. (1999). Factors associated with skin cancer prevention; practices in multi-ethnic population. *Health Education, 26*(3), 344–359.

Glanz, K., Patterson R. E., Kristal, A. R., Feng, Z., Linnan, L., Heimendinger, J., et al. (1998). Impact of work site health promotion on stage of dietary change: The working well trial. *Health Education and Behavior, 25*(4), 448–463.

Glanz, K., Rimer, B. K., & Lewis, F. M. (Eds.). (2002). *Health Behavior and Health Education* (3rd ed.). San Francisco, CA: Jossey-Bass.

Green, L. (1976). *Determining the Impact and Effectiveness of Health Education as It Relates to Federal Policy*. Washington, DC: Office of the Deputy Assistant Secretary for Planning and Evaluation/Health, Education and Welfare.

Green, L., & Kreuter, M. (2005). *Health Program Planning: An Ecological Approach* (4th ed.). New York: McGraw-Hill.

Green, L. W., & Iverson, D. (1982). School health education. *Annual Review of Public Health*, 3, 321–328.

Green, L. W., & Kreuter, M. W. (1990). Health promotion as a public health strategy for the 1990s. In *Annual Review of Public Health* (Vol. 11). Palo Alto, CA: Annual Reviews.

Green, L. W., & Kreuter, M. W. (1991). *Health Promotion Planning: An Educational and Environmental Approach*. Mountain View, CA: Mayfield.

Green, L. W., Kreuter, M. W., Deeds, S. G., & Partridge, K. B. (1980). *Health Education Planning: A Diagnostic Approach*. Palo Alto, CA: Mayfield.

Green, L. W., Levine, D. M., & Deeds, S. G. (1975). Clinical trials of health education for hypertensive outpatients: Design and baseline data. *Preventive Medicine, 4*, 417–425.

Green, L. W., Levine, D. M., Wolle, J., & Deeds, S. G. (1979). Development of randomized patient education experiments with urban poor hypertensives. *Patient Education and Counseling, 1*, 106–111.

Grimley, D., Prochaska, J. O., Velicer, W. F., & Prochaska, G. (1995). Contraception and condom use adaption and maintenance. A stage paradigm approach. *Health Education Quarterly, 22*(1), 20–35.

Grizzell, J. (2007). Behavior change theories and models. Retrieved May 15, 2008, from http://www.csup omona.edu/~jvgrizzell/best_practices/bctheory. html

Haire-Joshu, D., Auslander, W. F., Houston, C. A., & Williams, J. H. (1999). Staging of dietary patterns among African American women. *Health Education & Behavior, 26*(1), 90–102.

Harrison, J. A., Mullen, P. D., & Green, L. W. (1992). A meta-analysis of studies of the health belief model with adults. *Health Education Research, 7*(1), 107–116.

Herold, E. (1983). The health belief model: Can it help us understand contraceptive use among adolescents? *Journal of School Health, 53*, 19–21.

Hester, N., & Macrina, D. (1985). The health belief model and the contraceptive behavior of college women: Implications for health education. *Journal of American College Health, 33*, 245–252.

Howard, S. (1999). Guiding collaborative teamwork in the classroom. *Journal of Effective Teaching, 3*(1). Retrieved July 11, 2008, from http://www.uncwil .edu/cte/et/articles/Howard/

Jessor, R., & Jessor, S. (1977). *Problem Behavior and Psychosocial Development: A Longitudinal Study of Youth*. New York: Academic.

Jillson, I. A. (1985). The national drug abuse policy delphi: Progress report and findings to date. In L. A. Turoff (Ed.), *Delphi Method: Techniques and Applications* (pp. 119–154). Reading, MA: Addison-Wesley.

Kelly, G., Mamon, J., & Scott, J. (1987). Utility of the health belief model in examining medication compliance among psychiatric outpatients. *Social Science Medicine, 25*, 1205–1211.

Kerlinger, F. N. (1986). *Foundations of Behavioral Research* (3rd ed.). New York: Holt, Reinhart and Winston.

Kime, R., Schlaadt, R., & Tritsch, L. (1977). *Health Instruction: An Action Approach*. Englewood Cliffs, NJ: Prentice Hall.

King, K., Price, J. H., Tellojahann, S. K., & Wahl, J. (1999). High school teachers' perceived self-efficacy in identifying students at risk for suicide. *Journal of School Health, 69*(5), 202–207.

Kirscht, J. (1974). The health belief model and illness behavior. In M. Becker (Ed.), *The Health Belief Model and Personal Health Behavior* (pp. 403–418). Thoroughfare, NJ: Slack.

Kuhn, J. (1970). *The Structure of Scientific Revolutions*. Chicago: University of Chicago Press.

Levenson, H. (1974). Activism and powerful others: Distinction within the concept of internal-external control. *Journal of Personality Assessment, 38*, 377–383.

Levine, D. M., Green, L. W., Deeds, S. G., Smith, C., Chwalow, A. J., & Finlay, J. (1979). Health education for hypertensive patients. *Journal of the American Medical Association, 241*, 1700–1703.

Levine, D. M., Morisky, D. E., Bone, L. R., Lewis, C., Ward, K. B., & Green, L. W. (1982). Data-based planning for educational interventions through hypertension control programs for urban and rural populations in Maryland. *Public Health Reports, 97*, 107–112.

Maiman, L., & Becker, M. (1974). The health belief model: Origins and correlates in psychological theory. In M. Becker (Ed.), *The Health Belief Model and Personal Health Behavior* (pp. 336–353). Thoroughfare, NJ: Slack.

McGuire, W. (1981). Behavioral medicine, public health and communication theories. *Health Education, 12*, 8–13.

Montambeau, J., & Finch, J. (2008). Beyond bells and whistles: Affecting student learning through technology. The College of Charleston, South Carolina, Department of Academic Computing. Retrieved July 22, 2008, from http://www.cofc.edu/bellsand whistles/research/retentionmodel.html

Mullen, P., & Iverson, D. (1982). Qualitative methods for evaluative research in health education programs. *Health Education, 13*, 11–18.

National Cancer Institute. (2005). Theory at a glance: A guide for health promotion practice (2nd ed.). Retrieved June 1, 2008, from http://www.cancer .gov/theory.pdf

Oberteuffer, D., Pollock, M., & Harrelson, O. (1972). *School Health Education*. New York: Harper and Row.

Pajares, F. (2002). Overview of social cognitive theory and of self-efficacy. Retrieved June 12, 2008, from http://www.emory.edu/EDUCATION/mfp/eff.html

Parachini, L., & Covington, S. (2001). Community organizing toolbox: a funder's guide to community organizing neighborhood funders group. Retrieved April 20, 2008, from http://www.aecf.org/tarc/publications/pubs_toolbox.php

Parcel, G., & Meyer, M. P. (1978). Development of an instrument to measure children's health locus of control. *Health Education Monographs, 6,* 149–159.

Parcel, G., Nader, P. R., & Rogers, P. J. (1980). Health locus of control and health values: Implications for school health education. *Health Values, 4,* 32–37.

Parcel, G. S. (1984). Theoretical models for application in school health education research. *Special combined issue of Journal of School Health 54,* 39–49 *and Health Education 15,* 39–49.

Parraga, I. M. (1990). Determinants of food consumption. *Journal of the American Dietetic Association, 90,* 661–663.

Pike, R. (1994). *Creative Training Techniques Handbook* (2nd ed.). Minneapolis: Lakewood.

Pike, R. W. (2003). *Creative Training Techniques Handbook* (3rd ed.). Amherst, MA: HRD Press.

Prochaska, J. O. (1979). *Systems of Psychotherapy: A Transtheoretical Analysis.* Homewood, IL: Dorsey Press.

Prochaska, J. O. (1994). Strong and weak principles for progressing from precontemplation to action on the basis of twelve problem behaviors. *Health Psychology, 13*(1), 47–51.

Prochaska, J. O., Norcross, J., Fowler, J., Follick, M., & Abrams, D. (1992). Attendance and outcome in a worksite weight control program: Processes and stages of change as process and predictor variables. *Addictive Behavior, 17,* 35–45.

Prochaska, J. O., Redding, C. A., Harlow, L. L., Rossi, J. S., & Velicer, W. F. (1994). The transtheoretical model of change and HIV prevention: A review. *Health Education Quarterly, 24*(4), 471–486.

Rakowski, W., Dube, C., Marcus, B., Prochaska, J., Velicer, W., & Abrams, D. (1992). Assessing elements of women's decisions about mammography. *Health Psychology, 11,* 111–118.

Rogers, E. M. (2003). *Diffusion of Innovations* (5th ed.). New York: Free Press.

Rosenstock, I. (1974). Historical origins of the health belief model. In M. Becker (Ed.), *The Health Belief Model and Personal Health Behavior* (pp. 175–183). Thoroughfare, NJ: Slack.

Rosenstock, I., Stretcher, V., & Becker, M. (1994). The Health Belief Model and HIV risk behavior change. In R. J. DiClemente & J. L. Peterson (Eds.), *Preventing AIDS: Theories and Methods of Behavioral Interventions* (pp. 5–24). New York: Plenum Press.

Rosenstock, I. M., Stretcher, V. J., & Becker, M. (1988). Social Learning Theory and the Health Belief Model. *Health Education Quarterly, 15,* 175–183.

Rotter, J. B. (1954). *Social Learning and Clinical Psychology.* Englewood Cliffs, NJ: Prentice Hall.

Rubinson, L., & Alles, W. F. (1984). *Health Education: Foundations for the Future.* Prospect Heights, IL: Waveland.

Rubinson, L., & Baillie, L. (1981). Planning school-based sexuality programs utilizing the PRECEDE model. *Journal of School Health, 51,* 282–287.

Stainbrook, G., & Green, L. W. (1982). Behavior and behaviorism in health education. *Health Education, 13,* 14–19.

Stewart, K. L., & Felicetti, L. A. (1992). Learning styles of marketing majors. *Educational Research Quarterly, 15*(2), 15–23.

Strauss, A., & Corbin, J. (1990). *Basics of Qualitative Research: Grounded Theory Procedures and Techniques.* London: Sage.

Tarabokia, J. R. (1985). *Forecasts by Selected Professional Health Educators and Their Implications for Health Education: A Delphi Application.* Unpublished doctoral dissertation, Brigham Young University, Provo, UT.

Toohey, J. V., & Shireffs, J. H. (1980). Future trends in health education. *Health Education, 11,* 15–17.

Travis, R. (1976). The delphi technique: A tool for community health educators. *Health Education, 7,* 11–13.

U.S. Department of Health and Human Services. (1979). *Principles of Community Engagement.* Atlanta, GA: U.S. Public Health Service.

Velicer, W. F., Prochaska, J. O., Fava, J. L., Norman, G. J., & Redding, C. A. (1998). Smoking cessation and stress management: Applications of the Transtheoretical Model of behavior change. *Homeostasis, 38,* 216–233.

Wallston, K. A., & Wallston, B. S. (1978). Preface to health locus of control. *Health Education Monographs, 6,* 101–105.

Wallston, K. A., Wallston, B. S., & DeVillis, R. (1978). Development of the multidimensional health locus of control scales. *Health Education Monographs, 6,* 160–170.

Wallston, K. A., Wallston, B. S., Kaplan, G. D., & Maides, S. A. (1976). Development and validation of the health locus of control scale. *Journal of Consulting and Clinical Psychology, 44,* 580–585.

Wirz, D. (2004). Students' learning styles vs. professors' teaching styles. *Inquiry, 9*(1). Retrieved July 15, 2008, from http://www.vccaedu.org/inquiry/inquiry-spring 2004/i-91-wirz.html

Wodarski, J. (1987). Evaluating a social learning approach to teaching adolescents about alcohol and driving: A multiple variable evaluation. *Journal of Social Science Research, 10,* 121–144.

Wolfgang, J., & Dennison, D. (1981). The effects of a heart health education workshop. *Journal of School Health, 51,* 356–359.

Methods of Instruction/Intervention

Entry-Level and Advanced 1 Health Educator Competencies Addressed in This Chapter

Responsibility II: Plan Health Education Strategies, Interventions, and Programs
Competency F: Select appropriate strategies to meet objectives.
Competency G: Assess factors that affect implementation.

Responsibility III: Implement Health Education Strategies, Interventions, and Programs
Competency A: Initiate plan of action.
Competency C: Use a variety of methods to implement strategies, interventions, and programs.

Method Selection in Health Education

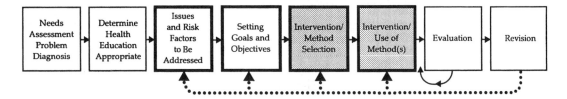

Heavy-bordered boxes indicate subjects addressed in this text; shaded boxes indicate subject(s) of current chapter.

Note: The competencies listed above, which are addressed in this chapter, are considered to be both entry-level and Advanced 1 competencies by the National Commission for Health Education Credentialing, Inc. They are taken from *A Framework for the Development of Competency Based Curricula for Entry Level Health Educators* by the National Task Force for the Preparation and Practice of Health Education, 1985; American Association for Health Education, National Commission for Health Education Credentialing, & Advanced I (1999). *A Competency-Based Framework for Advanced 1 Health Educators.* Allentown, PA: The National Commission for Health Education Credentialing, Inc., American Association for Health Education, and the Society for Public Health Education; and *A Competency-Based Framework for Health Educators—The Competencies Update Project* (CUP), 2006.

OBJECTIVES   After studying the chapter, the reader should be able to verbally:

- Describe the major advantages and disadvantages of using each method.
- Describe how to use each method.
- Provide a rationale for using each method.
- Match methods with objectives.

KEY ISSUES   Method description   Disadvantages
When to use   Method implementation
How to use   Examples
Advantages

Using Methods as a Framework

An arsenal of methods is available to us in health education. It is important that we consider the objectives first and then focus on the methods to meet those objectives within the context of the resources we have at our disposal. This chapter will focus on the many methods available to the health educator, some of which are as follows:

1. Getting acquainted (icebreakers)
2. Audio
3. Audiovisual materials
4. Brainstorming
5. Case studies
6. Computer-assisted instruction
7. Cooperative learning and group work
8. Debates
9. Displays and bulletin boards
10. Educational games
11. Experiments and demonstrations
12. Field trips
13. Guest speakers
14. Guided imagery
15. Humor
16. Lecture
17. Mass media
18. Models
19. Music
20. Newsletters/flyers
21. Panels
22. Peer education
23. Personal improvement projects
24. Problem solving
25. Puppets
26. Role plays
27. Self-appraisals
28. Service learning
29. Simulations
30. Storytelling and literary venues
31. Theater (using scripts)
32. Value clarification
33. Word games and puzzles

Each method should be considered a "framework." Every possible method should be considered for each objective to be achieved. An important step in making the decision is to use the preceding list of activities/methods and consider how each might conceivably be employed to meet your objectives. This will force you to consider the many options available for achieving your objectives and make it less likely you will pick a method for inappropriate reasons.

Objective: After reviewing the case study, the reader will compare and evaluate whether using a small-group discussion or a lecture is more appropriate to achieve the objective.

Case Study: Pam   Pam has been asked to develop a health education program for the local community in an affluent suburb just outside of a major metropolitan area. During her years in college the only teaching method she experienced was lecture. She therefore develops and emulates an intellectual lecture presentation on the evils of drugs for the five parents of adolescents who are believed to have drug problems. When the parents seem uninterested in her approach, she is disappointed. One of the parents suggests she just sit down and talk with them. Another parent, who is a physician, says they are all aware of the evils of drugs but need help in relating to their children. (See Case Studies Revisited page 181.)

Questions to consider:

1. Which method—lecture or small-group discussion—is most appropriate for Pam's lesson? Explain why.
2. How might the demographic make-up of the target population influence the selection of a method to address the objective?

This chapter will present a variety of methods and one or more examples of the application of the method. The reader should remember that the methods presented can be converted to other subject matter with relative ease. To reiterate, each method is a framework that can and should be adapted to meet your needs. Always think of how each method might be applied to meet your objectives. Health educators often "crash" into a method without thinking through what is the best method to achieve the desired outcome. Table 4-1 presents a matrix helpful in method selection. We will examine each of the methods listed there in detail. Note the varied roles of the **facilitator**.

Of all the beasts in the jungle, we most often resemble the crashing boar.
—Mohan Singh

Method/Intervention 1: Getting Acquainted (Icebreakers)

Getting-acquainted activities, also called *icebreakers*, can be used to set the tone for a workshop or class. These activities should be easy to follow and fun. They range from having participants introduce themselves to more complex activities designed to show what will be covered or why the lesson is being presented. They should be selected very carefully, with the objectives and **target population** characteristics in mind. It is often said that the first 15 minutes of any presentation sends a message of what is to follow. Send a positive message

Table 4-1 Methods Selection Matrix

Method	Cognitive Objectives	Affective Objectives	Psychomotor Objectives	Time Required (Minutes)	Ages/Years	Size/Suggested Max	Budget	Community Setting	School Setting	Comments
1. Getting acquainted (icebreakers)	X	P	P	15+	All	None	Low	X	X	
2. Audio	X	P	P	15+	All	None	Low	X	X	Equipment required
3. Audiovisual materials	X	P	P	15+	All	None	Mod	X	X	Equipment required
4. Brainstorming	X			20+	All	20	Low	X	X	
5. Case studies	X	X		30+	All	20	Low	X	X	
6. Computer-assisted instruction	X	P		30+	10+	Ratio	High		X	Equipment required
7. Cooperative learning	P	P	P	30+	All	20	Low	X	X	
8. Debates	P	P		30+	All	30	Low	X	X	
9. Displays/bulletin boards	X			30+	All	None	Low	X	X	Special materials required
10. Educational games	X			20+	All	30	Low	X	X	
11. Experiments and demonstrations	X		X	30+	All	Ratio	Mod+		X	Equipment required
12. Field trips		P		60+	All	Ratio	Mod	X	X	
13. Guest speakers	X	P		30+	All	None	Low+	X	X	
14. Guided imagery		X	P	30+	All	None	Mod	X	X	Equipment required
15. Humor	X	X		2+	All	None	Low	X	X	
16. Lecture	X			5+	All	None	Low	X	X	
17. Mass media	X			5+	All	None		X	X	Access required
18. Models	X		P	5+	All	None	Low+	X	X	Equipment required
19. Music	P	X		5+	All	None	Low	X	X	Equipment required
20. Newsletters/flyers	X			120+	All readers	None	Mod	X	X	Equipment and duplication required

continued

Table 4-1 *continued*

Method	Cognitive Objectives	Affective Objectives	Psychomotor Objectives	Time Required (Minutes)	Ages/Years	Size/Suggested Max	Budget	Community Setting	School Setting	Comments
21. Panels	P	X		30+	All	None	Low	X	X	
22. Peer education	P	X		120+	All	Ratio	Mod	X	X	Special training needed
23. Personal improvement projects		X	P	600+	10+	None	Low+	X	X	Requires adequate time
24. Problem solving	P	P		30+	All	25	Low	X	X	
25. Puppets	X	X		30+	All	25	Low+	X	X	Equipment required
26. Role plays		X	P	30+	10+	25	Low	X	X	
27. Self-appraisals		X		15+	10+	None	Low	X	X	Handout or computer required
28. Service learning	X	X	P	120+	All	None	Mod	X	X	Consider insurance
29. Simulations	X	X	X	30+	10+	25	Mod+	X	X	Special materials required
30. Storytelling and literary venues	P	X		15+	10+	None	Low	X	X	Abstract thought required
31. Theater/scripts (memorized/readers)	X	X		30+	All	None	Mod	X	X	Scripts required
32. Value clarification		X		30+	14+	30	Low	X	X	
33. Word games and puzzles	X			10+	10+ readers	None	Low	X	X	Handout required

X = Yes, common use.
P = Possible.
Blank = Uncommon.

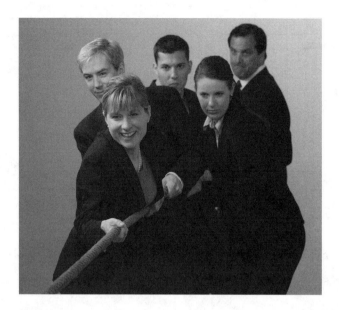

Icebreaker activities can be a helpful way to begin a workshop with a positive tone.

that this will be a good presentation! Start on time, and be enthusiastic. Always be polite and interested in the people present. Try to address people by name. Encourage all to participate, and participate as much as possible yourself. Your active participation sets the tone for the group.

Advantages and Disadvantages

Advantages of getting-acquainted activities are that they:

1. Can serve to create an atmosphere of mutual trust and respect.
2. Can help the facilitator learn the names and interests of participants.
3. Can promote and set the ground rules for participant interaction.
4. Can truly energize participants.
5. Can put participants at ease.

Disadvantages are that they:

1. Can be time-consuming, reducing time for more important needs.
2. Can make participants uncomfortable.

Tips for Effective Implementation

1. These activities have the potential to make participants either comfortable or uncomfortable. Choose them wisely, considering participant characteristics.
2. Explain clearly the rules or what is expected of the participants prior to beginning the activity. Participants are more likely to engage in an activity when they are confident they are doing it correctly.

Example 1: The Name Game

1. Sit in a circle so that all faces can be seen.
2. Reviewing the rules: All will participate in associating names with faces without writing down names.

3. First person says his or her own name (generally only first name).
4. Second person says first person's name and then adds his or her own.
5. Procedure is repeated until the final person says all names plus his or her own.
6. Reverse directions and have the first person say all names in reverse order.
7. After several persons have completed game in reverse, change places and pick several people to say names.
8. Repeat until all are comfortable saying all names.

Example 2: Get It Off My Back

Purpose
1. To introduce a new area of instruction
2. To get a group better acquainted
3. To review
4. To determine the knowledge of the group

Background
The facilitator must do background work on the topic to be covered and identify key vocabulary words. Examples include drug names, nutrients, diseases, and pollutants.

Player Objective
To identify the word on your back.

Materials
Three-by-five-inch cards and masking tape. (Self-adhesive mailing labels may also be used.)

Rules of Play

Participant Information

1. The objective of this activity is for you to identify the term or phrase written on the label attached to your back. You may not look at your label.
2. You can ask only yes-and-no questions of other people in the room as you simultaneously attempt to identify your mystery term or phrase.
3. You can ask each person only one question. If you have asked a question of all participants, you may repeat the process.
4. You must get at least three yes answers to your questions before you can make a guess at the word on your back.
5. The first person to guess correctly is the winner. Continue the game until at least half of the group has been successful.
6. Instruct participants to answer "I don't know" or "I am not certain" rather than taking a chance on giving the wrong yes or no answer, because wrong answers will ruin the game. If no one is certain of the correct answer, the facilitator should give the answer.

Facilitator Information

1. After reviewing all rules, the facilitator places a 3-by-5-inch card (or a self-adhesive mailing label) with a word on it on the back of each

participant. It is important that no one sees the card placed on his or her own back.

2. The facilitator should mingle among the participants to provide help if needed.
3. In the cases where the correct answer is uncertain, the facilitator should provide the answer.
4. Repeat the game if there is time. Consider using different cards for the next round.
5. Debrief by discussing the logic followed in discovering the words being guessed.

Example 3: Special Name Tags   Construct special name tags to include information that will open up common ground and put the group at ease. Figure 4-1 shows an example.

After completing the answers to the questions posed on the name tag, each person should pair up with another and ask clarifying questions. Participants can decline to answer any question but generally find these questions nonthreatening. This is a good beginning activity to promote some safe self-disclosure that contributes to a positive atmosphere.

Other Examples   Two other examples of getting-acquainted activities follow:

1. Pair up participants and give them 2 minutes to interview each other to find five unique things they have in common that they can share with the larger group.
2. Ask each participant to reveal a personal trait of which they are proud.

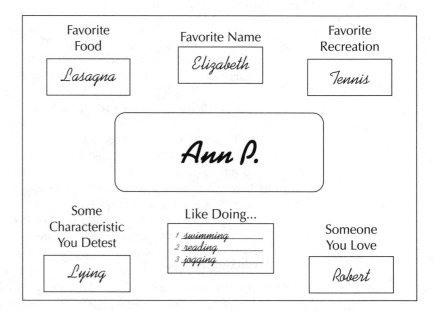

Figure 4-1
Name Tag Serving as an Icebreaker

Method/Intervention 2: Audio

Audio methods such as tapes, compact discs (CDs), and sound bites can be used in many creative ways throughout a program and are often combined with other methods. You can **simulate** situations or play real voices.

Advantages and Disadvantages

Advantages of audiotapes are that they:

1. Are fairly low in cost.
2. Provide a structured and controlled experience.
3. Can allow for self-paced learning when listening independently.
4. Are easy to use.
5. Can provide excellent feedback.

Disadvantages are that they:

1. Appeal to only one sense.
2. Require equipment.
3. Require special equipment for large groups.
4. Can be boring.
5. Have a high risk for equipment malfunction.

Tips for Effective Implementation

To avoid awkward transitions when using audio techniques, the facilitator should cue up the audio materials and assess the volume prior to delivery of the method.

Example 1: Interviews with Experts

Interviews with experts on the subject involved can be played back for the group. Try to select charismatic leaders or voices.

Example 2: Self-Interview

Participants may conduct a self-interview by pretaping questions to answer themselves. For example, propose a conversation with a crystal ball. The participant controls the on-and-off button and asks the crystal ball about his or her future if certain unhealthy behaviors are followed. (See also Chapter 7.)

Example 3: Development of Skills

Provide each participant with a practice CD containing step-by-step instructions to complete a task related to the content. An example might include deep-breathing exercises in a stress management program.

Method/Intervention 3: Audiovisual Materials

Audiovisual materials include such things as DVDs, presentation sofware, and Internet clips. Older means include videotapes, films, overhead transparencies, flip charts, and filmstrips. The use of audiovisual equipment will be discussed in detail in Chapter 7. Here we will just summarize the advantages and disadvantages and provide some brief examples of use throughout a program.

Advantages and   Advantages of audiovisuals are that they:
Disadvantages

1. Provide potential for variety.
2. Serve as an attention-getter.
3. Can be used to introduce, solidify, or reinforce a topic.
4. Can be a nonthreatening way to introduce issues.
5. Can provide a backdrop for discussion.
6. Are often relatively cheap and easy to use (as in the case of blank DVDs, presentation software, and media clips from the Internet.)
7. Can serve as a class or individual project (as in the case of making a video).

Disadvantages are that they:

1. Are unpredictable in outcome.
2. Require equipment that may be expensive (such as interactive videodiscs).
3. Can create a situation in which some are unwilling to participate and allow others to do all the work.
4. Can raise too many issues to have a focused discussion.

Tips for Effective   1. Prior to showing audiovisual materials, introduce the content and clarify
Implementation   the objective of the method. Asking participants to look for key pieces of information helps them to maintain focus and gives learners a more active rather than passive role.
2. Justify the credibility of the source for the learner and approximate the length of the presentation.
3. Cue up the audio materials and assess the volume prior to delivering the method.
4. Provide a closure to the audiovisual method by discussing or summarizing key concepts.

Examples   Following are some examples of how to use audiovisual materials.

1. As a supplement to lecture, provide real-life examples and experts.
2. Make tapes (audio or video) as a group. For example, a videotape could be made of community problems, using the approach of an investigative reporter.
3. Use previously recorded videotapes to monitor behaviors such as drug transactions. This practice can become a deterrent to such behavior.

4. Record by audiotape or videotape a confrontational situation, such as parents and child arguing over the use of a drug of interest to the group. Use actors to portray the wrong way and a better way of engaging in such a confrontation.
5. Download short topic-related clips from sources such as YouTube to introduce the content or to provide a foundation for discussion.

Method/Intervention 4: Brainstorming

Brainstorming, a method of eliciting ideas and information from a group, can be used anytime throughout an intervention. It can be used to define a problem or to consider possible solutions to a problem. It can be very effective in developing a positive group attitude since it recognizes the importance of each group member. It often provides a sense of group empowerment. Basically, it is a free-thinking forum with the facilitator working to elicit as many possible solutions to a problem as possible. This is followed by grouping and reorganizing ideas until they are well understood and all are considered.

Rules   Rules for brainstorming are as follows:

1. There are no bad ideas. Do not make negative remarks about ideas because this will stifle creativity.
2. All ideas/solutions will be considered (listed).
3. Go around the group in a circle and list ideas that are possible solutions to the problem or issue at hand. If possible, use large sheets of paper and hang them on the walls. Alternatively, use a chalkboard or dry erase board.
4. Individuals can pass on their turn if they feel they have no new idea to contribute.
5. Continue the process until people run low on new ideas. Make certain not to stop before all new ideas are presented.
6. The process can end here or can move to a second step.
7. The second step is to consolidate common themes and ideas. This must be done with the full consent of the group. It may be possible to consolidate the list to a more manageable list without losing the essence of the ideas presented.
8. The third step is to prioritize the ideas. This step may not be necessary, but if needed it should be done with ample time for discussion. If consensus cannot be reached, some form of voting may be necessary. Consider the group dynamics before deciding on an oral or secret ballot.

Advantages and Disadvantages

Advantages of brainstorming are that it:

1. Provides an opportunity for all to be important contributors.
2. Requires little equipment.
3. Builds a cooperative environment.
4. Sparks a variety of ideas as members build upon suggestions.
5. Creates a spirit of congeniality.
6. Draws on group members' knowledge and experiences.

Disadvantages are that it:

1. Is unpredictable in outcome.
2. Can make some individuals uncomfortable, feeling forced to contribute.
3. Can be time-consuming if taken through all steps.
4. Can fail if people refuse to participate.
5. Can be unfocused, especially if people have difficulty getting away from known reality.

Tips for Effective Implementation

1. The facilitator should emphasize the importance of generating ideas, not solving problems, and encourage participants to include all ideas, regardless of feasibility during the first step.
2. Indicate to the participants in advance the amount of time they will spend brainstorming. The unstructured nature of this method leads to off-task behavior if participants are not allotted time limits appropriate to the difficulty and complexity of the task. Strive to allot a maximum of 7 minutes during each brainstorming stage. The time limitation will motivate the participants to get to work quickly.
3. The facilitator should be prepared to provide suggestions to stimulate a stagnated group.
4. Allot time for all groups to report their ideas or samples of ideas if time is a concern. Groups that do not have an opportunity to share often feel unvalued and that their efforts were wasted.
5. Encourage groups to strictly adhere to the one conversation at a time rule to avoid distracting side conversations (Sutton, 2006).
6. Provide participants with a brainstorm prompt both orally and in a printed format.
7. Participants can be challenged to create more thorough lists by introducing an element of competition. For example, a statement may be included to indicate minimum standards. Figure 4-2 provides an example.

Sample Operational Procedures

Following is an example of operational procedures in brainstorming:

1. Brainstorm objectives and record them by using large wall charts.
2. After creating an exhaustive list, quickly review the intentions/wording of each stated objective.
3. Establish priority objectives.
4. Assign suggested implementation responsibility.

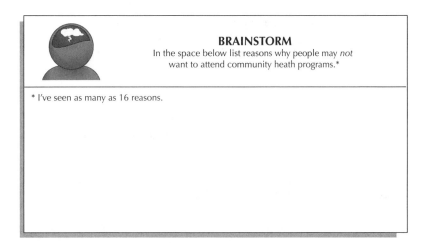

BRAINSTORM
In the space below list reasons why people may *not*
want to attend community heath programs.*

* I've seen as many as 16 reasons.

Figure 4-2
Brainstorm Template

Assumptions Effective brainstorming rests on certain assumptions that should be clarified for the group before beginning the operational procedures previously mentioned.

1. All contributions are welcomed and should be considered.
2. All suggested objectives will be reported unless withdrawn by the person making the suggestion.
3. It is permissible, in fact encouraged, to overlap with other groups.
4. Rotation input will be used, but anyone can decline to make suggestions.

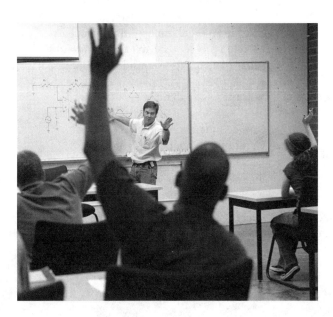

Solutions to many problems can be generated in brainstorming activities if the activity is conducted correctly. It is important to remember that no ideas are bad and to include everyone.

Examples   Use brainstorming to generate ideas on how to address such problems as:

1. School littering
2. Access to local services
3. Using condoms
4. Teenage pregnancy
5. Poor food selection
6. Drug sales in the neighborhood

Method/Intervention 5: Case Studies

A powerful tool for health educators is the **case study**, which presents situations for the sake of problem diagnosis and solution. The situations can be real and based on historical events, or they can be based on hypothetical events, structured to fit any content area. This method should be used after a foundation of trust and mutual respect has been developed among participants. This book is replete with case studies on a variety of issues. Entire textbooks in public health are written around collections of case studies (Kreuter, Lezin, Kreuter, & Green, 2003).

Advantages and   Advantages of case studies are that they:
Disadvantages

1. Generally require little equipment.
2. Are able to address difficult topics in a controlled manner.
3. Allow for good control over content.
4. Can be structured to appear realistic.
5. Provide an excellent opportunity to learn in a practical fashion.
6. Develop problem-solving and analytical skills.
7. Allow participants to consider multiple aspects and solutions to a problem.

Disadvantages are that they:

1. Can be time-consuming.
2. Can result in pooling of ignorance.
3. Can be an ineffective method if participants do not see the relevance to their personal situation.

Tips for Effective   1. Clearly indicate what the learner is expected to ascertain from the case
Implementation   study exercise by stating the objective. Consider listing the objective as an introduction to the case study.
2. Provide participants a list of questions to consider to encourage further exploration on the topic.

*Example 1: Case
Study of Diabetes
Prevention Program
in Charlotte, NC*

Objective: After considering the demographics of the population, the reviewer of the case study will recommend components for inclusion in a diabetes prevention intervention.

Your agency has received a large grant ($500K) to develop a diabetes prevention program in a predominantly Hispanic community (approximately 50% of inhabitants are of Mexican ancestry). You have been assigned the task of determining the components of the program. Consider how you would go about determining which intervention methods and teaching strategies to use. Ask yourself how you can be certain you are being sensitive to the needs of the community.

- What steps would you follow?
- Where would you physically locate the program?
- What specific teaching or other intervention methods might be productive, and why?

*Example 2: Case
Study of Problem
Pregnancy
Prevention Program
in Raleigh, NC*

Objective: After considering the demographics of the population, the reviewer of the case study will recommend components for inclusion in a pregnancy prevention intervention.

Your agency has received a large grant ($500K) to develop a problem pregnancy prevention program in a predominantly Chinese American community. The community comprises approximately 2,000 girls/young women ages 12–19. The pregnancy rate has been approximately 10% per year. Approximately 13% speak very little English. You have been assigned the task of determining the components of the program. Consider how you would go about determining which intervention methods and teaching strategies to use. Ask yourself how you can be certain you are being sensitive to the needs of the community.

- What steps would you follow?
- Where would you physically locate the program?
- What specific teaching or other intervention methods might be productive, and why?

*Example 3: Case
Study of AIDS
Prevention Program
in Washington, D.C.*

Objective: After considering the demographics of the population, the reviewer of the case study will recommend components for inclusion in an AIDS prevention intervention.

Your agency has received a large grant ($500K) to develop an AIDS prevention program for the deaf in your community. It is estimated you have approximately 2,000 **deaf** and **hard-of-hearing** adults ages 18–40 living in the community. Most live in the northwest and northeast part of the city. There is a large cluster near Gallaudet University. Approximately 40% are African

American and approximately 15% are Hispanic. You have been assigned the task of determining the components of the program. Consider how you would go about determining which intervention methods and teaching strategies to use. Ask yourself how you can be certain you are being sensitive to the needs of this community.

- What steps would you follow?
- Where would you physically locate the program?
- What specific teaching or other intervention methods might be productive, and why?

Method/Intervention 6: Computer-Assisted Instruction

Computer-assisted instruction can be used at any time and is generally best combined with other teaching techniques. The main issue is to find the software that meets your objectives and a setting that has the hardware to implement the program. The possibilities are exciting, but the costs can be high. The use of such technology is currently much more common in school settings but could be used in community settings. Many people have computer and Internet access at home, and if the program can be shared, this can be a major way to reach large numbers of people.

Health education software has been slow to develop because it is often difficult to make a profit on software that can be very high in developmental costs. The market is often small, and unfortunately much of the software has been the object of software pirating.

Other possible approaches to gain access to adequate hardware are to use local community colleges or to purchase portable machines. Libraries generally have computers for public use and often lend public domain software. Public domain software can also be obtained over networks and public systems via the Internet. In the future such applications will probably be even more feasible.

Portable projection systems are now available, making use of a large screen. This means one computer can be used to reach a large audience. Changes can be made on the spot, and new technology permits on-screen movement and sound. Custom lessons/presentations can be developed that are very professional attention-getters. (See also Chapter 6.)

Advantages and Disadvantages

Advantages of computer-assisted instruction are that it:

1. Can provide an element of fun.
2. Is considered innovative.
3. Provides variety.
4. Can involve participants actively in the learning process.
5. Provides almost immediate feedback.

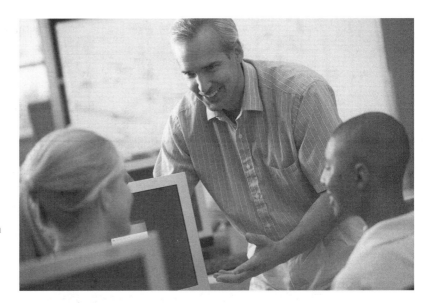

Computer use in health education can provide an element of fun and variety to a lesson or workshop.

6. Makes self-pacing exercises possible.
7. Requires higher-level thinking in some applications, such as simulations.
8. Can provide individualized programs.
9. Can be used to reinforce other lessons.
10. Is professional in appearance.
11. Is effective for large or small groups.
12. Is easy to integrate with classroom discussion.
13. Is easy to update and incopraorate up-to-date information.

Disadvantages are that it:

1. Can be expensive.
2. Requires special equipment.
3. Requires special software.
4. Requires special training in computer use.
5. Can be frightening to someone new to computers.
6. Can be time-consuming to create.

Tips for Effective Implementation

1. Create an electronic document that contains all the necessary URL addresses for the activity. This will allow the participants to click directly on the link and avoid the possibility of mistyping the URL address.
2. Demonstrate how to use the features of the designated website while having participants mirror your actions on their own computers.
3. Provide participants with a printed copy of step-by-step instructions that include screen snapshots to ensure they are following directions accurately.
4. Check all links to ensure they are available prior to the use of computer-assisted learning.

Examples   Following are some examples of applications of computer-assisted instruction.

1. Dietary analysis programs
2. Health risk appraisals
3. Health games
4. Monitoring compliance, such as with medications
5. Simulations
6. Expert system applications
7. Using computers to plot trends such as birth rates or violent acts
8. Automatically sending reminder notices using computer voice messaging
9. Providing a visual outline of the topic for participants

(See also Chapter 6.)

Method/Intervention 7: Cooperative Learning and Group Work

Cooperative learning is a broad category of learning experiences that center on learning from fellow participants. Generally participants are working toward a common goal. It includes group work such as brainstorming but can be as straightforward as permission to share personal experiences. Cooperative learning differs from group work in that members are typically intentionally selected to complete a task, with individual learners being held accountable for their own performance as well as the performance of the group. The element of accountability, "we sink or swim together," makes cooperative learning unique from group learning. Both, however, have the potential to enhance group spirit and can be very important in group situations.

When to Use   Working in small groups can be an effective strategy in both the school and community settings. The health educator must first establish some very clear behavioral objectives before deciding whether or not small-group work is even appropriate. There are many reasons for incorporating group work into the learning process. Group work can facilitate cooperative learning, problem solving, the sharing of ideas, brainstorming, or be nothing more than a device to allow the members of the group to get to know one another. The ability to use group work may be driven by the overall number of participants, their willingness to participate, facilities that allow for small-group setup, and the health educator's aptitude for running small-group exercises.

Advantages and Disadvantages   Advantages of cooperative and group learning are that they:

1. Can provide an element of fun.
2. Potentially create an atmosphere of cooperation.

3. Utilize multiple thinkers and therefore can create high-quality, innovative answers.
4. Allow participants to learn in a more active and involved manner, therefore decreasing the potential for boredom.
5. Encourage cooperation and collaboration that a large group setting might inhibit.
6. Stimulate innovation in thought, which again might not be encouraged in a large group.
7. Allow participants to quickly become acquainted with each other. This is particularly useful in making people feel at ease in a new situation.
8. Expose individuals to a variety of viewpoints and ideas that might not surface in a large group setting.
9. Can foster an acceptance of differences in heritage, socioeconomic status, disabilities, and so forth.
10. Can foster mutual responsibility for learning.
11. Provide immediate feedback and provides the facilitator information about learner motivation (Wehrli & Nyquist, 2003).

Disadvantages are that it:

1. Is unpredictable in outcome.
2. Has the potential for being very disruptive in the school setting. School health educators must be very clear about their expectations regarding behavior and noise levels and be prepared to end an activity prematurely should the students get out of control.
3. Can sometimes be dominated by overassertive individuals. In both school and community settings, facilitators need to circulate among the groups to minimize the effects of such behavior. In the school setting, if there are tasks to be performed within groups (such as recorder or reporter), the health educator should appoint these individuals before the groups begin work to avoid disruptive arguments.
4. Has the potential to wander off the track of the activity, particularly in the school setting. Again, the health educator can minimize this problem by regularly checking in with individual groups and bringing them back on task.
5. Can be uncomfortable for individuals who prefer to work independently.

Tips for Effective Implementation of Group Work (Wehrli & Nyquist, 2003)

1. Develop questions in a clear sequence to address objectives while stimulating learners to move to the next higher level of thinking.
2. Avoid questions that result in single answer responses. Challenge the learner to think critically. Most questions can be elevated to a higher level of thinking if you ask the participant to "explain why" or "justify your response."
3. Apply group facilitation skills to manage interactions and time.

Tips for Effective Implementation of Cooperative Learning (Kagen, 1999)

1. Implement team-building and class-building activities prior to moving to academic tasks, which will create the will to work together.
2. Begin with brief and highly structured cooperative tasks.
3. Avoid moving to unstructured interaction until participants have acquired the skills and will work together effectively.

Examples

Examples of cooperative learning or group work follow:

1. Brainstorm on how to prevent drug sales on certain street corners.
2. Share personal experiences.
3. Make individual presentations, assigned by the instructor. The instructor reviews the format prior to presentation and ensures that a quality experience will be provided.
4. Plan an environmental day such as Earth Day.
5. Design an antismoking ad poster or 30-second videotape.
6. Form dyads or triads for problem-solving tasks.
7. Prepare and practice delivery of a report (small-group practice and critique).

Method/Intervention 8: Debates

Debates are organized discussions of differing points of view, basically arguments with rules. By providing structure we hope to achieve better understanding of multiple points of view and perhaps some wisdom. Debates also can potentially develop skills in oral persuasion. To effectively debate a topic the participant must have a substantial knowledge base; therefore, this method is often reserved for a culminating activity.

Advantages and Disadvantages

Advantages of debates are that they:

1. Can provide an element of fun.
2. Can develop many skills.
3. Provide variety.
4. Can expose a group to many diverse opinions.
5. Can function to solidify the debater's opinion on the subject.

Disadvantages are that they:

1. Require careful controls.
2. May reinforce current positions.
3. May develop into controversy.
4. Can make some people uncomfortable.
5. Can fail if people refuse to participate.
6. Can create hostility among opponents, fostering a negative environment.

Tips for Effective Implementation

1. Limit the topic to a two-sided debate that has a controversial topic with opposing views. Debate topics that elicit strong emotions are more powerful.
2. Chose topics that are demographically and developmentally appropriate for your target audience.
3. Provide both sides a common reputable source of information to keep the debate points focused.
4. Keep participants from knowing which side—pro or con—they will present until the last minute. This forces them to consider and prepare for both sides of an issue.
5. Set a structured time frame in advance—for example, 3 minutes for each side's opening arguments followed by 3 minutes rebuttal and 3 minutes closing.
6. Have the order of arguments drawn at random.
7. Consider ascertaining the participants' position on an issue and assigning them to debate the opposite side.

Debates can be inspirational events or the dull sharing and reinforcement of opinions. What happens is a result of organization and planning. First, you must review your objectives and determine if a debate will be helpful in achieving them. Do you wish to bring in outside debaters, use a debate team, or plan a notable debate and invite the community? What would be useful? If you wish to use your group or class, it is important to structure the debate so you can be certain to achieve your objectives. Since you are not teaching debate, remember that debate skills are an important secondary benefit but not the primary objective. The primary objective is usually the knowledge gained from preparation and observation of the debate or considering an issue from an alternative viewpoint.

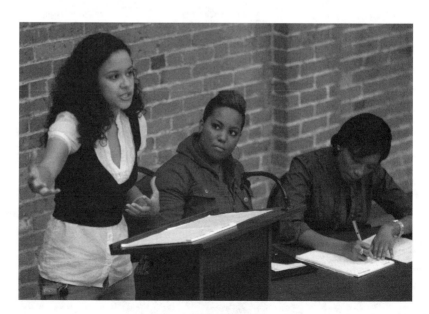

Debates help students practice oral skills and look at issues from alternative perspectives.

Examples   Examples of debate issues in health education follow:

1. Should helmet laws be mandatory?
2. Should condoms be provided to minors on demand?
3. Should parents be notified of all medical procedures (sexually transmitted infection [STI] treatment, abortion, etc.)?
4. Should abortion be legal?
5. Should free needles and sterilization kits be provided to drug users?
6. Who is responsible for the problem of pollution, violence, poverty, etc.?

Objective: After reviewing the case study, the reader will discuss two or more problems related to Pat's debate topic that possibly contributed to the activity's ineffectiveness.

Case Study: Pat   Pat Thomas, a school health educator, decides to have a debate on the issue of abortion. She asks for volunteers for the debate from the class. They select their position, and the debate follows in 1 week. The students provide excellent arguments on both sides of the issue. Pat feels good about the experience until she notices hostility among the students following the debate. Upon questioning the class she learns almost no one changed his or her position in any way, and many feel upset that others will not change their position given the righteousness of their cause. What happened? What could improve the chances that learning will take place and students consider both sides? (See Case Studies Revisited page 182.)

Question to consider:

Do you believe the topic selected is developmentally appropriate for high school students? Why or why not?

Method/Intervention 9: Displays and Bulletin Boards

Displays and bulletin boards are graphics and text combined in formats to attract attention. They can provide a positive educational environment and reinforce important points. They can also reach groups not attending any formal presentation or course.

Advantages and   Advantages of displays and bulletin boards are that they:
Disadvantages

1. Can set a positive environment.
2. Can be an ongoing educational tool.
3. Can reach special populations such as "walk-bys."
4. Provide variety.

Disadvantages are that they:

1. Can be expensive.
2. Require special materials.
3. Can be time-consuming.
4. Can raise the concern of vandalism.

Tips for Effective Implementation

Good bulletin board planning begins by analyzing its various elements: the title materials to be used, their arrangement, lettering, and color choices. Interest will be aroused by attention-getters such as puns, riddles, exaggeration, associations, comic strip figures, and other familiar figures. Elements to be used should be considered in terms of the following variables:

1. **Topic selection:** Focus attention on a single theme or subject. The message should be short and to the point. Select a brief catchy caption to draw attention while conveying the subject at a single glance using imaginative words, a question, current advertising slogans, or humorous television jargon.
2. **Materials (background):** The best materials will vary with the theme or subject. Once you have a rough sketch, take time to decide which materials will create the desired effect. You can use construction paper, white newspaper print, burlap, wallpaper, newspaper, gift-wrapping paper, or corrugated paper.
3. **Display materials:** Use actual objects and three-dimensional objects whenever possible. You can also use drawings, cartoon and stick figures,

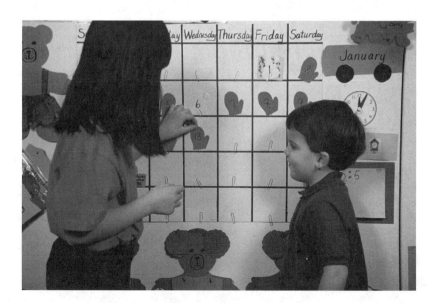

A well-organized bulletin board can add to a positive classroom environment.

pictures, or cotton roving (this can be used to tie the board together, indicate direction, or add a decorative touch). Next best to real objects are drawings, pictures or cartoons, and stick figures.

4. **Arrangement:** A formal arrangement with two sides balanced allows all items to be quickly seen but may tend to be boring. It is best suited for complicated arrangements. An informal, or unbalanced, arrangement is more interesting and eye-catching (see Figure 4-3). Key elements should dominate. With either arrangement, use captions employing the left-to-right principle. Place these at the bottom only if the bulletin board is at eye level. Frames give an appearance of completeness. Use construction paper corners or paper strip corners for a final touch. The arrangement should guide the eye from one element to another with stopping places to emphasize key points.

5. **Lettering:** A bold, even stroke of about ⅙ of a letter is the most legible lettering. It must balance yet not overshadow the rest of the board. Capital letters, manuscript letters, or fancy or textured letters can be used. Use felt-tip pens, rope, paint, cutouts, ribbon or yarn, spray paint, stencils, twigs, popsicle sticks, and so on.

6. **Color:** Attention, force, and meaning are obtained through skillful contrasting of color. Choose colors that catch attention and not those that blend into the background. You can pick colors for shock effect. Red, green, and blue are good at all times, but dark and light tones add a dramatic and pleasing effect. *Contrast makes the difference!*

Formal Balance   **Informal Balance**

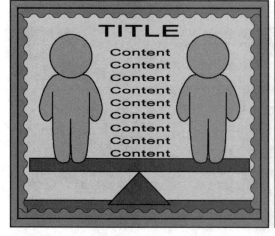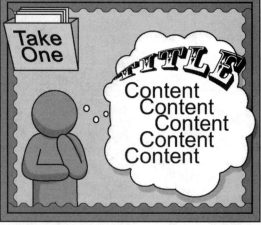

Figure 4-3
Bulletin Board Layouts

Method/Intervention 10: Educational Games

Educational games are activities that utilize an element of fun and competition. They differ from other games in that the educational objectives are clear and are the main focus of the activity. Games are generally competitive activities, and the user should consider the effects on all participants of using such a format.

Often participants can design their own games and rules. Utilizing existing frame games is a good way to develop interest. Use the format followed in current popular TV game shows. There are many computer programs that allow the facilitator to apply content-specific information to popular games such as *Jeopardy, Who Wants to Be a Millionaire?, Deal or No Deal,* or *Wheel of Fortune.*

Advantages and Disadvantages

Advantages of educational games are that they:

1. Provide an element of fun by actively involving learners.
2. Provide competition that can be motivating.
3. Provide variety.
4. Provide opportunities for repetition of important information.
5. Can be excellent introduction activities or good reviews.
6. Can encourage and enhance teamwork.
7. Provide feedback.

Disadvantages are that they:

1. Tend to focus on cognitive information for the most part.
2. Can be embarrassing for individuals who know little about the topic.
3. Can place too much emphasis on competition.
4. Can become disruptive if enthusiasm gets out of control.
5. Can fail if winning becomes more important than learning.
6. Can degenerate into off-task or social conversations (Wehrli & Nyquist, 2003).
7. Can reduce valuable learning time through explanation of directions/rules.

Tips for Effective Implementation

1. Select games at an appropriate level that will achieve the learning objectives.
2. Introduce the game and make clear the objective.
3. Do not assume the participants know the rules of the game. Give clear, thorough directions and adhere to the stated rules. Changing the rules during the game or vacillating on the application of rules fosters negative emotions of one group having an advantage over another. Whenever possible, provide written copies of the rules.
4. The facilitator should remain neutral, showing no partiality.

5. When providing token reinforcements such as prizes, consider having something for all but something a little extra for the winner. If you are handing out promotional key chains as incentives, you could allow the game winners to have first pick. This will recognize the efforts of the winners while reinforcing the efforts of all. Another thing to consider is the use of candy as a token reinforcement. As health educators we must be cognizant of sending contradictory messages. If you believe candy is appropriate, strive to provide sugarless items.

6. In order to maintain enthusiasm, limit the length of game play. No more than 30 minutes, including the time it takes to explain the rules, is recommended.

Example 1:
Football Game

The Football Game can be adapted to baseball, basketball, and so on.

Purpose

1. To review (could be used as a means of oral evaluation)
2. To start a card file collection of good testing items for future tests, reviews, and oral evaluations

Background

Facilitator must make up a large number of appropriate questions. Questions should be categorized according to difficulty to create five different piles of cards.

Rules of Play

1. Divide into two teams.
2. Flip a coin to see which team will be on offense first.
3. First offense begins from the team's own 40-yard line.
4. Questions are asked in rotating order among team members. If the answer is correct, the team advances 10 yards.
5. If the first person fails to answer the question, the next member is permitted to answer the question but a down is lost. If the first question was a true-false question, a new one is asked.
6. If the question is missed by the fourth person, the ball is lost on downs.
7. Questions are asked from pile 1 down to the 30-yard line.
8. Questions are asked from pile 2 between the 30-yard line and the 10-yard line.
9. Pile 3 contains the touchdown questions when the team reaches the 10-yard line.
10. Pile 4 contains the point after touchdown conversion.
11. From the 20- or 10-yard line, a field goal may be attempted from pile 5.
12. After a touchdown and conversion attempt, the team scored on starts a new offensive from its own 40-yard line.
13. If a field goal attempt is successful, the team that kicked starts a new offensive from its own 40-yard line. If unsuccessful, the defense takes over on its own 20-yard line.

14. A 5-minute halftime is taken in the middle of the period for consultation with team members and references on questions missed during the first half. Change possession of ball for second half.

15. In case of a tie score, the team with the most first downs (in this case the most correct answers) shall be the winner.

Materials Needed

1. A series of questions on 3-by-5-inch cards or cards that look like footballs, separated into piles.
2. Place cards showing numbers of piles.
3. Representative football field—could be a model or magnetic board, or you could draw one on a whiteboard, showing line divisions.
4. Whiteboard or scoreboard display of team scores and first downs.
5. Method of showing progress of ball. Three possibilities are
   a. Mark the whiteboard with dry erase markers.
   b. Use a model, moving a small indicator of some kind back and forth on top of it.
   c. Use a magnetic board.

Example 2:
Baseball Game

The Baseball Game is another sports-oriented educational game.

Rules of Play

1. Allow three outs to a side (three misses).
2. Limit singles to a maximum of three per inning. This will keep one team from dominating time.
3. Score by force-in only. This will prevent arguments. Be certain to explain that a runner can score at home plate if a new runner arrives to occupy third base. No base stealing (advancing to the next base without a runner arriving to occupy the space) is permitted.
4. Play as many innings as time permits (not more than nine).
5. If question is correctly answered, runner advances the corresponding bases.
6. Singles are easy questions, doubles harder, and so on.
7. If game ends in a tie, decide winner by total number of correct answers.

Alternate Rules of Play

1. Divide into two teams.
2. Make up a series of questions: true-false for singles, easy questions for doubles, harder questions for triples and home runs.
3. Runner must be forced in to score. No base stealing is permitted.
4. Limit three singles and three doubles per inning.
5. Talking by team at bat results in an out; talking by team on defense results in an out for the next inning.
6. Winner scores most runs.
7. Add third-inning stretch for study.
8. Missed questions may be used again later.

Example 3:
Hollywood Squares

Hollywood Squares is a cognitive (knowledge) oriented game that uses a tic-tac-toe framework for competition. It is especially suitable as an introductory game or as a review activity. The basic design (frame) is taken from the television game of the same name, and questions may be based on any desired content area. The instructor can make up questions or have students develop them as an assignment. Consider using another more current TV game show format.

Setting

1. Select nine people to act as celebrities, and ask them to leave the room. They might be selected earlier and come prepared, including appropriate costume.
2. Arrange chairs in the front of the class.
   a. Put three chairs in a straight row facing away from the blackboard toward the rest of the class. Allow room for three persons to stand behind and three to sit on the floor in front.
   b. Put a lectern at the back of the class as shown in Figure 4-4, with two captains.
3. Prepare a scoreboard to one side of the whiteboard in case there is time for more than one game.
4. Divide remainder of class in half alternately.
   a. Advise (name: _____) that she is captain of team X and seat her.
   b. Advise (name: _____) that he is captain of team O and seat him.
   c. Be sure to seat X on the right of the lectern, O on the left.

Celebrities Briefing

Celebrities wear tags and take on the role of famous people, or they can just be themselves. Celebrities step outside of the classroom and are provided the following instructions:

1. Questions will be directed to you; answer independently.
2. If you do not have a good answer, alibi or bluff—but make up your mind quickly, because there will be a time limit.

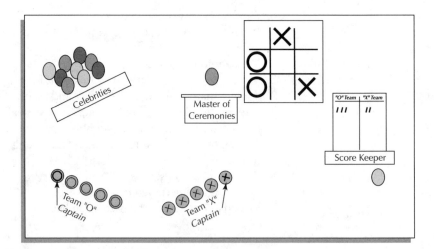

Figure 4-4
Room Setup for
Hollywood Squares
Game

3. When you come back into the room, situate yourselves in the front of the room as I direct you.
4. Please, no conversation, except to answer or bluff.
5. Do not be afraid to ask for a question to be repeated.
6. Any questions?

Return to Class
1. Celebrities are seated.
2. Check to see that teams are situated.
3. Brief class on the game.
   a. The object of the game is to get three squares in a row either up and down, across, or diagonally. To do this, the team must decide whether or not a celebrity is giving the right answer or making one up.
   b. Each completed game is worth 250 points. The team with the most points at the end of class will win a fabulous prize. The winning team will be given some prize, perhaps be allowed to leave first. If used with a community group, provide a tee-shirt or other incentive.
   c. Since we are deviating from the original format of *Hollywood Squares* in that teams will compete instead of single contestants, it is necessary to set a time limit of 30 seconds on deliberation between captain and team. Final decisions on how to answer each question will be left to the captain of each team. Please answer as quickly as possible.
   d. The facilitator will be the final judge of whether an answer is correct.
   e. If the captain's answer is correct, the team will be allowed to place their mark on the celebrity claiming the spot. Incorrect answers leave the celebrity open.
4. Are there any questions?

Begin
1. X, you start by choosing a square.
2. Question 1.

Questions
Questions should be based on important concepts and stated objectives. They should also be asked in such a way that they lend themselves to bluffing.

Materials Needed
Nine large cards with "X" on one side and "O" on the other side are needed. Two cards are used to designate teams—one "O" card and one "X" card.

Example 4:
Health Bingo
The Health Bingo Game uses a card like that shown in Figure 4-5.

Purpose
1. To review information
2. To introduce information
3. To evaluate workshop or class

Background   Facilitator must make up a list of questions suitable for the game. Each round requires 24 questions.

Player Objective   Achieve "bingo" by getting five correct answers in a row or column or diagonal line.

Materials   Bingo cards and pencils.

Rules of Play
1. Each person randomly assigns numbers (1–24) to the small corner boxes of his or her bingo card.
2. Facilitator begins game by drawing or otherwise randomly selecting the first number and reads a question.
3. Players locate the square and write the correct answer (if they know it).
4. The process is repeated until someone calls "bingo."

Health Education
B   I   N   G   O

22	2	11	5	13
1	17	20	9	7
4	8	Free Space	3	14
24	10	6	19	21
18	15	23	16	12

Figure 4-5
Health Bingo Card

5. The facilitator then checks the card to ensure there are five correct answers. If one or more is incorrect, play resumes; otherwise, the person is named the winner.
6. At this point the facilitator reviews the questions and answers.

Example 5:
Educational Relay   The room setup for the Educational Relay is shown in Figure 4-6.

Purpose
1. To introduce a new area of instruction
2. To get people up and active
3. To review material

Background   The facilitator must prepare a set of cards for each team (usually there are three teams with 15 to 20 cards each). Each set of cards should be the same except for a mark identifying each team. Three different-colored sets of cards could be used, for example. Cards each have a word appropriate to the topic being covered. Each container is labeled with the name of the category. An example would be containers labeled with food groups and cards with names of foods.

Player Objective   To get the cards in the correct container and to complete the task first.

Materials
1. Three sets of 3-by-5-inch cards. Sets are designated by common color.
2. Three labeled containers (large brown bags work fine).

Rules of Play
1. Teams are selected, and the room is cleared to allow running a relay.
2. Each member must start behind a line, pick up a card, run and place it in the correct container, and return to tag the next person in line. The next person repeats until all cards are used.

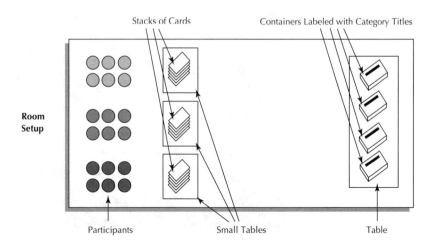

Figure 4-6
Room Setup for
Educational Relay

3. The winning team (first team to deposit all cards) receives 5 points for best speed; the second team receives 3 points; the third team receives 1 point.
4. The facilitator moves to the containers and removes the cards, checking with the group for correct answers. Each *correct* answer is worth 1 point.
5. The team with the highest point total is the winner.
6. Be extra careful with safety. Make certain the room is safe for a relay. Encourage people to walk or hop if appropriate or have a "designated runner" assigned for anyone uncomfortable or unable to run.

Method/Intervention 11: Experiments and Demonstrations

Experiments and demonstrations can serve as important tools for the health educator. Providing a factual demonstration is important for presenting information, reinforcing information, and enhancing recall. Demonstrations allow the learner to observe how something is done in order to transfer theory into practical applications (Wehrli & Nyquist, 2003). Experiments allow application in a control setting. Experiments and demonstrations can be used in community settings with careful planning. They are often remembered for a long time.

Advantages and Disadvantages

Advantages of experiments and demonstrations are that they:

1. Are visual and often hands-on.
2. Can serve to teach the scientific method.

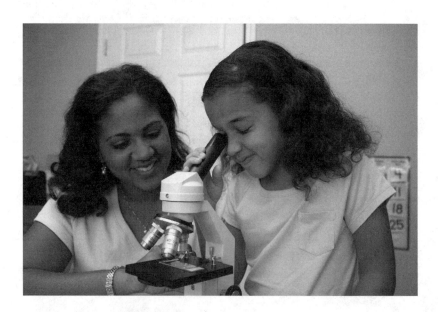

Active participation promotes learning.

3. Usually have a high interest level.
4. Reinforce theoretical aspects of a topic.
5. Promote self-confidence.
6. Facilitate individuals who learn best by modeling or active participation.

What I hear, I forget.
What I see, I remember.
What I do, I learn.
—Chinese proverb,
author unknown

Disadvantages are that they:

1. Can be costly.
2. Require time-consuming setup.
3. Require special equipment.
4. Are unpredictable in outcome.
5. Without proper controls and setup, can be dangerous.
6. May not be appropriate for the different learning rates of participants.
7. Require facilitator to have specialized expertise when highly technical tasks are involved (Wehrli & Nyquist, 2003).

Tips for Effective Implementation

1. The facilitator should be accomplished at what is being demonstrated/experimented upon. A smooth demonstration fosters a mental confidence promoting the idea: "If he can do it, I can too."
2. Carefully plan and practice the demonstration/experiment sequence prior to presentation.
3. Have all necessary materials at your fingertips, allowing you to transition smoothly from one step to another.
4. Keep your objective in mind as you execute the demonstration/experiment. When feasible, allow participants to practice what has been demonstrated or attempt the experiment independently.

Example 1: Fish Tank Ecology Demonstration

The Fish Tank Ecology Demonstration requires clearance and may evoke emotional responses. You must be prepared to deal with these issues from animal rights groups and others. Be certain this activity is appropriate for the age group involved. Seek permission and endorsement from your supervisor for such an activity.

Materials Required

1. Fish
2. Fish tank
3. Small fishnet
4. Litter, assorted sizes
5. Appropriate story
6. Clearance of agency or school to conduct activity (human subjects clearance may be required)

Description

One medium-sized fish tank is set up in plain view of the audience. Inside the tank is a goldfish. Next to this tank is a smaller tank or large jar with clean water. A fishnet is evident and in plain view.

Procedures

1. The facilitator sets up the demonstration without explanation but makes certain the audience sees all components, especially the fishnet.
2. The facilitator introduces someone to present a story. An excellent choice would be the Dr. Seuss story, *The Lorax*. The story is then read to the group.
3. Every so often the facilitator adds a piece of litter to the fish tank. This is done in full view of the audience. Hold up the litter item and examine the label before placing it in the tank.
4. As the story goes on, the litter becomes increasingly toxic. Progress from solid objects such as cans to soap products and oil.
5. If someone says to stop littering, ignore that person, but if someone takes action, allow that person to put the fish in the clean tank.
6. The activity ends when the story is over and the tank is thoroughly polluted or someone saves the fish.
7. The story reader usually leaves after reading the story.
8. Debrief the group as follows:

> *Question:* What happened?
> The usual response is, "You killed the fish."
> *Question:* Who killed the fish?
> *Response:* You all the killed the fish. You all knew what was happening but did nothing to save the fish. That is exactly what is happening to our environment. We talk a lot but do nothing. Every one of you could have saved this fish but you all made excuses and did nothing.
>
> If someone saves the fish, present the fish to that person and commend him or her for taking action.

Discovery is learning.
—Francis Bacon

Example 2: Smoking Experiment (Accumulation of Tar 1)

This Smoking Experiment is the first of two showing accumulation of tar, both taken from a Public Health Service book by G. G. Gilbert and M. Ziady (1986). Figure 4-7 illustrates the experiment.

Purpose

To show the accumulation of tar in water by change of color and smell.

Appropriate Age Group

Middle through secondary school.

Materials

1. Gallon jar with a two-holed stopper
2. Cigarettes and matches
3. Delivery tubes (glass, plastic, or rubber hose)
4. Cigarette holder
5. Hand squeeze pump or vacuum pump

Procedure

1. Assemble cigarette tar separating apparatus as shown in the diagram.
2. Fill the gallon jar half full with water.

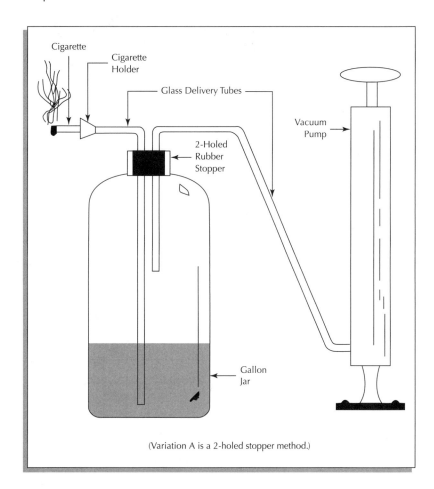

Figure 4-7
First Smoking
Experiment Showing
Accumulation of Tar

(Variation A is a 2-holed stopper method.)

3. Place cigarette in intake and light.
4. Using vacuum pump, draw smoke from cigarette into gallon jar and water.
5. Pump until cigarette is burned completely. Replace with additional cigarettes until tars can be seen in water.
6. Examine color and smell of water.

Key Points for Discussion

1. What happens to your lungs when you smoke?
2. What are the similarities between this experiment and what happens to your lungs?
3. What chemicals are in the water?
4. Where can we find out more about the effects of smoking?
5. How does your body rid itself of these tars?

Example 3: Smoking
Experiment
(Accumulation of
Tar 2)

This Smoking Experiment is the second of two showing accumulation of tar, both taken from a Public Health Service article by G. G. Gilbert and M. Ziady (1986). Figure 4-8 illustrates the experiment.

Purpose   To show the accumulation of tar in cotton balls.

Appropriate
Age Group

Primary school.

Materials   1. Plastic window cleaner container or other empty plastic container, transparent if possible

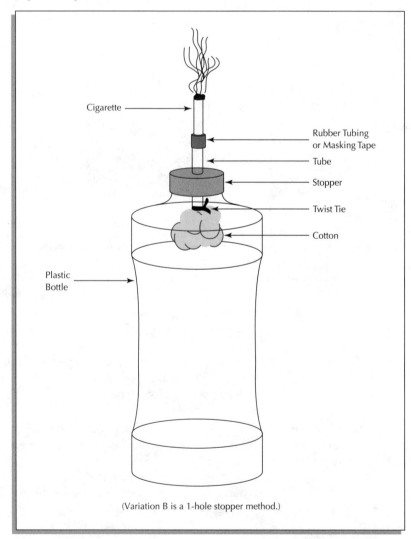

(Variation B is a 1-hole stopper method.)

Figure 4-8
Second Smoking
Experiment Showing
Accumulation of Tar

2. Ballpoint pen barrel or other tubing approximately the size of a cigarette
3. Cotton
4. Cigarettes and matches
5. Ashtray or other item to catch ashes

Procedure   You may wish to conduct the experiment outside or with the windows open to avoid side-stream smoke.

1. Rinse the container thoroughly.
2. Make an opening in the cap of the container to fit the tubing into the cap.
3. Place the tubing in the opening and seal tight with cement or clay if needed.
4. Insert loosely packed cotton ball into tubing.
5. Insert cigarette into open end of tubing.
6. Press firmly on the plastic container to force air out, light the cigarette, and then proceed with slow and regular pumping action.
7. Withdraw cotton from tubing to show accumulation of tar.
8. Pass container around for individuals to smell and to observe that smoke continues to be expelled for a period of time.

Variation   1. Divide into groups and conduct several experiments, keeping a close watch for safety.
2. Try the same experiment with a filter cigarette.
3. Compare filter and nonfilter cigarettes.

Key Points for Discussion   1. What happens to your lungs when you smoke?
2. Is this experiment similar to what happens to your lungs?
3. Consider this effect multiplied by 20 or 30 times per day for 5, 10, or 20 years.

Other Examples   Three other examples of experiments follow:

1. Put powder that is visible only under a blacklight on a doorknob. Use the black light experiment to discuss transmission of germs.
2. Test local streams for contaminates.
3. Test wall paints for the presence of lead.

Method/Intervention 12: Field Trips

Field trips are visits with individuals, to sites of interest, or both. Such visits provide special opportunities to put people or activities in the context of the environment. Such activities are common in many schools but should also be considered in community health programs. If you expect individuals to use services, for example, it would be a good idea to visit the site and get acquainted with the personnel. Chances are then much greater that these services will be utilized.

When to Use   It is appropriate to use field trips when you believe the trip will actually help meet your objectives. Being on-site affords special opportunities not found elsewhere, and visiting a site can often have a demystifying effect. If you want to ensure that your group is more comfortable in using a facility, for example, a field trip would be a good idea. Knowing how to get there can be an important issue. Which bus to take or where to park can be important considerations. These issues have been shown time and again to be major barriers for action.

You may gain access to special expertise or equipment that is important to reaching your objectives only through field trips. Prior planning is most important if you want to ensure a successful trip. Field trips typically function as an effective culminating activity. You should always personally visit the site first before taking a group. Take only those groups that you are certain you can handle. This is especially important with any group that will be in a potentially dangerous area. One method often used is to establish a list of questions to be answered by each visitor and collect the responses following the trip. Always conduct a debriefing session after the visit.

Advantages and   Advantages of field trips are that they:
Disadvantages

1. Can be structured to address difficult objectives.
2. Are often very entertaining and enjoyable.
3. Put people in the context of their environment.
4. Often have models and materials not available elsewhere.
5. Provide opportunity to learn through multiple senses.

Disadvantages are that they:

1. Usually require transportation and can be costly.
2. Can be very time-consuming.
3. Are unpredictable in outcome because of uncertainty of interaction.
4. Often raise the concern of liability coverage.
5. Often require elaborate planning.

Tips for Effective   1. Prepare an agenda for the trip indicating the times and objectives of the
Implementation   activities to be completed. The agenda should also include the leader's contact information and procedures for emergency situations.
2. Divide the larger group into subgroups to ensure all participants are accounted for during the trip. Consider rotating groups among the various areas or staggering the start to avoid overcrowding.

3. Avoid attempting to "see it all" and pressing learners to hurry. It is better to cover less but cover it well.
4. Intentionally overestimate the amount of time it will take to execute the trip and allow for unexpected delays.
5. Consider making arrangements for first aid and other emergencies.

Objective: After reviewing the case study, the reader will state two obvious mistakes of Meshah's and offer suggestions to improve the outcome of the field trip experience.

Case Study: Meshah   Meshah took a group of high school students to a comprehensive community health clinic to meet with the staff. The agenda was so full the students had little opportunity to ask questions. On the bus home Meshah engaged the students in discussion about the football season. Unknown to Meshah, the students still had many questions about privacy issues, access to care, and the qualifications and training of staff. Many students left with incorrect assumptions because of the lack of follow-up. How could Meshah have structured this visit more effectively? (See Case Studies Revisited page 182.)

Questions to consider:

1. How has over-planning the agenda negatively impacted the field trip experience?
2. What do you consider to be the objective of the field trip?

Health Museums or Health Education Centers   Several centers around the country specialize in health education activities. These are very exciting places that have a wealth of materials on display. Most are hands-on places that schedule group visits. Generally, they have specially trained staff who will lead tailormade sessions. Examples of such centers include:

1. Center for Health Education in Indianapolis
2. Poe Center for Health Education in Raleigh, North Carolina
3. National Health Museum at Walter Reed Hospital in Washington, D.C.
4. Denver Museum of Natural History: Hall of Life Health Education Center

Examples   Four examples of field trips follow:

1. Visit an emergency room.
2. Visit a public health clinic and take on the role of a client.
3. Ride with a police officer for an evening.
4. Interview individuals who have experienced a health problem of special interest.

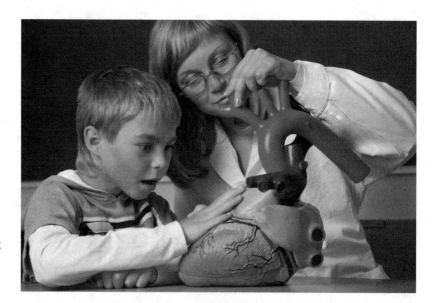

Health education centers are entertaining places to bring students for a hands-on learning experience.

Method/Intervention 13: Guest Speakers

Guest speakers can be a tremendous resource in both the school and community settings. Many individuals have knowledge or experiences that make them uniquely qualified to add a great deal to health-related topics. Individuals who have experienced or are experiencing health problems can help bring alive and personalize what might be viewed as dull and irrelevant health information. Other speakers might be experts in a field who can bring up-to-date information about topical health issues. Be aware that in community settings, the health educator is often considered a guest speaker during the early stages of multisession programs. It is wise to establish yourself as a credible source within the program prior to bringing in a guest speaker.

One caution must be made, however. Health educators must think carefully about what they are trying to achieve before using guest speakers (see the information on constructing behavioral objectives in Chapter 2). It is the health educator's responsibility to ensure that the speaker provides factual information that promotes positive health attitudes and behaviors. He or she must also avoid inadvertently teaching participants how to perform undesirable behaviors. For example, all too often school and college health educators, in an attempt to increase the students' awareness of their own susceptibility to HIV, will bring in a guest speaker who is HIV positive. The speaker is a middle-aged man who discusses how he contracted the virus through homosexual sex. The students usually feel moved by the tragedy of the situation and the courage of the individual, but leave the presentation with their stereotypical view strongly reinforced, that HIV is still really a gay disease.

Objectives must be clearly defined before utilizing a speaker, and the health educator should avoid the trap of using someone simply because "it seemed like the right thing to do!"

Advantages and Disadvantages

Advantages of guest speakers are that they:

1. Allow groups access to experts in the field and the opportunity to obtain up-to-the-minute information.
2. Enable participants to personalize, or put a face to, a health issue that up to this point might have seemed abstract.
3. Give participants a "break" from the regular presenter or teacher.
4. Allow participants to meet individuals who might be influential at the local, state, or even national level. This opportunity can facilitate networking.

Disadvantages are that they:

1. Can be ineffective if the speaker is poor. Many individuals have some good information to share, but because their speaking skills are so poor, their presentations are boring and thus ineffectual. Every effort should be made to hear a speaker before extending an invitation.
2. Can present an unbalanced picture of an issue. The single guest speaker tends to bring one viewpoint to an educational setting, which, of course, is not always a bad thing. However, care must be taken to at least consider this factor, and, when discussing controversial issues in particular, make an effort to present the opposing viewpoint.
3. In a school setting, will require notification and permission from the administration. It is of particular importance to obtain such permission when "sensitive" issues such as human sexuality or drug education are being addressed.
4. May not be the kind of person to whom participants can relate. Issues such as the speaker's race, gender, age, and national origin are all important factors to consider when bringing in a guest speaker to a community. Close consultation with community leaders is an effective way to facilitate the choice of speaker.
5. May charge a speaking fee. Although many speakers will not charge any type of fee, those individuals who have a particular expertise, who are regular speakers, and who have a good reputation will invariably charge a speaking fee. This can range from a few hundred to a thousand or more dollars per engagement. Always be sure to ask about a fee before arranging a presentation!

Tips for Effective Implementation

1. Enthusiastically introduce the guest speaker by providing his or her credentials. When possible, promote the guest speaker's event in a meeting prior to the occasion.

2. Prepare a contingency plan in the event of a last-minute conflict resulting in the speaker's inability to be present.
3. Establish a nonverbal cue that can be used to indicate time constraints.
4. Close the guest speaker's presentation by thanking him or her and reiterating specific insights.
5. Always send a thank-you note.

Example: Eating Disorders Unit

Assume that you have been asked to teach a small unit on eating disorders to college students. You have covered the "theory" of the issue, but it is clear to you that despite the statistics you have given related to the prevalence of this problem, the students are having a difficult time understanding how individuals become involved with eating disorders. After a little research on your part, you discover that the campus has an eating disorder support group that provides students who are willing to share their stories with other students. A student from the group attends your class, and suddenly eating disorders has a face and a personality . . . and because the face and personality probably look very similar to those of the regular class members, the effects of using such a guest speaker can be profound.

Method/Intervention 14: Guided Imagery

Guided imagery as a method involves experiencing through a guided sensory journey some health-enhancing behavior or potential outcome. It generally involves closing of the eyes and being guided through some experience. It is commonly used in stress management and sports psychology.

When to Use

It is appropriate to use guided imagery when you believe the experience will actually help meet your objectives.

Advantages and Disadvantages

Advantages of guided imagery are that it:

1. Can positively influence attitudes and values such as efficacy.
2. Can be entertaining and enjoyable.
3. Is low in cost.
4. Can be motivational.

Disadvantages are that it:

1. Requires some training and practice.
2. Can be time-consuming.
3. May be uncomfortable for some participants who feel overly vulnerable.

Tips for Effective Implementation

1. It is important to establish a conducive environment to effectively execute guided imagery. Excessive noise and termperature, uncomfortable

seating, and inappropriate lighting can act as distractions, thereby interfering with the learners' ability to concentrate.

2. Remind learners that guided imagery is a personal experience with no correct or incorrect way to experience the method.
3. Practice reading your script to become fluid and to identify natural pauses.
4. Monitor the participants' responses and be sensitive to issues that elicit a highly emotional response.
5. Guided imagery can be enhanced by stimulating multiple senses such as hearing (by adding soft background music) or smell (by burning scented candles).

Examples   A variety of scripts on multiple topics is available commercially. For example, if a health educator were to type "guided imagery scripts pain control" into a search engine on the Internet, over 149,000 sources would be available to view. The following are some examples of guided imagery:

1. **Pain control:** Participants are to contract and relax muscles in sequence while applying deep breathing techniques.
2. **Stress education:** Soft music such as sea sounds is accompanied by directions to imagine walking on a beach.
3. **Weight control:** The participants are directed to imagine themselves at their ideal weight and how good it feels and looks.
4. **Procedure anxiety:** The participants are asked to imagine the steps for a medical procedure such as a mammogram or a testicular exam.

Method/Intervention 15: Humor

Humor can be used as an attraction or a reinforcing activity. It is an important tool for health educators. It can liven up a meeting and help to establish rapport with an audience. However, it is important to note that people differ in what they find humorous. Be certain to avoid humor that may offend. For example, the bumper sticker proclaiming, "Support Mental Health or I Will Kill You" is funny to many but upsetting to others. Likewise, "How in the Health Are You?" may offend some people. Also, it is important to keep humor focused on objectives.

Advantages and   Advantages of humor are that it:
Disadvantages

1. Provides an element of fun.
2. Is a good attention-getter.
3. Provides variety.
4. Can address affective information or issues in a palatable format.
5. Can provide new perspectives.

Disadvantages are that it:

1. Is unpredictable in outcome because everyone has a different sense of humor.
2. May require special setup, such as props or special characters to act as a standup man.
3. May require permission to use.
4. May be viewed as a waste of time by some participants.

Tips for Effective Implementation William and Pauline Carlyon (1987) have some good suggestions for using humor:

- Remember, humor is not just a joke. It is one of a range of positive emotions you want to evoke.
- Do not assume that others share your sense of humor and its underlying social attitudes.
- Beware of satire and irony. They are easily misread as sarcasm or ridicule.
- Do not tell jokes, unless they are "on you." Save your standup comedy for your family and friends, who are familiar with your eccentricities.
- Avoid ethnic humor and dialect imitations particularly. You will almost always sound insulting.
- Do listen to your clients/patients/students and encourage their humor by participating in its enjoyment. Only they know the humor that's best for them.

Examples Some examples of how to use humor follow:

1. Ask the group to design cartoons that would influence a target group.
2. Use cartoons on a overhead projector with text removed and ask the group to write new text that would influence the target population.
3. Ask the group to write humorous health sayings.
4. Photocopy cartoons or humorous health sayings and make transparencies from them to spice up a presentation.
5. Tell a funny story. This could be a story about yourself and the health issue.
6. Show a humorous commercial related to the topic.
7. Tell a joke related to issues.

Method/Intervention 16: Lecture

Lecturing is a primary tool of the health educator. It is often maligned as a method, but in fact it is the most common tool in health education although it is often poorly utilized. Good lecturing requires practice and organization. Most of us will not become world-class orators, but we can become competent speakers. We strongly urge you to enhance your speaking skills by reading some books on public speaking, taking a course, or joining a Toastmasters club to improve your skills. You will constantly be called upon to make presentations as a health educator. Whether you are in school or community health education, you must develop skills in making presentations. Your presentations may be to small or large groups, but the basic principles are the same.

Any time you must lecture for over 20 minutes, utilize some of the other methods or prepare a truly stirring presentation. It is unlikely that you can keep the attention of your audience much beyond this time frame unless audience members are personally highly motivated (i.e., graduate students or victims of the disease you are discussing, who perceive you to clearly have information they want) or you are charismatic. Preparation is the key to a successful presentation. (See also Chapter 5.)

Advantages and Disadvantages

Advantages of the lecture style are that it:

1. Allows you to cover large amounts of information in a short time.
2. Can be used with very large groups.
3. Requires little equipment, although a microphone is important for large groups.
4. Presents factual information in a logical sequence.
5. Can stimulate thinking to open discussion.
6. May be recorded for future use.

Disadvantages are that it:

1. Can be a difficult method for holding the attention of an audience.
2. Requires a very high level of expertise on the topic to do well without other aids.
3. Is not a good way to attract an audience unless the speaker is well known and respected.
4. Is generally effective only for short periods of time.
5. Is difficult to assess the degree of learning taking place.
6. Is passive versus active learning, placing the burden of promoting learning fully on the lecturer (Wehrli & Nyquist, 2003).

Tips for Effective Implementation

Prepresentation Tasks

Preparation for presentation, or *prepresentation* tasks, include the following:

1. Select or write objectives (see Chapter 2).
2. Analyze the audience—needs assessment (see Chapter 2).
3. Develop appropriate content for lecture. Be careful not to cover too much material at one time. The lecture should contain an obvious introduction, include examples and anecdotes, and have a clear conclusion. Consider providing a handout to reinforce important points.

4. Develop lecture notes as part of your lesson plan (see Chapter 5). This preparation should be done well before the presentation. Knowing you are prepared is a great confidence builder. Preparing the night before often gives you the jitters and is self-defeating.

5. Develop an alternate plan in case something does not work right. What do you do if the audiovisual equipment does not work or the participants do not ask questions when you want them to?

6. Practice making your presentation. If you have the time and resources, video- or audiotape it and play it back. Practice keeping your hands at your side. Do not hold your notes or read directly from them. It is okay to glance at them when needed, but do not be tied to them. This concept also applies when using presentation software; the audience is usually capable of reading a slide. Allow the information on the slide to act as a backdrop clarifying the point you are making in the lecture. If this is a topic you do not know well, use overheads or some other visual aid. This will ensure you do not miss any key points, and people will look at your visual aid a good part of the time, taking some of the pressure off you.

The Presentation

Guidelines for presentation follow:

1. Clarify what you will cover—what are your objectives? Students or clients will learn more if you make it clear what you want them to get out of your presentation. Your participants should be fully aware of what they should know, feel/believe, or be able to do when you are finished speaking. Speak at an appropriate level, but do not be patronizing.

2. Present your information clearly, repeating important points.

3. Whenever possible check to be certain the audience is understanding your message. Always remember you are lecturing to reach your objectives. You are not there to only entertain. You are a health educator hoping to influence lives. Use humor if it helps achieve your objectives.

4. Summarize frequently and use indicators to identify major points, such as, "the key is to remember," "there are three things you should consider," and "in conclusion" (Wehrli & Nyquist, 2003).

5. Manager your time and allow for questions prior to your planned conclusion (Wehrli & Nyquist, 2003).

6. Review key points and prepare for the next step in your program. What do you want participants to do? What is the next step?

7. Finally, review these "Dos" and "Do Nots" of presentation:

The "Do Nots" of Presentation

- Do not play with chalk like dice.
- Do not put your hands in your pocket or use some other distraction with your hands.

- Do not say "I don't know this area very well" or "I don't know why I was asked to cover this."
- Do not get tied to a podium or your notes.
- Do not use filler words such as "ah," "um," or "you know."

The "Dos" of Presentation
- Do smile and move about.
- Do reinforce key points.
- Do let the audience know you are a credible speaker on the topic.
- Do use visual aids as appropriate.
- Do show an aura of confidence.
- Do make eye contact.

Method/Intervention 17: Mass Media

The term **mass media** refers to the use of media to reach large audiences or the use of available mass media materials to educate a target group. These materials include television, newspapers, magazines, pamphlets, billboards, and radio. Be certain to consider local media such as ethnic publications and community-based publications. Developing your own mass media program is generally expensive and requires special skills. Most venues of mass media offer public service announcements (PSAs) or will provide free access for worthy causes and may even make their professional staff available. Generally, we recommend the use of specialists for such work. These specialists need not be Park Avenue firms, but can be local businesses or local community college or university staff personnel.

Another way to use media is to utilize available media examples through videotaping or copying. Often formal permission can be granted for educational programs. Many of the **voluntary health organizations** such as the American Cancer Society have high-quality materials.

An important issue is often preparing groups to analyze media messages and to examine fallacies.

Advantages and Disadvantages

Advantages of the mass media are that they:

1. Can reach a large number of individuals.
2. Can reinforce important ideas.
3. Can create a positive environment for change.

Disadvantages are that they:

1. Are usually inadequate to change complex behaviors because of the brevity of the messages.
2. Can be very expensive.
3. May require special personnel.

Whom to Contact   Here are some guidelines on whom to contact:

1. For newspapers, contact the education or medical science editor if they have one; otherwise, the appropriate news editor.
2. For television, contact the public service director or the program director.
3. For radio, contact the public service director or the program director.

Example: Local Media Campaign   Conduct a mass media campaign for a health fair. Contact the local television station regarding what it needs. It may wish to conduct live interviews for its public service programs or as part of local news segments. The key is to be cooperative and flexible about air time. Generally stations are very cooperative in providing some time. The following media kits can give you ideas about putting together a campaign to support school health education or other health topics.

1. American School Health Association, Marketing Kit—A Healthy Child: The Key to the Basics, available from ASHA, P.O. Box 708, Kent, OH 44240. 330-678-1601 or http://www.ashaweb.org.
2. Health Education Advocacy Kit, available from American Association for Health Education, 1900 Association Dr., Reston, VA 22061. 703-476-3437 or http://www.aahperd.org/AAHE.

Method/Intervention 18: Models

Models are useful visual aids for instruction. Examples of models include anatomical facsimiles, breast models for self-examination practice, model communities, car models, and any variety of materials to make a point or draw people visually into a discussion.

Advantages and Disadvantages   Advantages of models are that they:

1. Can provide variety.
2. Can be used to provide "hands-on" experiences.
3. Are very attractive and good attention-getters.
4. Can be much more meaningful than a picture in a text.

Disadvantages are that they:

1. Require equipment.
2. Can be expensive.
3. Require extra setup.

Tips for Effective Implementation   1. Display the models in clear view to spark participant interest.
2. The model should be significant in size so that it is easily seen by all learners.

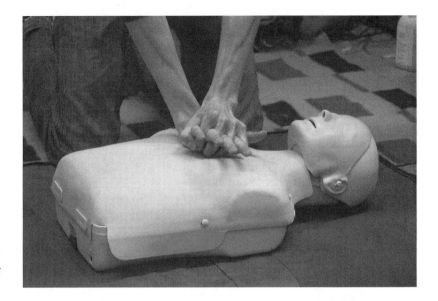

Models offer a more interactive approach to learning than photos or illustrations can offer.

3. If using a model to support a lecture, avoid passing the item while the lecture continues; instead, leave the model displayed for individuals to view following the presentation.
4. Present your content prior to distributing models to participants. The models may act as a distraction if available to participants prior to instruction.

Examples   Some examples of how to use models follow:

1. Use mannequins to teach CPR.
2. Use a heart model for teaching heart attack prevention and care.
3. Use a breast model for teaching breast self-examination.
4. Use a testicle model for teaching testicular self-examination.

Method/Intervention 19: Music

Music can be used in several ways to achieve objectives. It can be used as a method or as part of a method. Music is a powerful mood setter. Music can be used in the background as a way of setting the mood for a skit or role play. It can be used to draw attention to the message found in the lyrics. Participants can make up their own lyrics. Music affects us all. We can select music to help us create a special mood or capture the interest of a group.

Advantages and Disadvantages

Advantages of music are that it:

1. Can be low in cost. You can always sing without any equipment.
2. Often can be used to help discuss affective issues.
3. Is excellent for setting a mood.
4. Can allow for individual expression.

Disadvantages are that it:

1. Often requires equipment, such as a piano, which may be difficult to obtain and move.
2. Is sometimes difficult to find correct music.
3. Poses difficulty in appealing to a variety of tastes.

Tips for Effective Implementation

1. Always review the music prior to its use to assess appropriateness/suitability.
2. Cue up the music and assess the volume before you present.

Examples

Some examples of the use of music follow:

1. Sing songs with health messages.
2. Develop songs to reinforce health messages.
3. Start a group chant: "No matter what you say about me, I'm still a worthwhile person." While the group is chanting, walk around the room making negative statements about each person. Have the group continue chanting, ignoring the negative statements.
4. Use chants to reinforce various messages.
5. Play a funeral march to lead into a discussion about funeral customs and the purposes of a funeral.
6. Ask participants to make up health lyrics to popular songs.
7. Ask participants to bring in a sample of music that expresses something personal or special to them.
8. Ask participants how relationships are depicted in popular songs. Bring in examples to discuss.

Method/Intervention 20: Newsletters

We are all familiar with newsletters but often do not realize that they can be an important component of an educational intervention. They can provide vital information to target groups, such as location; set a climate for an upcoming workshop or class; serve to reinforce concepts presented in a workshop; or act as a reminder for action. The newsletter is often a very cost-effective way to deliver and reinforce information, encourage compliance, and increase the likelihood of attendance. The availability of personal computers makes this method accessible to most groups today. Figure 4-9 shows an example of a newsletter.

Advantages and Disadvantages

Advantages of newsletters are that they:

1. Have the potential for providing a considerable amount of information at relatively low cost.
2. Can target specific needs.
3. Can reinforce information presented in a program.
4. Can serve as a reminder to take action (often referred to as a bolster).

Disadvantages are that they:

1. Have high mailing costs and production costs.
2. Require some equipment—for example, they generally require access to a personal computer.
3. Can be very time-consuming to construct.
4. Require at least a minimal level of expertise.

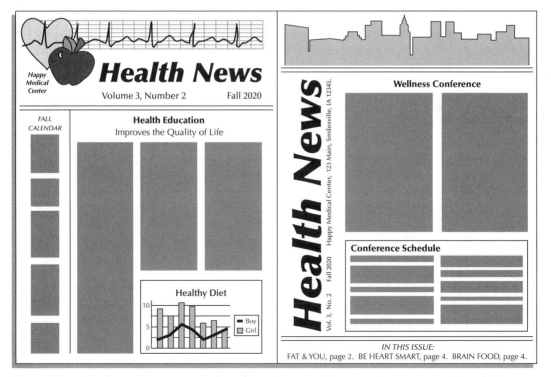

Figure 4-9
Example of a Newsletter

<table>
<tr><td>

Tips for Effective Implementation

</td><td>

1. When distributing a newsletter as part of a program, highlight an interesting aspect of the newsletter to entice participants to read or share the information.
2. Deliver your newsletter as a single item. Bulking newsletters with other materials to be distributed reduces their importance.

</td></tr>
</table>

Method/Intervention 21: Panels

A **panel** is a useful way for an audience either to explore differing opinions about the same topic or to examine varying issues within the same subject area. A panel can be used in both the school and community settings, made up of members of the local community (or class) or "experts" brought in from outside agencies. In the school setting a panel is an innovative way to motivate students to research an area and present their findings to the class. The school health educator should always ensure that the school administration has full knowledge of any panels that include outside speakers.

Using a panel in the community is a little more complicated, and great consideration must be given to certain factors when matching panel members with the community setting. For example, will the community members view the panel members as legitimate? Will the community give credence to "outside opinions"? Can the community members relate to the panelists in any way? These are all basic questions that must be considered with great care by the community health educator.

Advantages and Disadvantages

Advantages of panels are that they:

1. Allow the audience to hear a diversity of opinions about the same subject.
2. Have the potential for critical debate among panelists, allowing the audience to learn about the issues in greater depth.
3. Allow the audience to hear more than one speaker, decreasing the likelihood of boredom.

Disadvantages are that they:

1. Are often difficult to compile with just the right "mix." For example, one of the panelists might dominate the proceedings, or the members might be so antagonistic toward one another that nothing meaningful gets accomplished.
2. Have the potential to lack closure. A good moderator can prevent this problem. In the classroom setting a moderator might ask the students to write a paragraph about what they have heard or their feelings about a topic in light of the panel discussion. In the community setting a moderator might

briefly summarize the discussion or allow a few minutes for each panelist to review his or her position.

3. Allow participants (moderator and/or panelists) to get off track, either individually or collectively. Rules, such as allowed time to speak, opportunities for questions, and so on, should be considered before beginning.
4. Can dilute the content when personalities overshadow the information.
5. Have the potential to be or feel disorganized if the content presented does not follow a logical sequence.

Tips for Effective Implementation

The focus of a panel discussion can be enhanced by providing the panel members with a list of questions from you or generated from the program participants. One effective method for providing panel members insight on the knowledge base and concerns of the audience is to have the participants create a K-W-L (know/want to know/learned) chart (Ogle, 1986). This type of chart is an organizer that mirrors the process of scientific inquiry by identifying K "what the participant *currently knows*," W "what he *wants to know*," followed by a measurement of L "what he *learned* after the discussion" (Frey & Fisher, 2007, p. 57).

Example:
Supplements

Participants:

A group of college student athletes will be hearing a panel discussion on the use of performance-enhancing supplements in professional sports.

Materials:

- Three sets of three different colored sticky-back papers (e.g., Post-it Notes)
- Pencil
- Whiteboard and dry erase markers

Procedure:

1. Prior to the panel discussion, draw the K-W-L chart (Figure 4-10) on the whiteboard.
2. Provide each participant with three (or more) sticky-back papers of each color.
3. Instruct participants to use a designated note color to record the requested information.
4. Provide the sticky-back notes with the questions from the K and W sections to the panel to review.
5. Following the presentation, have participants record "What I learned" statements and place them in the L section of the K-W-L chart. The facilitator may review the sticky-back notes placed in the L section to assess student learning.

Instructions for Participants:

1. Write down one thing you know about performance-enhancing supplements on each of the #1 color (e.g., yellow) sticky-back papers.
2. Write down one question you have about performance-enhancing supplements on each of the #2 color (e.g., blue) sticky-back papers.
3. Stick your yellow notes in the "What Do I Know" section and the blue papers in the "What Do I Want to Know?" section on the whiteboard.
4. Your K and W notes will be shared with the panel members prior to their presentation.
5. After the panel discussion you will record one thing you learned about performance-enhancing supplements on each of the #3 color (e.g., pink) sticky-back papers and then place them on the whiteboard in the space "What I Have Learned."

Example: Teenage Pregnancy A panel to help expectant teenage mothers and fathers anticipate problems they may encounter might include the following individuals:

- A teenage mother and father who have already been through the process and can describe their experiences.
- A representative of a local agency who can explain the available program resources, both financial and otherwise.
- A member of the local school system who can give information related to finishing school.

This list is not exhaustive, yet even a panel limited to these few people would be much more useful than a lecture from a single "expert" who has probably never experienced this particular problem. A link to local resources alone would make this panel a worthwhile and valuable health education strategy.

What Do I KNOW?	What Do I WANT to Know?	What have I LEARNED?

Figure 4-10
K-W-L Chart

Method/Intervention 22: Peer Education

The **peer education** approach of presenting health education information has become very popular over the past few years. This approach, which consists of individuals or groups presenting workshops for their peers, can be a very effective and productive means by which to disseminate information. Peer teaching has been reported as a significant strategy for promoting active learning (Fuchs et al., 2001; McLauchlan, 2002; Thrope & Wood, 2000). This method is commonly used on college campuses and in school and community settings. Peer education is a particularly useful method to use when funding for professional personnel is limited or when it is particularly important for the audience to be able to relate to the presenters. (See the example at the conclusion of this section.)

Advantages and Disadvantages

Advantages of peer education are that it:

1. Provides a modeling experience. Individuals often learn through modeling. Because peer educators are extremely similar to their audiences, the opportunity for modeling to occur is enhanced.
2. May have a greater effect than a solitary health educator. The peers have many more points of entry into a population than a professional and can thus reach more people.
3. Has the potential for providing continuing, informal education. Peers will become known in the community as sources of information and referral and will therefore have the opportunity to educate even when they are not offering a structured presentation.
4. Can influence people that professionals cannot. Peers can be "gatekeepers" to a population that would otherwise be unreached. The peers' values and interests are similar to those of their potential clients, and this can provide an effective entrée.
5. Affords an incredible opportunity for the personal growth and development of the peers themselves. We should not ignore this benefit by focusing exclusively on the recipients of the programming efforts (Goodhart, 1993).

Disadvantages of peer education are that it:

1. Might sometimes lack credibility in the eyes of the audience because peer educators are not perceived as "experts."
2. Could provide inaccurate information or poor performance, resulting in the loss of program credibility, unless the peer educators are well trained and their programming is closely monitored.
3. Could be dangerously inadequate for programs requiring a high degree of sophisticated and technical information. Peer educators should not be asked to do more than they are capable of doing.

Tips for Effective Implementation

1. When recruiting peer educators determine your criteria for the skills and qualities needed, and then select volunteers based on these guidelines.
2. Involve peer educators in the planning process to ensure that they understand the program objectives.
3. Provide training and opportunities for peer educators to practice prior to delivery during your program.

Example: Alcohol Abuse, Sexuality, and Stress Management Programs

Assume you have just been appointed community health educator at a college with an enrollment of 15,000. You are the only health educator on staff, and your supervisors would like you to begin implementing programming around the issues of alcohol abuse, sexuality, and stress management as soon as possible. After educating your supervisors as to what is humanly possible, you set about planning your strategy, which includes peer education.

Peer education can be an incredibly valuable programming strategy, particularly when staffing levels are low. Although finding interested, enthusiastic students to help is not usually a problem, training them to high standards of performance can be demanding. High standards, however, are crucial in order to avoid fellow professionals questioning the wisdom of using "mere students" in a paraprofessional role. Once the programs are up and running, an additional suggestion would be to formalize the program by investigating the possibility of obtaining course credit for the students. Independent studies or internships (through sympathetic academic departments) are possibilities,

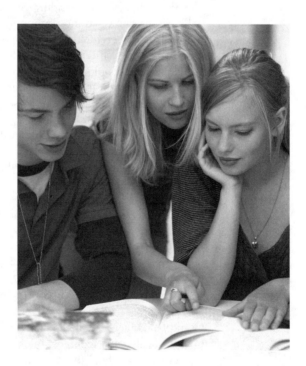

Peer education is a method that can solve low staff problems for administrators and can help students get extra credit for their efforts.

but the health educator must ensure that the programs are sufficiently well developed to survive academic scrutiny and sometimes cynicism!

Method/Intervention 23: Personal Improvement Projects

Personal improvement projects can serve as incentives to make positive personal changes in a targeted health behavior. The objective is to provide clients with an opportunity to learn proper techniques for changing health behaviors such as those involved in nutrition and enable them to incorporate these new skills into a **healthy lifestyle**.

Components of a personal improvement project are to:

1. Establish a contract with realistic objectives.
2. Chart these realistic objectives.
3. Chart actual progress.
4. Maintain some type of diary to explain progress.

Advantages and Disadvantages

Advantages of personal improvement projects are that they:

1. Are low in cost.
2. Have the potential for actually influencing directly health behavior.
3. Can target specific needs, including behavioral objectives.
4. Can reinforce information presented in a program.
5. Require active application of principles.
6. Personalize health practices for every participant.

Disadvantages are that they:

1. Require considerable individual attention.
2. Can be difficult to achieve.
3. Require considerable paperwork.
4. May not sufficiently motivate some participants. If this is a course, you may wish to provide an alternate assignment.

Tips for Effective Implementation (Wehrli & Nyquist, 2003)

1. Provide adequate instruction and outline in writing the objective of the project as well as the requirements for completion.
2. Provide adequate time to complete the project.
3. Supply each participant with a means to analyze his or her own results from the project. Select instruments for measuring success that are valid and reliable.
4. Encourage, but do not require, participants to share their outcomes.

Examples   Examples of personal improvement projects follow:

1. Weight reduction—see Figure 4-11 for a sample project.
2. Regular exercise.
3. Increasing fruit and vegetable consumption.
4. Regular mental health breaks.
5. Smoking cessation.
6. Consistent seat belt use.

It is not the intention of this project merely to provide incentive for another crash-diet program. The objective is to provide you with an opportunity to gain a good knowledge of proper diet and nutrition practices and to enable you to incorporate them into your chosen lifestyle.

In order to ensure this, it is part of this assignment that you read proper background material and determine a course of action that fits your needs (this should include consultation with your physician if possible and for certain if any major weight reduction is contemplated). In your paper you should explain your selection of a diet plan, your goal, and any problems you encountered, and include a graph of your progress as shown here. Weight data must be made on the same scales and measured at the same time of day to be "officially accurate." Before undertaking this project you must have a conference with your instructor.

Progress toward the objective should be charted. A personal computer can make charting progress easy.

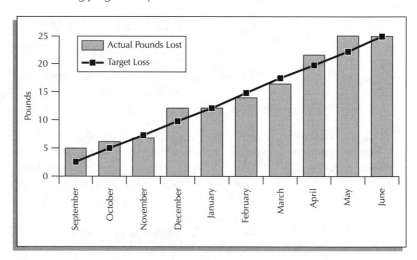

Figure 4-11
Personal Improvement
Project for Weight Loss

Method/Intervention 24: Problem Solving

The **problem–solution technique** requires scenarios that need a solution. These can be written or oral. Given the circumstances described, participants are asked to determine the best answer. Often there is no one, guaranteed acceptable answer. The purpose is to stimulate discussion and to expose participants to multiple points of view.

Advantages and Disadvantages

Advantages of using a problem–solution technique are that it:

1. Can serve to create a questioning atmosphere.
2. Can demonstrate that often there is no one certain correct answer.
3. Sets the ground rules for participant interaction.
4. Develops questioning strategies.
5. Promotes higher thinking by exploring pre-existing knowledge and then building upon it (Kellough & Kellough, 2007).

Disadvantages are that it:

1. Can be time-consuming.
2. Can make participants uncomfortable as they realize that there may be no clearly correct answer.
3. Increases the potential for interpersonal conflicts (Wehrli & Nyquist, 2003).

Tips for Effective Implementation

1. Provide participants with a list of quiestions to be considered for the group's discussion.
2. Select problems that support your objective and are relevant to the participants.

Examples

Two examples of problem solving follow:

1. A scenario such as that shown in Figure 4-12 can apply problem solving to a health problem such as cardiovascular disease.
2. A scenario such as that shown in Figure 4-13 can apply problem solving to a social and community problem such as gang violence.

It is important to note these problem—solutions are designed so that there is no clear answer to most questions posed. An important component of the activity is this planned disagreement that generally gives rise to a fairly heated discussion. It is possible to make assumptions and then make an argument for agreeing or disagreeing with statements. The whole point of the activity is the discussion that follows. This element will make some participants uncomfortable. Many participants insist on getting the "right answer" and are distraught when told there could be many correct answers depending on assumptions.

Harvey Schwartz, a fat middle-aged diabetic, was seated in front of the TV smoking and feasting on a meal of french fries, shrimp, strawberry shortcake, and beer when his wife Hilda came in screaming about his lazy habits. He jumped to his feet and began shouting in return, then collapsed on the floor holding his chest. His funeral was the following Monday. He was buried alongside his father and brother, who died of heart attacks and strokes.

Which of the following do you feel contributed to Harvey's demise? Check the statements you agree with.

_____ 1. *His understanding wife, Hilda Schwartz.*
_____ 2. *His obese body.*
_____ 3. *His culinary habits.*
_____ 4. *His choice of beverage.*
_____ 5. *His fine physical conditioning.*
_____ 6. *His use of tobacco products.*
_____ 7. *His genetic background.*
_____ 8. *His youthful appearance.*
_____ 9. *His foul-functioning pancreas.*
_____ 10. *His job as a taxi driver in Brooklyn, New York.*

Figure 4-12
"The Demise of Harvey Schwartz," a Problem–Solution Scenario

Lamon Thomas and Bruce Chen, wearing their gang colors, are attending a high school dance together when Lamon gets into a verbal argument with another student. The other student is offended when Lamon asks the other student's girlfriend to dance. All participants have been drinking. Bruce comes over to aid his friend when a gun appears. In the struggle, Bruce is shot twice and later dies.

Which of the following do you feel contributed to Bruce's death? Check the statements you agree with.

_____ 1. *Lamon's asking the young woman to dance.*
_____ 2. *Bruce's getting involved with something that was not his business.*
_____ 3. *The way the young men were dressed.*
_____ 4. *Bruce's choice of beverage.*
_____ 5. *Lack of metal detectors at the entrance.*
_____ 6. *The availability of handguns.*
_____ 7. *Poor supervision.*
_____ 8. *Lack of parental control.*
_____ 9. *Lack of stated policies.*
_____ 10. *No police protection.*

Figure 4-13
"The Wrong Place at the Wrong Time," a Problem–Solution Scenario

Method/Intervention 25: Puppets

Puppets can be a very powerful tool in health education, particularly with the young. They can be purchased or made at low cost. An easy-to-make puppet is the finger puppet, which consists of a small paper drawing that is cut out of paper and attached to a finger. The drawings, or paper dolls, can also be attached to long sticks. Making puppets can be used as an icebreaker or team builder. Alternatively, a doll can be used as a puppet, or the educator can simply draw on their own hand.

Advantages and Disadvantages

Advantages of puppets are that they:

1. Are entertaining.
2. Can address difficult topics and the affective domain.
3. Allow participants to act out feelings without reprisals.
4. Can promote creative thinking and oral communication skills.

Disadvantages are that they:

1. Will not be effective if people refuse to participate.
2. Can bring out unintended emotions or outcomes.

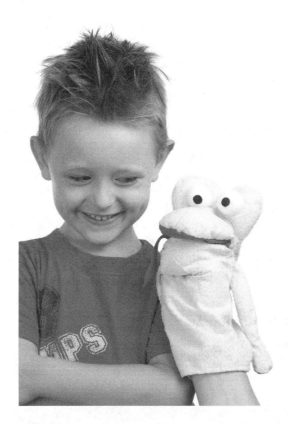

Puppets are inexpensive to create and a fun learning tool for children.

3. Require the facilitator to be well prepared because of the uncertainty of outcome.
4. Can be threatening to some individuals.
5. Can be used effectively with adults but are better suited for younger learners—up to age 8.
6. Can be difficult to manipulate (moving the puppet in time with speech) while maintaining focus on the script.

Tips for Effective Implementation

1. Bring the puppets to life for the audience by giving the puppets names and creating voices to match the puppets' size and personality.
2. Use exaggerated movements and voice inflection.
3. The script should clearly define the problem, situation, and roles of each puppet character.
4. In some cases the facilitator may act as a narrator to control the pace and content of the performance.
5. All puppeteers are to read the script and practice matching puppet movements to the content prior to delivery of the show.
6. Set a stage for the show; this can be as simple as a large floor rug or as elaborate as a puppet theater.
7. Repetition is a critical aspect of learning for children. Repeat songs and key concepts throughout the skit.

Examples   Examples of ways to use puppets follow:

1. Puppets are effective in working with children to express feelings. Young children will often talk to a friendly puppet when they would not talk to an adult. This technique is used extensively with victims of child sexual abuse to elicit responses, a fact that indicates how powerful a tool puppets can be. Be certain you choose your questions carefully.
2. Puppets can be used to bring some entertainment to an adult group. Have a debate with your puppet. Tape a conversation, and then play the tape as you provide the answers.
3. Puppets can be used to represent an organ or other body part in a demonstration of the effects of healthy and unhealthy practices or to explain a surgical procedure.
4. Purchase a ready-made program with puppets and scripts.

Method/Intervention 26: Role Plays

Role plays are acting out assigned roles. There is no script as in a play, but participants are *not* free to act in any way they wish. They are assigned parameters with limited flexibility.

Advantages and Disadvantages

Advantages of role plays are that they:

1. Require no equipment.
2. Can address difficult topics and the affective domain.
3. Can allow participants to act out feelings without reprisals.
4. Are interesting and entertaining.

Disadvantages are that they:

1. Will fail if people refuse to participate.
2. Can bring out unintended emotions or outcomes.
3. Require that the facilitator be well prepared because of the uncertainty of outcome.
4. Can sometimes be difficult to control.
5. May not be taken seriously by participants.
6. Can provide inaccurate or inappropriate content.

Tips for Effective Implementation

Rules

Certain rules should be established for role plays:

1. Actors are acting out *assigned* roles. It must be understood that they are not playing themselves.
2. No putdowns of actors should be allowed.
3. Do not stereotype casting.
4. Establish parameters for roles.
5. It should be understood that in real life it is rare that there is one clear-cut correct answer or role.

Setup and Performance

1. Provide role players props, such as sunglasses or hats, to help them disguise themselves and get into character.
2. Limit the role play to 3 minutes and watch for signs that it may be dissolving. Long pauses, glances at the facilitator, and manipulation of props indicate the players are running out of content.
3. Provide the role players a few minutes to prepare prior to the performance.
4. A role reversal technique that asks the players to switch roles in the middle of the role play can expand the drama and provide different perspectives (Meeks, Heit, & Page, 2007).

Debriefing

Debriefing is particularly important after role playing. It is critical to tactfully correct any misinformation immediately following the role play. Be sure to analyze the roles for realism and most common responses. Ask participants what are appropriate and realistic ways to handle the problems posed. Explore alternatives, asking for the likely consequences of each alternative. Finally, promote discussion on how we can achieve positive outcomes.

Sample debriefing questions (that should be outlined by facilitator before role play) follow:

1. Was the situation realistic?
2. What would be the likely outcome of the actions of the big brother/sister?
3. What are other options?
4. What are the issues here (drug use, dating older man, some unknown, sexuality, no supervision, etc.)?
5. What are realistic objectives?
6. How can we reach these objectives?

Example 1: Drug Prevention/ Education

Following are several possible role plays for the subject of drug prevention/education:

1. Two parents discuss the marijuana joint one parent has found in their son's room. They must decide what action to take.
2. You (age 21 and a college student) walk into your home unexpectedly and find your younger sister (age 15) home alone with an older (age 19) boy. The couple is in the kitchen drinking beer, and there are some red capsules on the table that are obviously illegal drugs. When you walk in, they both act nervous and try to hide the drugs. Your mother (a single parent) is working and will not be home for several hours.
3. Parents are teaching their child about drug abuse. You are sitting in the kitchen at home.
4. You find someone in the next dorm room smoking marijuana.
5. An intoxicated date wants to drive you home.
6. You are at a party where two friends urge you to try pot, LSD, cocaine, methamphetamine, or some other illicit drug.
7. Your friend gives you his locker combination so you can retrieve the book you loaned him last night. While getting the book you notice several bags of drugs in his locker. This guy has been a pretty good friend and has never offered you or sold you drugs. What do you do?

Example 2: Violence Prevention

Following are two possible role plays on the subject of preventing violence:

1. A friend who lives in a very tough part of town has brought a handgun to school for protection. You spot it when you are having lunch together, and he explains he needs it for protection. He says he does not

need it at school but has nowhere else to hide it. You often bring your mom's car to school. He suggests leaving it in the trunk of your car during the day.

2. A good friend of your son is arrested for assault and carrying a concealed weapon (knife).

Example 3: Sexuality Education

Following are three possible role plays on the subject of sexuality education:

1. Parent finds diaphragm belonging to 16-year-old daughter
2. Parent discovers condoms in purse of 14-year-old daughter
3. Parent discovers condoms on dresser of 14-year-old son

Example 4: Ecology Social Responsibility

Following are two possible role plays on the subject of ecology social responsibility:

1. Your son or brother pours oil into the street drain after changing your oil
2. Your friend dumps trash out of the car window

Method/Intervention 27: Self-Appraisals

Self-appraisal is a technique to encourage personal assessment as an important step in personal behavior change. It involves some form of personal assessment, which can range from a checklist of a few items to a diary and computer analysis kept for a long time. The key element is to encourage self-inspection as a first step in behavior change. Self-appraisal is sometimes coupled with personal improvement projects. Figures 4-14 and 4-15 present forms for self-appraisal.

Self-appraisal can be used effectively as an evaluation tool for a **community health education** program. We can label an anonymous assessment a self-appraisal and make it acceptable. If we call it a test, participants may walk out.

Advantages and Disadvantages

Advantages of self-appraisals are that they:

1. Allow individual assessment.
2. Are an important first step in personal behavior change.
3. Provide excellent focus to start a workshop or class.
4. Are interesting and entertaining.

Disadvantages are that they:

1. Require development of instruments.
2. Can be misinterpreted.
3. May require medical testing.
4. Can be expensive if using a commercial vendor.
5. Are self-reported and, therefore, only as valid as the learner is honest.

> **SELF-ASSESSMENT OF PRESENTATION (REVIEW OF VIDEOTAPED PRESENTATION)**
>
> Name: _____
>
> Date video reviewed: _____
>
> Overall impression of presentation:
> _____
> _____
> _____
> _____
> _____
>
> Some things I did well:
> _____
> _____
> _____
> _____
> _____
> _____
>
> Some things I should work on:
> _____
> _____
> _____
> _____
> _____
> _____
> _____

Figure 4-14
Example of Self-
Appraisal Form for
Video Presentation

**Tips for Effective
Implementation**

1. Encourage participants to summarize what they have learned from the assessment.
2. Follow the self-assessment with goal-setting activities to facilitate behavior maintenance or change as needed.

Examples   Examples of ways to use self-appraisals follow:

1. Use to test health education knowledge.
2. Use to appraise health risks.
3. Use to evaluate food intake—24-hour recall.
4. Use as a post-workshop assessment.
5. Use as a stress audit.

NEEDS ASSESSMENT SELF-ASSESSMENT

Name: _____ Year in school: _____

Local phone: _____

Specialization? School, community, worksite, or other: _____

If a grad student, degree program and major interests: _____

Are you currently employed? Yes No
If yes, approximately how many hours do you work a week? _____

TEACHING/PRESENTATION EXPERIENCE (PAST 5 YEARS)
1. Teaching or working with children _____ (Contact hours with you as the primary instructor)

2. Teaching or working with adults _____

LESSON/PRESENTATION PLANNING
1. How many lesson/presentation plans have you personally written? _____

2. Have you been trained in writing behavioral objectives? _____ If yes, what system was used? _____

EQUIPMENT USE
Have you successfully used (feel comfortable in using) the following?
_____ 1. Overhead projector
_____ 2. E-mail
_____ 3. Film projector
_____ 4. DVD player
_____ 5. Computer projection system
_____ 6. Videotape camera and recorder
_____ 7. CD-ROM and computer
_____ 8. Slide projector
_____ 9. Personal computer model _____
              Preferred word processing software _____
_____ 10. Internet—finding health information

Figure 4-15
Example of Self-
Appraisal Form for
Needs Assessment

Method/Intervention 28: Service Learning

Service learning is the notion that one learns through doing and can acquire good personal values through service to others. This method also provides real service to the community. Some school districts require such service of all students and have even gone so far as to make it a graduation requirement. East Carolina University, through its Department of Health Education and Promotion, has operated a large service learning program for many years. The program is promoted through many courses on campus. An amazing 9,000 of the total 18,000 students on campus in a recent year provided service to local groups and agencies through the program. All participants are covered by insurance, and only agencies with negotiated contracts ensuring supervision and an appropriate experience are included.

Service learning is not a new notion, of course, but it has been gaining popularity at many institutions of learning. Not that long ago educational institutions were encouraged to be value-neutral, but often today they are actively encouraged to teach basic values such as treating others with respect and responsibly giving back to the community.

Advantages and Disadvantages

Advantages of service learning are that it:

1. Generally requires little equipment.
2. Is able to address affective objectives.
3. Provides real service to the community.

Disadvantages are that it:

1. Is often unpredictable in outcome.
2. Can place participants at risk and often requires insurance.
3. Requires close supervision and time-consuming cooperation with community agencies.

Tips for Effective Implementation

1. Provide participants with printed agendas and instructions that summarize their roles and responsibilities.
2. Provide participants with the supplies and materials necessary to complete the project.
3. Host a debriefing session after the project to allow participants to share their experiences.

Example: Big Event

Joe Nussbaum, former Vice President of the Student Government Association at Texas A&M University, began The Big Event in 1982 as a way for students to say thank you to the surrounding community. Nussbaum envisioned a one-day service project where community residents surrounding the university would be shown appreciation for their support for the health and well-being of the students at Texas A&M University. A&M students did this by completing various tasks (e.g., changing air filters, cleaning windows, picking up trash) to improve the quality of life of its community members. The annual event fosters both unity and improved health in the community (Texas A&M University, 2008).

Other Examples

1. Require a given number of service hours in a health-related agency before being eligible to graduate from high school.
2. Require a given number of service hours in a specific agency as part of a health education course.

Method/Intervention 29: Simulations

Simulations are activities that take on the appearance of some real-life phenomenon. They allow participants to observe and even participate in an event without the risk of injury that would occur in the real event and in a very controlled manner. An example would be an injury simulation kit, providing realistic-looking blood and ways to make people look wounded. Participants can treat injuries as they would in real-life situations.

According to Cruickshank (1972), a simulation is "the end product, the model resulting from the process of simulating. The simulation is contrived experience used to expose someone to a certain prescribed set of circumstances based on a model. It is usually to teach a role, function, or operation. By using simulation, it is possible to attain the essence of something without its reality."

The open-ended nature of a simulation promotes the use of critical thinking as participants evaluate and respond to the ever-changing situation (Jansiewicz, 2004). The artificially induced reality allows the participants to experience the emotions one might feel in a real situation.

Rationale   The common application of simulations to emergency care such as first aid is useful for the following reasons:

1. They provide examples of real-life emergency care situations.
2. They provide an opportunity for the practical application of skills covered in the classroom.
3. They provide practice in the analysis and evaluation of emergency situations without the risk of injury resulting from judgment errors.
4. They provide an alternative teaching strategy for the instructor.
5. They provide an evaluation technique for the instructor.
6. They provide students with practice in performing skills under stress and thus increase self-confidence.

Advantages and
Disadvantages   Advantages of simulations are that they:

1. Provide an element of realism.
2. Can address some difficult-to-teach issues such as comfort levels of performance.
3. Provide variety.
4. Can provide opportunities for repetition of important skills.

Disadvantages:

1. Generally are time-consuming.
2. Can be expensive.
3. Are often difficult to use with large groups.

See Figures 4-16 through 4-20 for information on first-aid instruction.

1. You must treat this **like a real-life situation**. Nothing will be assumed—you must do all that you would in a real-life situation. To receive credit for any procedure, it must actually be completed. The only exceptions to this are procedures that cannot be done in the classroom such as making a phone call, and they must be explained.
2. You may use only material **provided** in the testing area.
3. You may not use any notes or cards.
4. For assistance you may use only those people provided, and you **must give them explicit directions** for any aid they administer. No undirected assistance or information is to be given by other students or victims.
5. **Time will be an important factor in life-threatening situations**. A reasonable time will be allowed for less severe injuries, but do not waste time. (After using a situation several times, an instructor will have an idea of how long it should take to complete and may wish to set a time limit.)
6. In situations where you want to take a pulse, you must actually take a reading. (Victims will also be taking their own pulse so that assessment can be properly made.)
7. Bleeding tags will be marked mild, moderate, or severe. Mild bleeding will require direct pressure and elevation for credit. Moderate bleeding will require the same plus proper use of pressure points where appropriate. Severe bleeding will require the use of all three aforementioned techniques plus proper use of a tourniquet. This is done only as a grading convention and is not meant to imply that proper first aid would be guided only by estimates of blood flow.

Figure 4-16
First Aid Instructions for Participants

From Gilbert, G.G. (1981). *Teaching First Aid and Emergency Care*. Dubuque, IA: Kendall/Hunt.

Tips for Effective Implementation

1. Minimize uncertainties that will frustrate participants by providing a detailed explanation of the procedures for the simulation. Knowing what to expect will build the participants' self-efficacy in their ability to perform.
2. Keep the pace of the simulation as true to life as possible.
3. Know what you wish to accomplish and make participants aware of the specific outcomes you expect of them.

Examples   Some examples of simulations follow:

1. Fire alarm and building evacuation.
2. Application of CPR.
3. Simulation games in which community member roles are simulated.

Information Supplied to First-Aider.
Situation:
    You are home with your younger sister (age 11) when you hear her crying. You
    find her on the front porch.
Where:
    Your home.
Miscellaneous Information:
    No one else is home.

Position of Victim:
    Seated.
Special Instructions for Victim:
    Cry, but answer questions. You fell and scraped your knee. You have no other
    injuries.
Supplied Materials:
    Home materials box.
Tags:
    1. Moderate bleeding (1)–knee.

Figure 4-17
Sample Simulation
Situation 1

Scraped Knee

Name of First-Aider

Grader

	Yes Well Done	Yes Adequate	No
1. Was the victim properly examined and questioned for all possible injuries?	4, 3	2, 1	0
2. Was the victim given verbal encouragement?	2	1	0
3. Was moderate bleeding controlled and bandaged properly? a. Direct pressure (2) b. Elevation (2) c. Proper bandage (3)	7, 6, 5, 4	3, 2, 1	0
4. Was proper shock treatment given?	2	1	0
Comments:			

Add _____
Deductions _____
Total _____
Possible _____15_____

The evaluator circles the appropriate point value and adds the points up for grading.
These can be used to determine pass or failure or a letter grade. Multiple situations must
be developed prior to class (see Gilbert, 1981) so all participants have different situations.

Figure 4-18
Sample Simulation
Evaluation 1

Information Supplied to First-Aider.
Situation:
    You are the first to arrive at the scene of a single-car automobile accident.
Where:
    Freeway (interstate).
Miscellaneous Information:
    Several other people stop, but no one has first-aid training. There appears to
    be no danger of fire.

Position of Victim:
    Victim is face down on front seat (use two chairs).
Special Instructions for Victim:
    You are unconscious and will remain so.
Supplied Materials:
    1. Coats.
    2. Bandaging materials.
    3. Water.
    4. Splints.
Tags:
    1. Moderate bleeding (1)–forehead.
    2. Moderate bleeding (1)–nose (nose bleed).

Figure 4-19
Sample Simulation
Situation 2

Bleeding

Name of First-Aider   Grader

	Yes Well Done	Yes Adequate	No
1. Was the victim examined carefully for all injuries?	4, 3	2, 1	0
2. Was moderate bleeding of the forehead controlled properly? a. Direct pressure (4) b. Bandaged properly (3)	7, 6, 5, 4	3, 2, 1	0
3. Was victim removed from the car? (If removed, give credit if good explanation for removal given and proper technique applied.)	0	0	4
4. Was note made of possible head injury (medical personnel notified and movement minimized)?	5, 4, 3	2, 1	0
5. Was proper aid sent for?	2	1	0
6. Was the victim treated for shock?	3, 2	1	0
Comments:			

Add _____
Deductions _____
Total _____
Possible _____25_____

Figure 4-20
Sample Simulation
Evaluation 2

Method/Intervention 30: Storytelling

Storytelling is one of the oldest methods of communicating ideas and images. Storytelling through the ages has been used as a teaching tool, whether for imparting the values contained in many of the folktales or for simply passing along information. Stories provide a venue to deliver information while engaging, entertaining, and challenging the listener through inferred meaning. "The imagination of each individual is free to create its own: drawing not only on the story, but on personal experiences of people and places, social interactions, sites, sounds, smells and sensations, dreams" (Haggarty & Norgate, 2006).

Folktales, myths, legends, hero tales, humorous stories, and realistic stories are especially suitable for storytelling. Literature is an under-utilized venue in health education. Poems, parody, and satire can be effective methods for alluding to poor health practices. Health educators can use stories to embed concepts related to health concerns. Facts embedded in a story are generally much easier to learn and recall than those presented in an informational format (Wagner & Smith, 1969). As the sequence of events unfolds, the listener will be able to see cause and effect relationships of behavior choices. The facilitator or participant can be the orator of a storytelling method.

Storytelling is becoming modernized with the addition of technology. Digital storytelling is the practice of combining narrative with digital content, including images, sound, and video, to create a short movie, typically with a strong emotional component (Educause, 2007). We live in a world that is increasingly interactive, communications intensive, and knowledge based; it would stand to reason that our methods of storytelling should evolve to keep up with the times.

Advantages and Disadvantages

Advantages of storytelling are that it:

1. Is interesting and entertaining.
2. Requires no equipment.
3. Can address difficult topics and the affective domain.
4. Is likely to be shared with others.
5. Reinforces speaking and listening skills (Caulfield, 2000; Grace, 2001).

Disadvantages of storytelling are that it:

1. Requires facilitator to have advanced speaking skills.
2. Can have unpredictable outcomes.
3. Is of limited value if participants do not make connections.
4. Can be time-consuming to create.
5. Is only as effective as the discussion that follows.

Tips for Effective Implementation (Bishop & Kimball, 2006)

1. Select stories with repetition and pleasing word sounds for younger children.
2. Adults prefer stories with action, humor, and suspense.
3. Develop a clear outline based on your objective and practice telling the story prior to delivery.
4. Speak distinctly with your natural voice using pauses and changes in pace and pitch to create moods.
5. Use appropriate gestures to enhance the story but avoid movement unrelated to the story.
6. Props can be used to emphasize key points.

Examples   Two examples of storytelling follow.

Storytelling example: Blood circulation—the story of the red blood cell's journey through the heart!

Objective

Using the paragraph provided, the learners will trace the circulation of blood through the heart by writing a story—to be read aloud—that describes the events in the life of a red blood cell as it circulates through the heart as well as a description of the four sections of the heart.

Prompt

You are a red blood cell traveling through the body. Write a story describing your adventure. Include descriptions using all the five senses: tell me what you see, smell, taste, feel, and hear as you journey through all four sections of the heart. Make your story interesting by writing about the troubles you may have on your journey or the things you might encounter. Use the information and diagram (Figure 4–21) to construct your story.

Path of Blood Circulation

Blood returns from the body in the **right atrium**. The blood has lost most of the oxygen it carries, and it is now **deoxygenated**. The right ventricle pumps (via contraction) the blood along the pulmonary artery to the lungs where it picks up fresh oxygen. It is now oxygenated. The oxygenated blood enters the left side of the heart and is pumped out through the aorta to the body. Once it reaches the capillaries around the body, oxygen diffuses out to the surrounding cells. The deoxygenated blood is carried back toward the heart in the veins. These join up to form the vena cava, which is the largest vein.

Interesting Facts About the Heart

- The heart is about the size of your fist.
- It generally only pumps about 50% of the blood that is in the chamber at the beginning of its pumping phase (this is called the "ejection fraction").

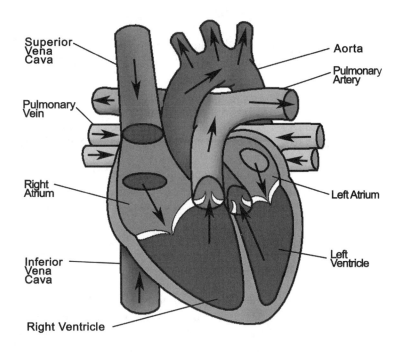

Figure 4-21
Blood Circulation Story

- It generally pumps about 5 quarts a minute.
- It can pump up to about 5 gallons a minute with exercise.
- It pumps about 4000 gallons of blood each day.

Storytelling Example: Poetry and Decision-Making Story   Adolescence is a time of tremendous confusion. As children progress from childhood to adulthood, they are faced with new challenges that often require them to make what could be life-altering decisions. Teaching students to recognize the importance of their decisions on future opportunities is a vital part of helping them become mature adults. Interdisciplinary teaching methods provide educators with unique ways to influence the behavior of adolescents. The use of literature in health education is one venue that allows the educator to address the affective domain while encouraging students to think on a higher cognitive level. This teaching technique allows students to analyze a famous piece of literature in an effort to discover implications related to decision making. The following example has been adapted to be used in conjunction with a unit on adolescent sexuality; however, it could be easily modified to address other important decisions.

Target Population

This activity is designed for adolescent students in grades 6–12 to reinforce the importance of thinking through important decisions.

Objective

At the end of the activity, students will be able to provide examples of inferences in the poem and describe how they relate to decision making.

Materials and Resources

- An enlarged copy, to be used in leading class discussion, of the poem "The Road Not Taken" by Robert Frost.
- Projection device.
- A student copy of the poem "The Road Not Taken" by Robert Frost (Figure 4-22).
- A student copy of the guided discussion sheet (Figure 4-23).

Procedure

1. Provide each student with a copy of the poem "The Road Not Taken" by Robert Frost.
2. Introduce the purpose of the activity to students by discussing the number of decisions they make each day. Emphasize the lack of thought that can go into making simple choices by providing examples of daily decisions (e.g., what to wear, where to sit at lunch, what to do about forgotten homework). Discuss the need for a greater amount of thought as decisions become more important.
3. Tell the students that the poem by Robert Frost stresses the importance of thinking through decisions before they are acted upon.
4. The instructor should begin reading the first stanza of the poem, stopping to ask questions 1–5 on the guided discussion sheet.
5. After discussing questions 1–5, continue reading stanza 2 and complete questions 6–7.

Two roads diverged in a yellow wood,
And sorry I could not travel both
And be one traveler, long I stood
And looked down one as far as I could
To where it bent in the undergrowth.

Then took the other, as just as fair,
And having perhaps the better claim,
Because it was grassy and wanted wear;
Though as for that the passing there
Had worn them really about the same.

And both that morning equally lay
In leaves no step had trodden black.
Oh, I kept the first for another day!
Yet knowing how way leads on to way,
I doubted if I should ever come back.

I shall be telling this with a sigh
Somewhere ages and ages hence:
Two roads diverged in a wood, and I—
I took the one less traveled by,
And that has made all the difference.

Figure 4-22
Robert Frost: The Road
Not Taken (1915)

Directions

As you answer the following questions think about how the poem relates to your decision about
_____ (fill in topic).

Today's Topic

Having sex for the first time with your partner.

STANZA ONE

1. What time of year is it? _____ How do you know?

_____

2. How does the season relate to the decision—what might be the symbolism?

_____

3. Where is the author standing? _____ What does this represent?

_____

4. Can he/she see the end of the road? _____ Why and how does this relate to your decision?

_____

STANZA TWO

5. Did he/she take the road most commonly chosen? _____ How do you know?

_____

6. Was he/she really sure the road taken was not the most frequently used? _____
   How do you know, and how might this relate to the phrase "everybody's doing it"?

_____

STANZAS THREE AND FOUR

7. Is the speaker happy with his/her choice? _____ Justify your answer.

_____

8. Why will the speaker be telling the story "with a sigh"?

_____

9. Do you agree with the statement Frost makes in the last two lines: "I took the one less traveled by, and that
   has made all the difference"? Explain your position.

_____

10. How does this poem apply to a person's choice about being sexually active?

_____

Figure 4-23
Frost Poem: Decision-Making Discussion Questions

6. Read stanzas 3 and 4 and then complete questions 8–10.
7. Alternate method: You may wish to have students read the poem and complete the study guide independently or in groups of three. The smaller venue might allow for more personalization of the activity.

Method/Intervention 31: Theater

Theater has been commonly used in many health education programs. It differs from role plays in that it employs a script that dictates all dialogue and action. These plays can be purchased or developed, and often professional actors or para-professional student actors are enlisted to make the presentation. The scripts can be memorized or directly read as in a reader's theater approach. Generally a follow-up discussion guide with questions for the audience is included.

Theater can be very powerful. Several plays have been developed in the AIDS/HIV prevention area (Denman, Davis, Pearson, & Madeley, 1996), and some university student health centers are using student actors to provide plays on date rape. Because there is an established script, presentations can be reviewed very carefully for content. It is therefore easy to determine if the play fits the objectives being sought and if it fits any model or theory being employed in reaching the target population.

Advantages and Disadvantages

Advantages of theater are that it:

1. Generally requires little equipment.
2. Is able to address difficult topics in a controlled manner.
3. Can address the affective domain.
4. Allows good control over content.

Disadvantages are that it:

1. Requires the use of actors, who may be difficult to find or afford.
2. May require a stage and related equipment.
3. May be ineffective if poor acting detracts from the message.

Tips for Effective Implementation

1. Purchase health-specific scripts.
2. Develop scripts as a classroom project. When allowing students/participants to write their own scripts, be very clear about your expectation for age-appropriate dialogue and behavior.
3. Use scripts constructed by a community group.
4. Provide actors with props to make the drama more engaging.
5. Consider hats or sunglasses that allow the actors to be behind disguises.
6. Ensure that the actors understand the objective of the drama and what the audience should learn from watching the performance.

Sample Script

Examples of theater use follow.

"The Babysitter's Dilemma"
Scene
Jane has been babysitting the Johnson children, who are now asleep. Jane is dressed like a typical teenager. Mr. and Mrs. Johnson return home from the

party they were attending. Scene takes place in living room and adjoining kitchen. Stage should include living room with couch and chair plus adjoining kitchen with counter, table, and chairs. Jane is sitting reading when Mrs. Johnson walks in the front door.

Mrs. Johnson: Hi, dearie. Sorry we're late, but the party was so much fun we lost track of the time.
Jane: The kids went to bed about 9:30, as you asked, Mrs. Johnson, but I don't think they fell asleep until much later.
Mrs. Johnson: Don't worry, dearie, they can sleep in tomorrow since it is Saturday. In fact, it *is* Saturday—what time is it?
Jane: It's almost 3 AM.

Mr. Johnson comes through the front door looking a bit disheveled and appears to have been drinking.

Mr. Johnson: Had a little trouble getting the car into the garage. Oh, Christ, I forgot the babysitter. Come on, cutie, I'll take you home. Where are my keys?

Mrs. Johnson: Maybe you left them in the car, dear. [*Mrs. Johnson takes off her coat and shoes.*]
Mr. Johnson: Oh yeah, that is probably where they are. Honey, you go to bed and I'll be right back. Come on, cutie—how old did you say you were?

Mr. Johnson looks her up and down with interest, in an inappropriate manner.

Jane: Maybe I should call my parents?
Mr. Johnson: Nonsense. It's too late, and I'm not tired. I'm feeling good.
Jane: My parents have a rule that if I work past 1 AM, they pick me up.
Mr. Johnson: That's a silly rule. You'll just wake them up for no reason.
Mrs. Johnson: We don't want to upset her parents. Let her call home if she wants.
Mr. Johnson: This is ridiculous! What do we have to drink? Do we have any bourbon?

Jane moves to the kitchen and calls her parents.

Jane: Mom, the Johnsons just got home from the party, and I need you to pick me up. Thanks, Mom. I'll be ready as soon as you can make it.
Mr. Johnson [using a stern, directive voice]: Why don't you call them back and tell them I can drive you home? I'm not going to give you a tip unless I drive you home. It isn't right for your parents to come.

Mrs. Johnson has moved to the kitchen and is cleaning up.

Jane: My Mom and Dad have strict rules, and I have to follow them since I'm only 15. Mrs. Johnson, let me help you clean up.

Jane moves to kitchen and begins cleaning. Mr. Johnson acts huffy, fixes himself a drink, and sits, watching the ladies clean up. A few minutes later Jane hears a car and moves to the window.

Jane: It's my Dad, and I have to go. [*She heads for the front door.*]
Mr. Johnson [*standing up and getting out his wallet*]: Here you go, Jane. There is a nice tip. I hope there are no misunderstandings. We may need you next week.
Jane: Thank you, Mr. Johnson. [*She hurries out the door.*]

Follow-Up Discussion
1. Did Jane do anything that contributed to the problem?
2. What other options did Jane have? What might be the consequences of these behaviors?
3. What if Jane did not have parents at home? What could she have done?
4. Should Jane return to babysit again?

Method/Intervention 32: Value Clarification

Value clarification is a method designed to help people understand how they have reached decisions. It has the potential of teaching *rational decision-making skills*. This method had great popularity in the 1960s and 1970s. It fell into disfavor under charges that it taught no values and allowed free choice even when the correct choice was clear to "any rational person." The method was often misused, and this contributed to its being banned in some settings. It is a useful tool if used properly. Many of the principles can be applied well under the title "developing decision-making skills."

Advantages and Disadvantages
Advantages of value clarification are that it:

1. Is low in cost.
2. Can deal with feelings and emotions.
3. Allows for individual and group expression.

Disadvantages are that it:

1. Can be controversial.
2. Requires that the instructor be prepared to deal with emotional responses.
3. Is unpredictable in outcome.
4. Can be dominated by over-opinionated individuals.

Tips for Effective Implementation
1. Emphasize the complexity of the issues and present multiple perspectives on the topic.
2. Encourage all to participate but do not demand it.
3. Encourage participants to use disagreements as a constructive method for learning.

Rules
Rules for value clarification should be established as follows:

1. No putdowns are to be allowed.
2. The rights of others to different opinions are to be respected.

According to Raths, Harmin, and Simon (1966, p. 30), true values are those which do the following:

Choosing:	The individual chooses what is valued according to the following criteria:
	1. It is chosen freely.
	2. It is chosen from alternatives.
	3. It is chosen after consideration of the consequences of each alternative.
Prizing:	The individual is proud of what is valued and is:
	4. Cherishing, being happy with choice.
	5. Willing to affirm the choice publicly.
Acting:	The individual is willing to perform behaviors that support what is valued by:
	6. Doing something with the choice.
	7. Repeating, in some pattern of life.

Example: Health Education Decision   Use value clarification to help participants make a health education decision by asking them to do the following:

1. List five major factors that influenced you to go into health education. These can be people, places, things, feelings, or desires.
2. Draw a large circle.
3. Divide the circle into pie slices for each of your "influencers," and make the proportion of each slice appropriate to the amount of influence (see Figure 4-24).

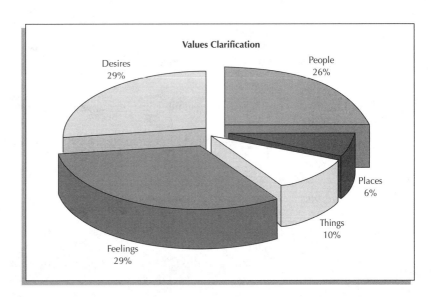

Figure 4-24
Pie Chart for Values
Clarification Exercise

Now lead a group discussion by asking participants these questions:

1. Are these rational and positive ways to make a decision?
2. How would the pie chart look if you went about this decision the most rational way?
3. Are you proud of your decision?

Method/Intervention 33: Word Games and Puzzles

Word games are entertaining and are very useful in increasing vocabulary. They are commonly used with elementary school children, with people studying English as a second language, or with any area that introduces a considerable number of new vocabulary words. These activities include crossword puzzles, anagrams, and other word games.

Advantages and Disadvantages

Advantages of word games are that they:

1. Are low in cost.
2. Are fun.
3. Serve as good productive filler for individuals who finish work fast or need additional stimulation.
4. Are excellent for improving vocabulary.

Disadvantages are that they:

1. Generally address only the cognitive domain.
2. Require time to develop. However, free or inexpensive software is now available that will construct puzzles from words you submit.
3. Require equipment to reproduce.
4. Are sometimes viewed as busy work.

Tips for Effective Implementation

1. Provide participants a mechanism for determining if their solutions are correct.
2. Consider using games/puzzles as a part of the competition among teams of participants to foster group comradeship.

Examples

Two examples of word games follow:

1. Crossword puzzle for health education methods and interventions—see Figure 4-25.
2. Anagram for drug classifications—see Figure 4-26.

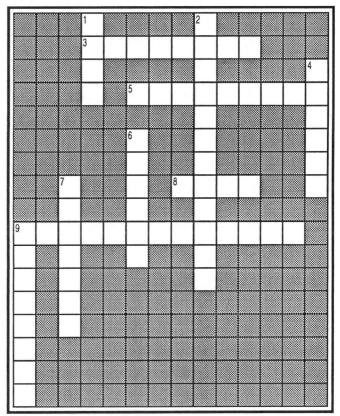

Created using Crossword Creator, Centron Software Technolgies, Inc., Version 1.12, 1992.

ACROSS

3 A classification of national background can be from any ethnic group.

5 A precise statement of intended outcome and must be stated in measurable terms.

8 An orderly self-contained collection of activities educationally designed to meet a set of objectives.

9 Belief or expectation by an individual that they can carry out the desired behavior.

DOWN

1 Certified Health Education Specialist.

2 The overall strategy to achieve stated objectives.

4 One component of intervention — can be used interchangeably with strategy.

6 Author of text.

7 Author of text.

9 One component of the intervention — can be used interchangeably with method.

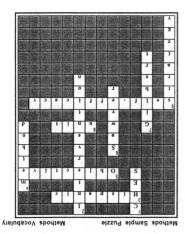

Methods Vocabulary   Methods Sample Puzzle

Figure 4-25
Crossword Puzzle on Health Education Methods/Interventions

> *Change the following names into drug classifications.*
>
> | Name | Drug Classification |
> | --- | --- |
> | *Minee Haptma* | *Amphetamine* |
> | *Bet Arbitura* | *Barbiturate* |
> | *Lum Stanti* | *Stimulant* |
> | *Ant Pedress* | *Depressant* |
>
> *See the methods selection matrix in Chapter 3.*

Figure 4-26
Anagram on Drug
Classifications

Promising Methods by Topic

As we have stated many times, we encourage you to consider all methods that might meet your objectives. Following is a list of methods by topic that have either had some success or the authors recommend the exploration of this method for the listed content area.

Drug Education
Debates
Experiments and demonstrations
Mass media
Panels
Peer education
Role plays
Value clarification

Human Sexuality
Debates
Guest speakers
Panels
Peer education
Puppets
Role plays
Value clarification

Environmental Health
Debates
Experiments and demonstrations
Field trips
Guest speakers
Panels
Storytelling

Consumer Health/Nutrition	Computer-assisted instruction
	Guest speakers
	Mass media
	Personal improvement projects
	Self-appraisals
	Storytelling
First Aid	Computer-assisted instruction
	Guest speakers
	Simulation
	Storytelling

For more information and tools related to this chapter visit http://healthedu cation.jbpub.com/strategies.

EXERCISES

Take a look at the following situations. Construct *one* behavioral objective for each situation, and then select *one* appropriate method to fulfill the objective. Give a brief justification as to why you selected a particular method, and explain how the method would facilitate achieving the objective.

1. You are teaching the first class in a five-part unit on nutrition for approximately 25 seventh-grade students.

2. You are conducting a 1-hour, once-only workshop for a community group of women (approximately 20 women ages 35 to 45) on the subject of menopause.

3. You are facilitating the first in a series of eight workshops on smoking cessation for a community group of 10 adults.

4. You are teaching the final class in a five-part unit on HIV/AIDS for a group of 25 tenth-grade students.

5. You are facilitating the second of six 1-hour workshops for approximately 10 college students on the subject of body image/weight management.

6. You are teaching the first in a three-part unit on environmental health for an eighth-grade class of approximately 20 students.

CASE STUDIES REVISITED

Case Study Revisited: Pam

Pam needs help in her method selection. She needs to consider the educational level of her participants, review her objectives, and select more appropriate methods. She has selected an inappropriate method for the target population and has failed to take advantage of an excellent opportunity for small-group techniques. If Pam had considered the characteristics of adult learners and the fact that her target population is well educated, she would have concluded that allowing the participants to identify common concerns and share ideas as they look for solutions is a better strategy.

There is an arsenal of methods available to us in health education. It is important we consider the objectives first and then focus on the methods to meet those objectives within the context of the resources we have at our disposal. (See page 99.)

Case Study Revisited: Pat

The fundamental question that should be asked is whether or not a debate on such a volatile subject as abortion should even be considered. High school students are notoriously opinionated and quite often totally unreceptive to opposing views, making an abortion debate a disaster waiting to happen. Pat was also incredibly naïve in thinking that a debate would change anyone's position on such a difficult and personal topic as abortion. One debate technique sometimes used is to have individuals research and present arguments that are diametrically opposed to their own viewpoint. This ensures that participants consider the "other side" in relation to their own opinions. However, abortion is such a personal and polarized issue that discretion, in the form of simply not debating such a topic, may indeed have been the better part of valor in this instance. (See page 118.)

Case Study Revisited: Meshah

Meshah could have done a couple of things to make the field trip more effective. Time could have been built into the day's events to allow for questions, although if someone on-site is coordinating the visit, that might prove difficult to control. Another strategy might be to provide the students with a list of questions that they need to have answered by the end of the visit. The design of the questions could require participants to meet specific people or experience targeted areas of the clinic. This could even be made into a type of informational scavenger hunt to encourage active participation. Clearly, Meshah could have used the bus ride home as a time to process the day's events and clarify any points of confusion, although in fairness to Meshah, a bus full of tired or boisterous students might not be the optimal place to process information! A football discussion might indeed be a sound plan, saving the post-visit processing or scavenger hunt analysis until the next class period. There is no one right way to implement strategies, but the likelihood of success with any single method relies heavily on the planning and thought that precedes the activity. (See page 135.)

SUMMARY

This chapter has reviewed over 30 categories of methods that can be employed by a health educator. Each has advantages and disadvantages that should be taken into account when making a selection for inclusion in any health education program.

REFERENCES AND RESOURCES

American Association for Health Education, National Commission for Health Education Credentialing, & Society for Public Health Education (1999). *A Competency-Based Framework for Graduate-Level Health Educators.* Allentown, PA: The National Commission for Health Education Credentialing, Inc., American Association for Health Education, and Society for Public Health Education.

Ames, E. E., Trucano, L. A., Wan, J. C., & Harris, M. H. (1992). *Designing School Health Curricula: Planning for Good Health.* Dubuque, IA: W.C. Brown.

Arends, R. I. (1991). *Learning to Teach.* New York: McGraw-Hill.

Bates, I. J., & Wider, A. E. (1984). *Introduction to Health Education.* Palo Alto, CA: Mayfield.

Bedworth, A. E., & Bedworth, D. A. (1992). *The Profession and Practice of Health Education.* Dubuque, IA: W.C. Brown.

Bishop, D., & Kimball, M. A. (2006). Engaging students in storytelling. *Librarian-Professional Development Collection*, 33(4), April.

Carlyon, W., & Carlyon, P. (1987). Humor as a health education tool. In P. M. Lazes, L. H. Kaplan, & K. Gordon (Eds.), *The Handbook of Health Education* (p. 115). Rockville, MD: Aspen.

Carroll, L. (1946). *Alice in Wonderland and Through the Looking Glass.* New York: Grosset and Dunlap.

Caulfield, J. (2000). The storytelling club: A narrative study of children and teachers as storytellers (Doctoral dissertation, University of Toronto, 2000). *Dissertation Abstracts International, 61*, 4273A.

Cruickshank, D. (1972). *Simulation and Gaming.* Unpublished mimeographed handout.

Davis, W., Feller, K., & Thaut, M. (1992). *Introduction to Music Therapy.* Dubuque, IA: W.C. Brown.

Denman, S., Davis, P., Pearson, J., & Madeley, R. (1996). HIV theatre in health education: An evaluation of *Someone Like You. Health Education Journal, 55*, 156–164.

Doyle, E. I., Beatty, C. F., & Shaw, M. W. (1999). Using cooperative learning groups to develop health-related cultural awareness. *Journal of School Health, 69*(2), 73–74.

Educause. (2007). Seven things you should know about digital storytelling. Retrieved August 2, 2008, from http://connect.educause.edu/Library/ELI/7ThingsYouShouldKnowAbout/39398

Feldman, R. H., & Humphrey, J. H. (1989). *Advances in Health Education: Current Research* (Vol. 2). New York: AMS Press.

Frey, N., & Fisher, D. (2007). *Reading for information in elementary school; content literacy strategies to build comprehension.* Columbus, OH: Prentice Hall.

Fuchs, D., Fuchs, L., Thompson, A., Svenson, E., Yen, L., Al Otaiba, S., et al. (2001). Peer-assisted learning strategies in reading: Extensions for kindergarten, first grade, and high school. *Remedial and Special Education, 22*(1), 15–21.

Galli, N. (1978). *Foundations and Principles of Health Education.* New York: Wiley.

Gilbert, G. G. (1981). *Teaching First Aid and Emergency Care.* Dubuque, IA: Kendall/Hunt.

Gilbert, G. G., & Ziady, M. (1986). *Experiments and Demonstrations in Smoking Education.* Washington, D.C.: U.S. Department of Health and Human Services, Office on Smoking and Health.

Gold, R. E. (1991). *Microcomputer Applications in Health Education.* Dubuque, IA: W.C. Brown.

Goodlad, J. I. (1984). *A Place Called School: Prospects for the Future.* New York: McGraw-Hill.

Goodwin, S. C. (1998). Bringing urban legends into the classroom. *Journal of School Health, 68*(3), 114–115.

Grace, R. D. (2001). An experimental study of elementary teachers with storytelling (Doctoral dissertation, Texas A&M, 2001). *Dissertation Abstracts International, 62,* 2346A.

Greenberg, J. S. (1988). *Health Education: Learner-Centered Instructional Strategies.* Dubuque, IA: W.C. Brown.

Greene, W. H., & Simons-Morton, B. G. (1984). *Introduction to Health Education.* New York: Macmillan.

Gronlund, N. (1991). *How to Write Instructional Objectives* (4th ed.). New York: Macmillan.

Haggarty, B., & Norgate, K. (2006). Storytelling in education. The Crick Crack Club, London Centre for International Storytelling. Retrieved August 2, 2008, from http://www.crickcrackclub.com/CRICRACK/EDUCF.HTM

Hellison, D. (1978). *Beyond Balls and Bats: Alienated (and Other) Youth in the Gym.* Washington, D.C.: AAHPER.

Hoff, R. (1988). *I Can See You Naked.* New York: Andrews and McMeel.

Jansiewicz, D. (2004, February). E=MC2: Teaching with Simulations. *Paper presented at the annual meeting of the APSA Teaching and Learning Conference, Washington, DC.* Retrieved August 2, 2008, from http://www.allacademic.com/meta/p117453_index .html

Joyce, B., & Weil, M. (1986). *Models of Teaching.* Englewood Cliffs, NJ: Prentice Hall.

Kagan, S. (1999). Cooperative learning: Seventeen pros and seventeen cons plus ten tips for success. *Kagan Online Magazine.* Retrieved July 28, 2008, from http://www.cooperativelearning.com/Kagan-Club/FreeArticles/ASK06.html

Kellough, R. D., & Kellough N. A. (2007). *Secondary School Teaching: A Guide of Methods and Resources* (3rd ed.). Columbus, OH: Allyn & Bacon.

Krathwohl, D. R., Bloom, B. S., & Masia, B. B. (1964). *Taxonomy of Educational Objectives: The Classification of Educational Goals. Handbook II: Affective Domain.* New York: David McKay.

Kreuter, M. W., Lezin, N. A., Kreuter, M., & Green, L. W. (2003). *Community Health Promotion Ideas That Work* (2nd ed.). Sudbury, MA: Jones and Bartlett.

Lazes, P. M., Kaplan, L. H., & Gordon, K. A. (1987). *The Handbook of Health Education.* Rockville, MD: Aspen.

Loya, R. (1984). *Health Education Teaching Ideas: Secondary.* Reston, VA: American Alliance for HPERD.

Mayshark, C., & Foster, R. (1966). *Methods in Health Education.* St. Louis: C.V. Mosby.

McLauchlan, D. (2002). Peers and PAL's: Student partnerships in a high school drama class. *Stage of the Art, 14*(2), 9–15.

Meeks, L., Heit, P., & Page, R. (2007). *Comprehensive School Health Education: Totally Awesome Strategies for Teaching* (5th ed.). New York. McGraw-Hill.

Ogle, D. (1986). K-W-L: A teaching model that develops active reading of expository text. *The Reading Teacher, 39,* 564–570.

Pfeiffer, J. W., & Jones, J. E. (1970). *A Handbook of Structured Experiences for Human Relations Training* (Vol. 2). Iowa City, IA: University Associates Press.

Pfeiffer, J. W., & Jones, J. E. (1971). *A Handbook of Structured Experiences for Human Relations Training* (Vol. 3). Iowa City, IA: University Associates Press.

Popham, W. J., & Baker, E. L. (1970). *Establishing Instructional Goals.* Englewood Cliffs, NJ: Prentice Hall.

Raths, L., Harmin, H., & Simon, S. B. (1966). *Values and Teaching.* Columbus, OH: Charles F. Merrill.

Read, D. A., Simon, S. B., & Goodman, J. B. (1977). *Health Education: The Search for Values.* Englewood Cliffs, NJ: Prentice Hall.

Rubinson, L., & Alles, W. F. (1984). *Health Education: Foundations for the Future.* Prospect Heights, IL: Waveland.

Scheer, J. K. (1992). *HIV Prevention Education for Teachers of Elementary and Middle School Grades.* Reston, VA: AAHE/AAHPERD.

Scott, G. D., & Carlo, M. W. (1979). *On Becoming a Health Educator.* Dubuque, IA: W.C. Brown.

Sculley, J., & Byrne, J. (1987). *Odyssey.* New York: Harper and Row.

Suess, D., Geisel, T. S., & Geisel, A. (1973). *The Lorax.* New York: Random House.

Sutton, R. (2006). Eight tips for better brainstorming. *Businessweek.* Retrieved July 28, 2008, from http://www.businessweek.com/innovate/content/jul2006/id20060726_517774.htm

Synovitz, L. B. (1999). Using puppetry in a coordinated school health program. *Journal of School Health, 69*(4), 145–147.

Taffee, S. J. (1986). *Computers in Education* (2nd ed.). Guilford, CT: Dushkin.

Texas A&M University. (2008). Student government, the BIG event. Retrieved July 31, 2008, from http://bigevent.tamu.edu/node/2

Thrope, L., & Wood, K. (2000). Cross-age tutoring for young adolescents. *Clearing House, 73,* 239–292.

U.S. Department of Health, Education, and Welfare. (1979). *Healthy People: The Surgeon General's Report on Health Promotion and Disease* (Publication 79-55071). Washington, D.C.: U.S. Public Health Service.

U.S. Department of Health and Human Services. (1980). *Promoting Health Preventing Disease Objectives for the Nation.* Washington, D.C.: U.S. Public Health Service.

Wagner, J. A., & Smith, R. W. (1969). *Teacher's Guide to Storytelling.* Dubuque, IA: Wm. C. Brown.

Wehrli, G., & Nyquist, J. (2003). Creating an educational curriculum for leaders at any level. AABB Conference. Retrieved July 30, 2008, from http://www.nhchc.org/TEACHINGSTRATEGIES_MET HODOLOGIES.pdf

Wilgoose, C. E. (1972). *Health Teaching in Secondary Schools.* Philadelphia: W.B. Saunders.

Zannis, M. A. (1992). *Health Educators' Use of Microcomputer Technology in Graduate Programs.* Unpublished doctoral dissertation, University of Maryland, College Park, MD.

Presentation and Unit Plan Development

Entry-Level and Advanced 1 Health Educator Competencies Addressed in This Chapter

Responsibility II: Plan Health Education Strategies, Interventions, and Programs
  Competency D: Develop a logical scope and sequence plan for health education practice.
  Competency E: Design strategies, interventions, and programs consistent with specified objectives.
  Competency F: Select appropriate strategies to meet objectives.

Responsibility III: Implement Health Education Strategies, Interventions, and Programs
  Competency A: Initiate plan of action.
  Competency C: Use a variety of methods to implement strategies, interventions, and programs.

Responsibility IV: Conduct Evaluation and Research Related to Health Education
  Competency A   Develop plans for evaluation and research.
  Competency B: Review research and evaluation procedures.
  Competency C: Design data collection instruments.
  Competency D: Carry out evaluation and research plans.
  Competency E: Interpret results from evaluation and research.
  Competency F: Infer implications from findings for future health-related activities.

Method Selection in Health Education

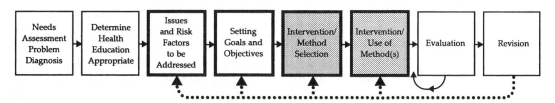

Heavy-bordered boxes indicate subjects addressed in this text; shaded boxes indicate subject(s) of current chapter.

Responsibility VI: Serve as a Health Education Resource Person
Competency C: Select resource materials for dissemination.

Note: The preceding competencies, which are addressed in this chapter, are considered to be both entry-level and Advanced 1 competencies by the National Commission for Health Education Credentialing, Inc. They are taken from *A Framework for the Development of Competency Based Curricula for Entry Level Health Educators* by the National Task Force for the Preparation and Practice of Health Education, 1985; *A Competency-Based Framework for Graduate Level Health Educators* by the National Task Force for the Preparation and Practice of Health Education, 1999; and *A Competency-Based Framework for Health Educators—The Competencies Update Project (CUP)*, 2006.

This chapter will discuss the components of lesson/presentation plans and unit plans in curriculum development.

OBJECTIVES

After studying the chapter, the reader should be able to:

- Develop an appropriate lesson/presentation plan for a given setting.
- Construct a unit of instruction for a given setting and population.
- Develop questions that promote discussion and higher-order thinking.
- Describe the strengths and weaknesses of using lesson/presentation plans for instructional organization.

KEY ISSUES

Preparing a unit plan
Preparing a lesson/presentation plan

Strengths and weaknesses of lesson/presentation plans and unit plans

---

Fundamental Principles

Presenting successfully requires the same skills as teaching successfully; it is simply the setting that is different. Should we assume that the community health educator who has to plan five 1-hour workshops on drug prevention will have to follow the same sound principles of planning and methods delivery as the teacher who has to prepare a five-lesson unit also on drug prevention? Yes, we should, because the principles of effective planning remain constant regardless of setting. True, the rules and constraints in the school classroom might influence the teacher's planning, but the fundamental principles remain the same in the school and community settings.

To be an effective health educator, particularly at the entry level, good presentation skills are essential. In order to optimize presentation skills, thoughtful planning must occur at both the individual lesson/presentation level and at the series or unit level. Anyone who has sat through a stunningly boring presentation in the classroom or in the community should consider how much time the presenter spent on thoughtful planning and method selection . . . probably very little! This important phase of preparation involves all health educators in this field, regardless of the setting.

The greatest medications are those swallowed by the mind.
—Mohan Singh

Planning the Intervention

An old saying states: "Those who fail to plan, should plan to fail." Like many old sayings there is a fair amount of truth in the statement. Spontaneity is valuable in teaching, but as the exception not as the rule. Without planning, education is less effective; it would depend completely on serendipitous events. Planning creates structure and helps ensure that each new piece of knowledge will fit into the framework of existing knowledge.

So how do you start? Unit plans and lesson plans are the maps that guide you as you design your intervention to achieve your goals and objectives. Imagine that you are going on a vacation. Simply jumping into the car and heading in a random direction may be exciting and free-spirited, but it may lead to an unpleasant get-away. Most vacation plans start with the selection of an ultimate location followed by an itinerary that outlines daily travel increments, selected sites, and experiences. Similarly, unit and lesson plans function as the itineraries for the health educator's intervention, giving an overview of what is to be accomplished en route to the designated goal.

Unit Plans

There are many ways to organize for instruction. Whenever you have more than a few hours of contact time with a target group, you should consider organizing for instruction in a unified manner. We will use the term **unit plan** to describe an orderly, self-contained collection of activities educationally designed to meet a set of objectives. Other terms for this are *curriculum*

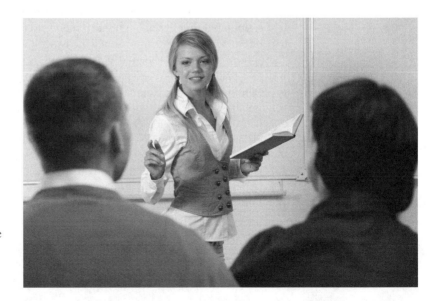

A thoughtful and prepared presentation style is the key to maintaining your audience's attention.

plans, modules, and *strands.* All such systems seek to organize materials so that they are more than the sum of their parts and have a high likelihood of achieving the stated objectives. They are meant to be more than a collection of lesson plans. As coordinated activities that build on one another, it is hoped they will be able to influence challenging issues such as attitudes or behaviors.

Depending on the time and other resources available, the unit plan can be a powerful tool if implemented as constructed. But there must be a significant amount of contact time allowed—usually more than 5 hours—and a fairly consistent participating group. A lesson/presentation plan (discussed later in this chapter) might be more appropriate than a unit plan if you are working with a group of people for only a short period of time. Whether you are planning a major 3-day community workshop or 20 hours of classroom contact time in a school setting, you need to provide for an adequate amount of contact time for your intervention so that you can build one component onto another.

Reinventing the Wheel

Unit plan construction is a challenging endeavor. Although good units already exist for a wide variety of health topics, the challenge is finding one that meets your particular objectives. Federal, local, and state governments have supported the development of many curriculum projects that include multiple units. Many of the voluntary agencies have curriculum materials designed to meet their health objectives, which are sometimes available free or at low cost. Others are more extensive and are sold by vendors, sometimes at considerable cost. If you are working on a curriculum development project, it is most helpful to review material that is currently available. Otherwise, you may needlessly be trying to reinvent the wheel. Try contacting local health educators for people who can help you. Professional organizations can also put you in touch with good contacts. Even if you decide your project or population group is distinctive enough that it requires a new unit, it is most helpful to review how others have approached the issues and objectives.

The health educator who plays roulette must first invent the wheel.
—Mohan Singh

Sources include professional organizations as well as vendors. Working with university health educators and reviewing Internet sites are good ways to locate material. Any national professional health meeting is replete with vendors showing their curriculum projects and related materials. Many vendors will sell copies of their curriculum guides or complete packages, which include all needed materials, such as videotapes, and some will develop custom units for you. Costs often are high, but you may acquire materials that are far better than you could develop on your own. If you wish to use part of the materials, you will need to negotiate permission from the vendor and generally a fee will be required.

Noteworthy Use of Your Tax Dollars

The federal government has supported the development of many curriculum projects over the years. These often cost taxpayers millions of dollars. Because of budget cuts and changing priorities, many of the projects have

The lotus, like health education, floats upon still waters; alas, while many admire their perfection, neither hath visible means of support.
—Mohan Singh

ended up in closets and are rarely used. Today most government agencies encourage vendors to take these projects and use them. The vendors turn them into marketable products and copyright the materials, sometimes making good profits. In one way this seems like a ripoff of public funds, but without such practice these good materials might well end up gathering dust. If you can find relevant government material, you can use it without violating any copyright law.

Unit Construction Guidelines

Possible components of a typical unit plan are as follows:

1. Overview
2. Statement of purpose
3. Long-range goals, general objectives, or key concepts
4. Behavioral objectives
5. Outline of content
6. Methods/strategies/learning opportunities
7. List of materials
8. Evaluation activities
9. List of available resources and materials
10. Block plan

Each component will be discussed in detail followed by an applied example from a variety of programs. Keep in mind that unit plans can be and often are hundreds of pages long. The examples provided are only representative of the type of information to be included and are incomplete for even a short unit plan. It is suggested that the reader review complete unit plans developed by professionals as well.

A unit plan is a vehicle for providing multi-faceted learning opportunities designed to enhance the delivery of instruction and assessment. The elements of the unit plan collectively provide a big picture of the health intervention. Just as the individual trees create a forest, the elements of the unit plan function to create a plan for health promotion. (See Figure 5-1.)

Overview   Begin with an overview, a paragraph or two describing the setting of where the unit will be offered. Include the ages of participants or grade level, number of meetings and duration, economic situation, and cultural environment. Identify the actual location(s) by name where the health education program will be conducted. Pertinent demographics should be included. (See Chapter 2 for information on needs assessment.) This overview section will generally be less than one page and will lay out the demographics of the group.

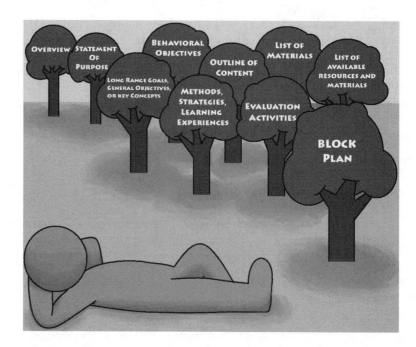

Figure 5-1
Unit Plans: Seeing
the Big Picture

Sample Overview (Well-Baby Program)

The unit plan for a Well-Baby Program is targeting pregnant women who have applied for the "HELP NOW" program of King Sam County of Anystate. The program will accept the first 50 women who sign up. Based on county statistics, it is estimated that the group will range in age from 13 to 40, with the majority of participants being under 20 years of age. Most will be English speaking, with approximately two thirds reading at above a fifth-grade level. Approximately half are expected to be African American and the other half white. Group size will be approximately 25, and participants will self-select their group according to their schedule. Only a small number of participants are employed, and the site is in the community, so transportation is not expected to be a problem. Day care, however, is an issue, since 50% of the participants have one or more children and less than 25% have a spouse or partner living with them.

Statement of Purpose

The *statement of purpose* is a description of why this content is part of the curriculum for this target population. Footnote any statistics or generalizations used to support the need for this unit. Write this section as if you were trying to convince an outsider of the need for this unit. Use statistics whenever possible to support the need for this specific target population. All statistics in the statement of purpose should be referenced and be as recent as available. Local statistics should be used when appropriate. The U.S. Health Goals for the Year 2020 are often helpful, as are local newspaper reports.

Sample Statement of Purpose (Drug Prevention Program)

The unit for a Drug Prevention Program was developed because of an identified need in the community. The program is modeled on one that has proved to be successful in other communities similar to "Anytown," USA, which has shown rather dramatic increases in drug use by school-age children. According to the Anytown Department of Health annual survey, the number of students using marijuana was as follows:

	2000	2004	2008
4th Grade	2%	6%	9%
6th Grade	3%	8%	9%
8th Grade	11%	13%	16%
11th Grade	14%	14%	18%
12th Grade	13%	16%	27%

Cocaine use has also shown a similar rising trend, as follows:

	2000	2004	2008
4th Grade	1%	2%	3%
6th Grade	1%	3%	3%
8th Grade	2%	5%	8%
11th Grade	1%	7%	10%
12th Grade	2%	8%	14%

Alcohol use has remained a serious problem:

	2000	2004	2008
4th Grade	11%	12%	13%
6th Grade	11%	13%	13%
8th Grade	22%	25%	38%
11th Grade	21%	27%	40%
12th Grade	32%	48%	64%

State studies indicate a strong relationship between the use of these drugs and the increase in violence, unwanted pregnancies, AIDS, and low school performance. Studies show that 90% of cases of unprotected intercourse occurred during the use of drugs, including alcohol, by both males and females. Last year three seniors scheduled to graduate died in an alcohol-related auto accident 3 weeks before commencement. This unit is needed in our schools and should be implemented as part of our comprehensive school health education program.

Long-Range Goals, General Objectives, or Key Concepts

The very broad outcome intentions for the unit may be expressed as *long-range goals, general objectives, or key concepts.* These are optimal behaviors you hope to achieve and need not be easily measurable. (See Chapter 2.) Three or four general goals are usually adequate to express the general nature of a program unless it is a very long unit. Many units are 10 hours or less in total contact time. Schools often have longer units that might average 20 contact hours each.

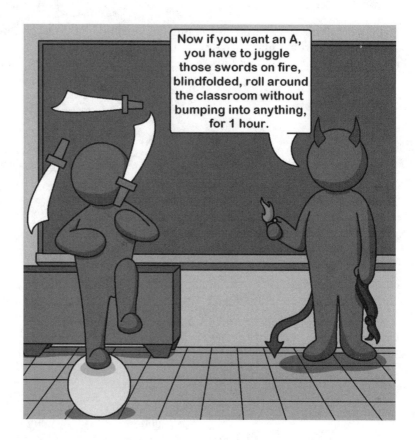

Your unit objectives must be reasonable in order to be effective.

Sample Goals (Child Abuse Prevention)

Goals for a Child Abuse Prevention Program are as follows:

1. Participants will acquire a set of workable and practical stress management techniques.
2. Participants will develop positive parenting skills.
3. Participants will develop efficacy in the presented parenting skills.

Behavioral Objectives

The *behavioral objectives* are stated in behavioral terms—that is, in cognitive, affective, and psychomotor domains—according to recognized authority or as covered by the instructor. Often your agency, hospital, or school will have a specific format. These are the specific objectives to be achieved and should include an indication of how they will be measured. (See Chapter 2.) The number of objectives will depend largely on the contact time and resources available. The number is not really important. The important consideration is that they be appropriate, achievable, and clearly stated. Most units of 20 hours or more have 15 or 20 objectives.

Sample Objectives (Stress Management) Objectives for a Stress Management Program are as follows:

Cognitive

Upon completion of the stress management workshop
1. Participants identify three personal sources of stress according to the guidelines presented in the program.
2. Participants will define stress, eustress, and stress management according to the handouts provided.

Affective

1. Participants will show a willingness to learn more about stress management by voluntarily signing up for future programs.
2. Participants will show an increase in self-efficacy about their ability to practice the presented stress management techniques, according to self-ratings on a post-evaluation instrument.

Psychomotor

1. Participants will demonstrate, to their group members, Jacobson progressive relaxation as shown in class.
2. Participants will demonstrate the Jones breathing techniques as presented in class meeting 4 during the simulation.

Outline of Content An *outline* of the content to be presented should include all items. This detailed outline can be supplemented by an appendix with more detail or photocopies of the PowerPoint to be used. The content in the outline should be presented in a logical order, though not necessarily in the order of presentation to be followed in the unit plan. If the contact time is about 20 hours, this section could be 30 or 40 pages.

Sample Outline (Nutrition) The outline for a Nutrition Program is as follows:
I. Dietary Guidelines for Americans
   A. Recommendations to help people maintain good health and/or improve it.
   B. A good diet is based on variety and moderation.
   C. Moderation means not eating large amounts of foods high in fat (saturated fatty acids and cholesterol).
   D. A risk factor is a condition that may increase the chance that something (usually negative) might be experienced by someone.
   E. For some people, certain types of diets are risk factors for chronic health conditions, such as heart disease, cancer, and high blood pressure.
   F. The Seven Dietary Guidelines
      (1) Eat a variety of foods.

      (a) No one food can supply all the essential nutrients needed for maintaining good health.

      (b) Should include foods from a variety of food groups.

      (c) Creates a balanced diet.

(2) Maintain desirable weight.

      (a) Desirable weight will vary according to many factors such as age, health, gender, and so on.

      (b) Avoid sudden, potentially dangerous, aggressive dieting.

      (c) Calorie intake and expenditure must be balanced to maintain weight.

(3) Avoid too much fat, saturated fat, and cholesterol.

      (a) A small amount of fat is needed in your diet.

      (b) Risk of heart attack is increased by diets high in fat.

      (c) How foods are prepared will influence the fat content of food.

(4) Eat foods with adequate starch and fiber.

      (a) Starch is a complex carbohydrate.

      (b) Carbohydrate-rich foods provide many essential nutrients and fiber.

      (c) Dietary fiber is plant material that humans cannot digest.

      (d) Grain products and starchy vegetables are good sources of starch.

      (e) Whole grain products, fruits, vegetables, nuts, and dry beans contain fiber.

      (f) How the food is prepared will affect the fiber content.

(5) Avoid too much sugar.

      (a) Sugars are carbohydrates; some are present in food naturally, some are added.

      (b) Added sugars provide calories/energy, but almost no nutrients.

      (c) High-sugar diets can increase the risk of developing tooth decay.

      (d) High-sugar foods often take the place of more nutritious foods in your diet.

      (e) Through careful food selection and preparation, you can control sugar levels.

(6) Avoid too much sodium.

      (a) Sodium is an essential nutrient.

      (b) Helps the body maintain normal blood volume and pressure, helps muscle function.

      (c) High sodium increases risk of hypertension, heart attacks, strokes, and so on.

      (d) Sodium is added to many foods as a flavor enhancer.

      (e) Food labels can help to identify high-sodium foods.

      (f) Through careful food selection and preparation, you can control sodium levels.

(7) For teens: avoid alcoholic beverages.
    For adults: if you drink alcohol, do so in moderation.
    (a) People who drink alcohol and drive increase their risk for un-
        intended injuries.
    (b) Heavy alcohol use can contribute to liver disease and some
        forms of cancer.
    (c) Alcohol can add calories to your diet, but almost no nutri-
        ents.
    (d) There are many nonalcoholic beverage alternatives.
II. Reading a Nutrition Label
    A. Found on food package/container.
    B. Calculate calories per container.

**Methods/Strategies/
Learning
Opportunities**

Methods (also referred to as *strategies* and *learning opportunities*) are the
component of greatest importance. Selection of the best methods to reach
one's objectives is essentially what this book is all about. Selection should
take place after reviewing all practical options (see Chapter 4). Each method
should be selected based on the objectives to be achieved, and each should
be named and described in detail in such a way that it could be utilized by
any health educator. All directions and rules should be included. Since these
directions may be lengthy, the details might be on attached photocopies.
Proper citations and permissions should be obtained. It is most important
that activities be selected based on achieving the desired objectives. This is
the most crucial component of a unit, assuming the objectives are appropriate and well stated. It is helpful to list after each method which specific ob-
jective(s) it is likely to achieve. This will help ensure that all objectives are
addressed and that methods are selected for the correct reasons. The number
of methods is dictated by the contact time and the objectives to be achieved.
A variety of learning styles should be addressed, as well as the characteristics
of the target population.

**Sample Application:
Methods (Nutrition)**

The methods for a Nutrition Program are as follows:
1. Lecture 1
   • Will cover outline parts I and II.
   • PowerPoint slides will be used for reinforcement.
   • Objectives addressed
     ○ Cognitive objectives 1, 2, 7, and 8
2. Lecture 2
   • Guest speaker (registered dietitian) will cover outline parts III and V,
     including food labeling.
   • Objectives addressed
     ○ Cognitive objectives 2, 3, and 4
     ○ Affective objective 1
3. Nutrition relay
   • See Appendix D for rules and questions.
   • Objectives addressed

- o Cognitive objectives 1, 2, 3, 4, 6, 8, 9, 10, 11, and 12
- o Psychomotor objectives 3, 4, and 7
4. Demonstration and cooking
   - Facilitator will demonstrate proper cooking of vegetables followed by an opportunity for all to enjoy a meal that they have prepared.
   - Prior notification is required, and special materials are needed.
   - See Appendix E for recipes and lists of ingredients.
   - Objectives addressed
     - o Affective objectives 4 and 9
     - o Psychomotor objectives 3, 4, and 5

List of Materials   A complete *list of materials* needed by the health educator (e.g., LCD projector) and those needed by each participant (e.g., paper) should be included. In many settings you cannot count on the participants arriving with anything, so it is necessary to provide all that is needed. It is a good safeguard to keep a few "extras" of your materials on hand to account for unexpected mishaps and shortages. Many activities can be ruined by three participants trying to share.

Sample Materials   Materials for an unspecified unit plan follow:
(Any Unit)

Facilitator

1. Extra pencils and paper
2. Dry erase board
3. Dry erase markers
4. LCD projector
5. Projection screen
6. Laptop computer/DVD player

Participant

1. Paper and pencil

Evaluation Activities   *Evaluation activities* are based on your stated objectives. For example, in a community setting you might use anonymous self-assessments. In a school setting you might include five quizzes, of 10 multiple-choice questions each, and one final, an essay variety worth 40%, and so on. Include activities to measure *knowledge*, *attitudes*, *skills*, and *behavior*. Use a variety of assessment techniques appropriate for the target population. Be certain to include *teacher/facilitator evaluation* activities for the assessment of the instructor. The quantity and to some extent the quality of evaluation strategies will depend on the contact time for the workshop and for evaluation. Evaluation strategies should be tied to the objectives.

Sample Evaluation   Evaluation for an HIV/AIDS Workshop is as follows:
(HIV/AIDS Workshop)

Outcome Evaluation

1. Pretest and posttest on content of workshop
2. Post-workshop survey of behaviors
3. Post-conference short survey of health behaviors in 6 months

Process Evaluation

1. Post-workshop evaluation of facilitator performance and daily rating of workshop components

List of Available Resources and Materials

A *list of resources and materials* should include only those materials (books, articles, films) that are available and known to be of good quality. Include complete titles, costs, and the Internet site or phone number at which prices and orders can be obtained. List only those materials you know to be useful and important to the success of the unit.

Sample Resources (First Aid)

Resources for a First Aid Program are as follows:

1. Doe, John. 2008. *First Aid.* J&J Publishers, Anytown. $79.95
2. American First Aid Society Film Series (five short DVDs)
   National Headquarters, Anytown, U.S.A.
   Cost $1,500 set or $25 for rental for each
3. First Aid Chart
   American First Aid Society Film Series
   National Headquarters, Anytown, U.S.A.
   800-222-2222
   $89.95

Block Plan

The term **block plan** comes from the days when teachers would divide the day into "blocks" of time. This item is a breakdown of your suggested sequence, specifying the amount of time to be spent on each activity. The block plan indicates how the total intervention fits together. Use of educational principles should be evident, including pacing, variety, and reinforcement. There is no need to review method or content in this section, for it will be developed in the outline and method sections of the lesson/unit plan.

An important distinction exists between an actual lesson plan and a block plan, because a block plan is most assuredly *not* a lesson plan. The layout provided in the block plan is useful for outlining the topics, activities, and assignments projected for the program, but it lacks the necessary details to fully execute an effective lesson. Educators who mistakenly believe the notations in a block plan are actual lesson plans are fooling themselves. Educators should not use block plans in lieu of authentic lesson plans (Kellough & Kellough, 2007).

Sample Block Plan (Any Topic)

The block plan is how the total intervention fits together. Use of educational principles should be evident, including pacing, variety, and reinforcement. There is no need to review method or content in this section, as it has already been developed in the outline and method sections. Figure 5-2 shows a block plan for an intervention to develop parenting skills for first-time fathers.

Block Plan D.A.D.S. Developing Awesome Daddy Skills (#) = Time allotted in minutes				
Session 1: Fathers, Families, & Finances	Session 2: What to Expect When Your Partner Is Expecting	Session 3: Baby Basics 101	Session 4: Building Better Fathers	Session 5: Partners in Parenting
Introduction (5)	Introduction (5)	Introduction (3)	Introduction (3)	Introduction (3)
Ice Breaker: Baby Bingo (10)	Ice Breaker: "Starburst" (5)	Self-appraisal: Rate Your Skills (5)	Brainstorm: Qualities of Fathers (7)	Ice Breaker: Two Truths & a Lie with Partner(10)
Expert Panel: Q&A Session (15)	Simulation: Empathy Belly (10)	Demonstration/ Practice: Diaper Changes (15)	Group Discussion: Building Better Fathers (20)	Experiment: Communication with Play-doh (10)
Media: Movie Clip (5)	Discussion: Feeling the Belly (15)	Project: Pack the Diaper Bag? (10)	Role Play: Baby Is Crying (15)	Lecture: Communication Skills (17)
Break (5)	Break (5)	Break (5)	Break (5)	Break (5)
Problem Solving: Budget Activity (20)	Lecture: We're Pregnant: What Now? (15)	Demonstration/ Practice: Holding, Handling, & Bathing (14)	Educational Game: Romancing the Mother (15)	Readers Theater: Keep Talking…(10)
Group Presentation Budget Plan (10)	Case Study: The Father's Role (15)	Guest Speaker: Baby Proofing Your Home (20)	Guided Imagery: Dating Your Baby's Mom (10)	Peer Education: Problem Solving with Partner (15)
				Self-Appraisal: Communication Skills (5)
Summary and preview next meeting (10)	Summary and preview next meeting (10)	Summary and preview next meeting (10)	Summary and preview next meeting (10)	Summary and post-workshop evaluation (10)

Figure 5-2
Block Plan: Developing Awesome Daddy Skills.
Source: Class project contributed by Mikka Basham, Lisa Belinowski, Krissy Noack, Jenna Sharer, and Annie Stoddard. Reprinted with permission.

Objective: After reviewing the case study, the reader will articulate a few similarities shared by community and school health educators when planning presentations.

Case Study: Michael   Michael, a young, enthusiastic health educator, had recently been hired by the local health department. His first assignment was to plan and implement a series of five 1-hour workshops on general health issues for a senior citizens' community group. In college Michael had taken a methods and materials course, but he had put little effort into studying the construction of lesson/presentation planning or unit development. He had argued that only school health majors needed that knowledge, and the last thing that Michael wanted was to be a teacher! Michael asked all the right initial questions related to group size, demographic background, location, time, available equipment, and so on. He then jotted down a few notes for the first meeting, grabbed an available DVD, arranged for the use of a player, and was on his way to the first workshop. Michael's first presentation left a lot to be desired. He lectured far too long, boring many of the participants, and he was unable to show the DVD on the player that the group had gone to great pains to borrow. When asked what the ensuing workshops would cover, Michael was unable to answer, mumbling something about covering whatever the group wanted. The following week only one of the group's members showed up, and eventually the series of workshops was canceled. Not surprisingly, Michael was asked to meet with his supervisor! (See Case Studies Revisited page 219.)

Questions to consider:

1. Are the initial questions asked by Michael the same questions a school health educator should also consider? Justify your response.
2. How might Michael's attitude about "not being a teacher" impact his effectiveness as a community health educator?

Lesson/Presentation Plans

Curriculum development involves much more than just the mere design of lesson/presentation plans and unit plans. The development of these types of plans, however, is the foundation of a comprehensive curriculum. Comprehensive curriculum development is outside the parameters of this text, and there are many outstanding books dedicated to the topic. This text focuses on just the plans, the starting point of curriculum development.

Preparing properly for a presentation requires careful organization. You must take into account all the issues used to select or write your objectives and carefully review what objectives are appropriate for your workshop, presentation, or class. **Lesson/presentation plans** should be written in a format that any health educator could use, given some preparation time, and present the materials well. If properly constructed, the presentation should capture the essence of what the author intended no matter who is the user. Figure 5-3 shows a recommended format.

There are many suggested formats for lesson/presentation plans. Check with your agency or school to see if there is a required or recommended format.

Lesson/Presentation Plan Format			
Name:			
Grade Level/Community Setting:			
Date:	Topic/Unit:		
Lesson Title:			
Age of Target Population :	Demographics:		
Standard(s) Code:			
Objectives:			
Cognitive-			
Affective-			
Psychomotor-			

Introduction (a statement of what you will be doing and what you expect the learner to know, be able to do, or believe when you are finished):

Developmental Section (*this may be several pages*):

Content	Method/Strategy	Estimated Time	Materials Needed

I. XXX
  A. XXXX
  B. XX
  C. XXXXXX
	Name Game	20 minutes	None

II. XXXXXXXXX
  A. XXX
  B. XXXXXX
  C. XX
    1. XXXXXXXX
    2. XXX
    3. XXXXX
	Lecture/Discussion	15 minutes	LCD projector
			Computer
			Screen

III. XXXXXXXXX
  A. XXX
  B. XXXXXX
    1. XXXXXXXX
    2. XXX
    3. XXXXX
    4. XXXXX
	Guided Imagery—
	  see attachment
		30 minutes	CD player
			CD of sounds
			Script—see
			  attachment

XX. XXX
  A. XXX
  B. XXXXXX
    1. XXXXXXXX
    2. XXX
	Game Bingo—
	See attached for rules
		20 minutes	Bingo Cards
			Pencils
			Questions
			Prizes

Culmination (Summary of key points for the lesson and what will happen next):

Anticipated Problems and possible solutions (Lesson extension and plan B):

Evaluation (How will you determine if you have been successful? Were your objectives met?):

Figure 5-3
Simple Lesson/
Presentation Plan
Format

All suggested formats include the basic components of background information, introduction, objectives, developmental section (body or core), conclusion/culmination, and evaluation. It is also recommended that you try to anticipate problems by preparing an alternative plan (often referred to as Plan B).

Objective: After reviewing the case study, the reader will suggest three or more planning tips that might prevent the negative outcome experienced by Shane, Mary, and Mr. Simpson.

Case Study: Shane   Shane is ill and asks a colleague at his agency to take over for the day. On his agenda is a presentation to Mr. Simpson's students at Hillsboro Public High School regarding HIV infections. Mary, the colleague asked to fill in, is well versed in HIV and AIDS issues, having formerly worked for the State Public Health Epidemiology Division. Mary can find only brief notes, so she grabs a flipchart on Kaposi's sarcoma and other diseases associated with AIDS and heads to the high school. She provides a very graphic presentation on sexual behaviors, including anal intercourse, and, of course, a very visual show on the effects of the diseases. Shane is surprised some days later when he is reprimanded for the presentation and told he is no longer welcomed at the high school. (See Case Studies Revisited page 219.)

Questions to consider:

1. What do you believe is the objective of the presentation?
2. Do you believe Mary's selected method and content to be appropriate? Explain.
3. What questions should have been asked of Mr. Simpson by the health educator prior to the presentation?

Elements of a Simple Lesson/Presentation Plan

Well-written lesson plans provide a blueprint to organize materials and indicate what will occur and why, while identifying potential gaps in the content. The remainder of the chapter provides an explanation of each of the components of a lesson/presentation plan followed by an example showing the application of the guidelines. The reader will also have the opportunity to critique a few additional examples.

Background   The initial section, which may be thought of as the background for the plan, includes basic information that will assist in determining strategy selection: the setting for the presentation (community or school), the presentation topic, the approximate number of participants, and as much demographic information about the participants as can be obtained (age, ethnicity, socioeconomic status, etc.). It may also include a numeric/letter indicator that correlates to state or national standards. For example, the National Health Education Standards are a list of competencies to be identified as the foundation for health education for students from pre-kindergarten through grade 12 (National Health Education Standards [NHES], 2007). It is common practice to include coding identification on lesson/presentation plans to act as evidence of meeting the outlined standards.

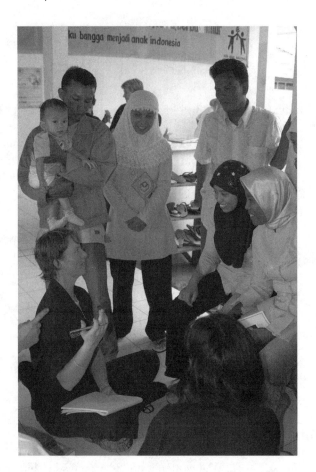

Your presentation will go smoothly and will hold your audience's interest if you have thoroughly researched the demographics of your participants.

Objectives   The objectives are the specific objectives you hope to achieve with this lesson/presentation. They must be stated in specific terms (see Chapter 2). You may have only one objective, or you may have several. However, contact time must be taken into account, since you cannot achieve some objectives in a short time frame. You must be realistic in what you set out to achieve. You might be able to achieve several cognitive objectives in a short time or one or two psychomotor objectives but generally not both. It is important to review educational principles and to remember the need to repeat key points and to use multiple approaches to accommodate differences in learning styles. A good rule of thumb is to cover less, but cover it well!

Introduction   The introduction is where you capture the interest of the target audience, give a welcome, and provide reasons for covering the information. From this introduction your audience should be able to identify what you expect them to know, be able to do, or feel after the lesson and how they will benefit from the experience. In other words, you should state your objectives. Include some local statistics, if appropriate, and logical statements regarding the issues addressed that will get the group enthusiastic about the topic.

Developmental Section   The developmental section is the core of the lesson plan and includes all strategies and the appropriate information to carry them out. Sufficient information must be supplied in outline or text format so *any health educator, given some preparation time, could conduct the lesson or presentation.* Time estimates and needed materials should be included. This section is often multiple pages. All the information needed for any health educator to conduct the lesson should be included.

Content materials such as handouts, discussion questions, or directions might be attached, especially if photocopying materials is easier than rewriting the information.

Some health educators find it helpful to include an outline of discussion questions in the lesson plan. Effective questioning is a skill that one must develop through practice. It is a good idea to develop discussion questions that call for high-level thinking skills. Though it is fairly easy to think up questions that require a simple one-word response, they do not facilitate thoughtful discussion of the content. Planning questions helps you move your participants from the lowest level of mental operations (simple recall) to the highest level of divergent thinking requiring application of thought (Kellough & Kellough, 2007). Benjamin Bloom (1984) created a taxonomy of questioning with six levels that progressively move learners to more complex reflection. For our purpose here, it may be more useful to think in terms of three levels of questioning: lowest, intermediate, and advanced.

At the lowest level of questioning, participants are asked to gather or recall information. Typically this is a regurgitation of what they have been given or what can be elicited from memory. A participant might be asked to count, define, recite, match, list, or restate information. Lower level questions are useful in establishing a foundation in the development of more advanced thought, but they do not facilitate it.

Examples of lowest thought level questions:

- Can you describe the common side effects of chemotherapy?
- If you were asked to explain the meaning of the acronym AIDS, what would you say?

At the intermediate level, participants are asked to process the information, thus they are developing intellectual skills. Intermediate questions challenge the participants to draw relationships of cause and effect, to synthesize, analyze, compare and contrast, rate, or classify data. "At the processing level, this internal analysis of new data may challenge a learner's perceptions (and misconceptions...) about a phenomenon" (Kellough & Kellough, 2007, p. 89). Increasing the mental challenge requires the learner's brain to draw upon previously stored data, resulting in addition to or a reshaping of mental concepts.

Examples of intermediate level questions:

- When attempting to lose weight, what are the advantages and disadvantages of fad weight loss diets?
- How would you organize an exercise regime to increase cardiovascular endurance?

Questioning at the highest level of thinking encourages learners to evaluate and apply the information to new situations. As participants apply, build, evaluate, hypothesize, imagine, predict, or speculate, they think intuitively and creatively to expose their own value system (Kellough & Kellough, 2007). According to Pike (2003), people do not argue with their own data; therefore, questions that require the participant to consider the information or make judgments are more likely to produce content retention.

Examples of higher level questions:

- What do you believe would be the outcome of imposing an additional "sin tax" on junk food?
- Why should industrialized nations such as the United States subsidize the AIDS prevention methods in under-developed nations?

Including a list of questions in the lesson plan will allow the health educator to evaluate the level of questions being asked throughout the presentation to ensure that learners are moved to higher levels of thinking.

Conclusion   The conclusion/culmination is the ending of the lesson/presentation and should include a summary of the key issues covered (reinforcement) and directions for the next meeting. If this is a one-time workshop or the final workshop of a series, it should include a thorough review of key points and an opportunity for feedback and questions. This would also be the time to administer an evaluation questionnaire.

Anticipated Problems   Obviously, we cannot anticipate every problem that might occur when making a presentation, but we can anticipate some common ones and plan to deal with them. It is important that we learn to do this as well as possible. This also is commonly called "turning to Plan B." Good planning will increase our self-confidence, allowing us to focus on the lesson. We should consider the possibility of running short or long on time, audiovisual failures, or a group's unwillingness to participate, for example, and develop an alternate plan for such events.

Some common problems often encountered in lesson/presentation preparation include the following:

1. Not enough material (people often speak faster when nervous, or anticipated group discussion does not materialize).
2. Methods inappropriate for group (group unwilling to participate).

3. Method is inappropriate to achieve the objective.
4. Little variety in methods employed (group acts bored and restless).
5. No evaluation or feedback system built in (no way to determine value or make improvements).
6. Overestimating or underestimating the amount of time it takes to execute the method.

One strategy to deal with problems is to plan a lesson extension or to have a Plan B. Lesson extensions are ideas to expand the method you are currently using. The health educator might suggest that the participants design an advertisement promoting healthy choices related to the content being covered as a method to fill excess time. The extension lets the participants expand upon what is already being covered.

A Plan B differs from an extension; it is a new method to replace an existing method or strategy that cannot be executed. Perhaps there is a scratch on the DVD you had planned to show or the computer lab gets flooded; a Plan B provides you with an alternate activity to replace what is planned. Ideally, lesson extensions and Plan Bs are methods that can be incorporated with minimal setup and supplies. It would be a waste of time and resources to prepare elaborate materials that may not be used.

Evaluation   The evaluation is an integral part of any lesson plan. If our objectives are well stated and achievable, evaluation should be straightforward. Short time frames influence evaluation in that we must often use the majority of time for the intervention. However, it is always important that we conduct as much evaluation as possible. Contact time will have a major impact on evaluation time. If this is a one-time, 1-hour presentation, a simple anonymous evaluation form or even a few oral questions may be all that is necessary. If this is the final presentation in a series, then a much more elaborate assessment tied to your objectives is in order. The type of evaluation techniques employed will be a function of the objectives, available time, type of group, and resources. Consider outcome and process evaluation techniques. As a general rule, 15% of time should be spent on evaluation.

Lesson Plan Example

Super Smiles is a program designed to be delivered to multi-ethnic males and females on Tuesdays and Thursdays in February to support National Children's Dental Health Month. The lesson plan—which is featured in this section—is part of a community intervention to improve dental hygiene among 6- and 7-year-old children participating in an after school program at the local youth community center. The intervention's block plan (Figure 5-4) follows.

The following sample lesson/presentation plan for Tuesday of week 2—from the block plan—shows in detail the elements used in such a plan (Source: Class project—Rachel Willmann, Sara Pennington, and Mandy Abrams):

Week #1		Week #2	
Tuesday	**Thursday**	**Tuesday**	**Thursday**
Pretest (10)	Experiment/ Lecture/Discussion *Identifying Plaque* (20)	Lecture/Discussion/ Educational Game/ Display *Sugar* (30)	Brainstorming/ Group Work *5 Food Groups* (40)
Brainstorming/ Discussion *Introduction Teeth* (20)	Discussion/ Demonstration/ Experimentation *Removing Plaque* (10)	Discussion/Puzzle *Snack Considerations* (15)	Demonstration/ Personal Improvement/Lecture *Brushing and Flossing* (20)
Discussion *Plaque Defined* (15)	Audio-video *Brushing* (20)	Personal Improvement *Brushing* (10)	Evaluation (10)
Experiment/ Demonstration/ Lecture *Plaque and Decay* (15)	Demonstration/ Audio-Visual/ Experiment *Flossing* (20)	Personal Improvement *Flossing* (5)	
Self-Appraisal *Gum Disease* (10)	Problem Solving *Signs of a Worn Toothbrush* (5)	Evaluation (10)	
	Evaluation (10)		

Week #3		Week #4	
Tuesday	**Thursday**	**Tuesday**	**Thursday**
Personal Improvement *Brushing and Flossing* (5)	Pretest (5)	Personal Improvement *Brushing and Flossing* (5)	Personal Improvement *Brushing and Flossing* (5)
Brainstorming/ Problem Solving *Functions of Teeth* (15)	Personal Improvement *Brushing and Flossing* (5)	Role Play/ Brainstorm/Models *5 Keeping Teeth Safe* (20)	Final Dental Exam Post-Program Evaluation (20)
Lecture *Parts of a Tooth* (10)	Field Trip Guest Speaker Demonstration *Dentist and Dental Helpers* (30)	Displays *Teeth and Gums Can Be Injured by . . .* (20)	Displays *Super Smile Fun* (25)
Lecture *Surrounding Tissue* (10)	Field Trip Guest Speaker Demonstration *Examining Teeth* (20)	Cooperative Learning *First Aid* (20)	Personal Improvement *Don't Forget* (5)
Experiment/Model/ Group Discussion/ Brainstorming *Specialized Teeth* (15)	Field Trip Guest Speaker Demonstration *Professional Teeth Cleaning* (10)	Evaluation (10)	
Model/Cooperative Learning *Primary Teeth* (10)	Evaluation (5)		
Evaluation (10)			

Figure 5-4
Block Plan:
Super Smiles
Source: Class project contributed by Rachel Willmann, Sara Pennington, and Mandy Abrams. Reprinted with permission.

Lesson/
Presentation Plan

Name: Super Smiles
Grade level/setting: Pebble Creek After School Program at the Youth Community Center
Date: Lesson Plan for Week #2 Tuesday   **Topic/unit:** Dental Health
Lesson title: Healthy and Unhealthy Snacks
Theory: Contemplation, Action, and Preparation
Age of Target Population: 6–7 year olds
Demographics: 11 girls and 9 boys, multi-ethnic
NHES: 1.2.2. Recognize that there are multiple dimensions of health (NHES, 2007).
2.2.1. Identify how the family influences personal health practices and behaviors (NHES, 2007).
3.2.1. Identify trusted adults and professionals who can help promote health (NHES, 2007).
7.2.1. Demonstrate healthy practices and behaviors to maintain or improve personal health (NHES, 2007).

Objectives
- **Cognitive:** By the end of the lesson, first-grade student will identify healthy snack foods by circling appropriate choices on the worksheet with 90% accuracy.
- **Psychomotor:** The participant will create a food collage to classify multiple examples of healthy food choices discussed in the lecture as high in sugar or not high in sugar.
- **Psychomotor:** By the end of the session, first-grade student will demonstrate plaque removal on tooth surfaces, to his or her partner, by removing 95% of the disclosing tablet stains using the method of brushing described.
- **Affective:** Following the discussion on healthy snacks, the learner will verbally justify which of the three foods he or she believes would be the best choice to promote dental health.

Introduction

We discussed last Thursday the importance of brushing and flossing. Remember that plaque can slowly destroy our teeth if we do not remove it by brushing and flossing. Today, we will be learning about healthy and unhealthy snacks. We will also be brushing and flossing our teeth at the end of class with disclosing tablets or plaque detectors. When we finish today, you will know which snacks are healthy choices for your teeth, so you can protect your dental health. You will also get to improve your brushing and flossing skills using special plaque detectors.

**Developmental
Section**

Content Outline	Method/ Strategy	Estimated Time Needed	Materials Needed

I. Sugar
  A. Common sources
    • Cookies
    • Cakes
	Lecture
	Discussion
		10 Minutes	Magazines
			Scissors
			Pictures of examples

• Sugared gum
  B. Harmful materials
    • Bacteria
    • Acid
	Educational game
	Display
	(see following pages)
		10 Minutes	Construction paper
			Glue

	Experiment Food tasting	10 Minutes	Assortment of healthy snack foods (see attached)

II. Snacks
  A. Considerations
  B. Healthy choices
    • Fruits
    • Vegetables
    • Nuts, etc.
	Discussion
	Puzzle
	(see following pages)
		15 Minutes	Worksheet: "Smart Snacks for Me"
			Colors

III. Brushing
  A. Surfaces to brush
  B. Thoroughness
	Personal improvement
	(see following pages)
		10 Minutes	Disclosing tablets
			Toothbrush
			Mirror
			Sink
			Water
			Tooth model (if needed)

IV. Flossing necessity	Personal improvement (see following pages)	5 Minutes	Floss
V. Evaluation	Recall (see following pages)	10 Minutes	None
Lesson Extension	Allow students to color the worksheet (II. Smart Snacks for Me)		
Alternative Plan B Healthy Snacks	Bulletin board (see following pages)	20 Minutes	Magazines Glue Scissors

Summary of Discussion Questions

Lecture/Discussion

- What are some of your favorite types of snacks?
- How long does it take for bacteria in plaque to make acid on my teeth?
- If I wanted to have something to drink, should I have a cola or a glass of water? Why?

Educational game, display

- Are most of your pictures falling into the sugary or non-sugary category? Why do you suppose this is happening?

Experiment

- What favorite healthy snack should I eat to help me have strong, healthy teeth?

Personal improvement/experiment

- Suppose you had a toothbrush in your hand; can you show me the direction you would brush your teeth to make sure you were getting the plaque off? Show me.
- Why do I need to brush that way?

Culmination

- Can someone tell me a healthy snack I should eat to help my teeth be strong?
- If your friend tells you flossing is not important, what would your say to convince your friend it is very important?

Culmination

Today we learned that when we eat sugary snacks, it only takes about 20 minutes for bacteria in plaque to make acid, which causes cavities. We learned about healthy snacks that are helpful to our teeth.

Question: Can someone tell me a healthy snack I should eat to help my teeth be strong?

We also practiced brushing and flossing properly.

Question: If your friend tells you flossing is not important, what would your say to convince your friend it is very important?

On Thursday, we will be learning about the basic food groups and proper proportions.

Anticipated Problems

Problems:

- Some students may have food allergies; check before allowing students to taste food items.
- Students may be reluctant to try the disclosing tablet—allow these children to practice brushing on the tooth model.

Lesson Extension: Allow students to color the worksheet (II. Smart Snacks for Me).

Plan B: Have students make a collage of healthy snack foods. Construct a "Smart Snacks for Me" poster or bulletin board display with pictures of no-sugar-added snack foods.

Evaluation

By the end of class, the students will have met the outlined objectives and be assessed via observation and questioning. The instructor will review and assess the worksheet Smart Snacks for Me, the collage, and the students' brushing/flossing techniques.

Supplemental Material to Support the Developmental Section

I. Sugar

Method/Strategy (Lecture, Discussion)

Discussion question: What are some of your favorite types of snacks?

A. Many common snack foods contain sugar. Show pictures of examples; include cake, candy, pie, sweet rolls, ice cream, cookies, doughnuts, sugared chewing gum, sugar-containing soft drinks, chocolate milk, and sugar-containing gelatin desserts.

B. Bacteria in plaque make acid when sugar is in the mouth. Each time food containing sugar is eaten, the bacteria continue to make acid (for about 20 minutes). Bacteria eat the surface of the tooth and leave holes in your teeth, called cavities.

Discussion questions:

1. If I wanted to have something to drink, should I have a cola or a glass of water? Why?
2. How long does it take for bacteria in plaque to make acid on my teeth?

C. When you eat sugary foods, you increase your chances of letting bacteria attack your teeth. This is why it is important to choose healthy foods that will not damage your teeth.

Method/Strategy (Educational Game, Display)

Give students magazines containing food items. Have students cut out pictures and separate them into food categories, sugary and non-sugary. Give each student two sheets of construction paper and label one sugary and the other non-sugary. Let the students glue their pictures on the appropriate page.

Discussion question: Are most of your pictures falling into the sugary or non-sugary category? Why do you suppose this is happening?

Method/Strategy (Experiment)

Discuss that snack foods need to be nutritious and do not have to be sugary to be good.

Have a tasting party. Blindfold students and have them eat small pieces of healthy snack foods and have them guess what it is according to taste, texture, and smell. Then have them rate the food as sugary or non-sugary. Emphasize that although fruits have sugar, they are a healthier choice when you want a sugary snack.

Discussion question: What favorite healthy snack should I eat to help me have strong, healthy teeth? *Note:* Some foods might include oranges, tangerines, apples, celery, carrots, cheese crackers, popcorn, pretzels, etc.

II. Snack Considerations

If an individual must snack, there are many nutritious non-sugary snack foods. They include meat, nuts, cheese, fresh fruits and vegetables, unsweetened fruit juices, sugarless soft drinks, milk, plain yogurt, hard-boiled eggs, popcorn, and pretzels.

Method/Strategy (Discussion, Puzzle)

Pass out the worksheet "Smart Snacks for Me" and have the students indicate those foods containing and not containing added sugar.

This section should take approximately 15 minutes. The material needed is the Smart Snacks for Me worksheet. Extend the lesson by allowing students to color, if necessary and time permits.

III. Brushing

Method (Instruction/Lecture)

Tooth brushing will remove plaque from the outer, inner, and chewing surfaces of the teeth. It is probable that the thoroughness with which one brushes is more important than the specific technique used. Use of toothpaste is not required for classroom plaque removal. However, use of a toothpaste containing fluoride is recommended for brushing at home.

Note: Some students may have been taught other cleaning methods by their dentists or dental hygienist. They should continue to follow the instructions they have been given.

Method/Strategy (Personal Improvement/Experiment)

Discussion questions:

1. Suppose you had a toothbrush in your hand; can you show me the direction you would brush your teeth to make sure you were getting the plaque off?
2. Why do I need to brush that way?

Remind students of proper brushing techniques discussed in Week #1/ Thursday (see notes).

Have a volunteer student or two demonstrate the correct brush position on the model.

Disclosing Tablets Experiment—explain how the disclosing tablets work and how to properly use them (see instructions on the package).

Practice: Now allow all students to brush their teeth with partners. After the students are finished brushing, have them disclose and see the areas they missed. Partners will check to make sure the plaque has been removed from the teeth after brushing. Allow them to go back and brush again until the remaining disclosing dye is gone.

This section is approximately 10 minutes. Materials needed include disclosing tablets, toothbrush, mirror, sink, and water.

IV. Flossing

Method *(Instruction/Lecture)*

Flossing is necessary to remove plaque from between the teeth and under the gum line. It is important to clean these areas thoroughly because dental cavities and periodontal disease often start in these areas where the toothbrush frequently does not reach.

Note: A method of holding floss, which may be easier for children, is to tie a knot in the ends of 12 to 14 inches of floss to form a circle. Hold with the third, fourth, and fifth fingers of each hand. Use thumbs and forefingers to guide the floss.

Method/Strategy *(Personal Improvement)*

Now allow the children to practice flossing by distributing floss to each student. Instruct the children to pretend that their partner's fingers are their teeth. Have the partner hold out his or her hand with fingers close together, representing the way your teeth are close together in your mouth. Have students floss between the fingers of their partner's hand, practicing the flossing guideline discussed Week #1/Thursday (starting with the backside of the back tooth and working around the arch in a regular pattern—see notes). Each child should have a turn practicing the flossing technique.

Note: For first-grade students, teachers should obtain the assistance of local dental professionals or parents when attempting in-class flossing.

After the students are finished flossing, have them disclose and see the areas they missed. Allow them to go back and floss again until the remaining disclosing dye is gone.

This section will take approximately 8 to 12 minutes. Materials needed include floss, mirror, sink, and water.

V. Evaluation

Each objective will be assessed according to the following technique:

Objective	Technique of Assessment
Cognitive: By the end of the lesson, first-grade student will identify healthy snack foods by circling appropriate choices on the worksheet with 90% accuracy.	Instructor will grade the worksheet.
Psychomotor: The participant will create a food collage to classify multiple examples of healthy food choices discussed in the lecture as high in sugar or not high in sugar.	Instructor will review the collages to ensure that foods are placed in the correct category.
Psychomotor: By the end of the session, first-grade student will demonstrate plaque removal on tooth surfaces, to his or her partner, by removing the disclosing tablet stains using the method of brushing described.	Instructor will observe the student activity and interaction between partners to ensure participants are properly brushing.
Affective: Following the discussion on healthy snacks, the learner will verbally justify which of the three foods he or she believes would be the best choice to promote dental health.	Instructor will randomly call upon participants to check for understanding.

A copy of the worksheet Smart Snacks for Me would also be found with the supplemental materials that support the developmental section. The thoroughness of this lesson plan enables any person to execute it with fidelity. If another educator can basically follow your plan and present the material as you would, you have a well-developed plan.

EXERCISES

Exercise 1: You Be the Judge!   Take a look at the following lesson/presentation plans and critique them. Consider the appropriateness and feasibility of the objectives, the variety of the teaching methods, and the general "completeness" of the lesson/presentation plan. (Please note that in the interests of time and space the "content" section of the plans are highly abbreviated. A greater depth of information would ordinarily be required.)

Lesson/Presentation Plan 1

Group: 25 seventh-grade students, mixed ability
Unit: Addictive behaviors (four sessions)
Topic: Cigarette smoking (first session)
Time: 50 minutes

Objectives

1. Students will understand that smoking is an unhealthy habit.
2. Students will understand the harmful effects of smoking.
3. Students will decide to stop or not begin cigarette smoking.

Introduction

Students will write down all the reasons why people their age begin smoking cigarettes.

Development

Content	Method	Time	Materials
1. Reasons why people begin smoking	Q & A	10 minutes	Pen/paper
2. Physical effects of smoking	Lecture	20 minutes	LCD projector, Computer screen
3. Smoking and addiction	Lecture	15 minutes	Posters

Note: Would include attachments with content details.

Conclusion

Verify that students have understood the basic concepts of the lesson by asking them questions about the material covered in class. Students will respond orally.

Critique of Lesson Plan 1

Objectives

The first problem with this lesson plan is that the objectives are poorly stated. The first two objectives are more like goals in that they are written in a very general and nonmeasurable sense. The verb *understand* is not appropriate for use in objective writing unless it is followed by another verb that reflects the degree or specificity of "understanding," such as *list* or *describe*. The problem with the third objective, "Students will decide to stop or not begin cigarette smoking," is that it is unrealistically optimistic. Again, as a goal for a lesson, this type of statement would not be out of place. However, to suggest that a 50-minute lesson could have such a dramatic, immediate impact on health behavior is to set up the health educator and the program for failure. When individuals begin smoking or fail to stop smoking, the behavioral objectives have not been met, and critics of the program might justifiably question the validity of continued support for such an ineffectual program. This objective could be made appropriate by qualifying it as follows: "Students will *be able to cite reasons* for stopping or not beginning cigarette smoking."

Development   The lesson has a promising beginning with quick involvement of the students in the learning process. They write down reasons why people their age begin smoking cigarettes and then, through question and answer, the responses are verbalized. Unfortunately for both the teacher and the students, that is the end of student involvement! For the majority of the lesson (35 minutes) the teacher intends to lecture to this class of seventh graders . . . good luck! In addition, the use of audiovisual equipment such as the LCD projector, which requires semidarkness and is not traditionally known for scintillating lessons, could exacerbate the problems. When developing a lesson/presentation plan, the instructor needs to pay particular attention to the target population. In this case, seventh-grade students require teaching methods far more diverse than simply lecture. Break up a 35-minute block by using methods that are more interactive and interesting and yet still permit the dissemination of important information (see Chapter 4).

Conclusion

The teacher has allowed for some type of summary, or wrap-up, in the form of verbal responses to questions. This conclusion may allow the teacher to get a sense of how effective the lesson has been. It is a method often used, yet it could be criticized as being somewhat haphazard. A better conclusion would be to allow a little more time so that teams could be organized and a game format could be utilized to review the information. Such a review could be followed by a brief pencil and paper test (see Chapter 4).

Lesson/Presentation   **Group:** 35 older adults (ages 60 to 65) in community group setting
Plan 2   **Topic:** Nutrition (one session only)
Time: 1 hour

Objectives

1. Participants will be able list the four major food groups.
2. Participants will be able to describe the contents of a well-balanced meal.
3. Participants will appreciate the relationship between nutrition and health and make a commitment to improve their diets.

Introduction

Facilitator will uncover four dishes (or photographs) at the front of the room to reveal four meals. Each dish will be described, and participants will be asked to rank-order each dish according to its nutritional value.

Development

Content	Method	Time	Materials
1. Describe the four major food groups	Lecture	15 minutes	Pictures of food
2. Discuss suggested daily caloric intake	Q & A	15 minutes	Pamphlets
3. Suggested healthy-food preparation	DVD	25 minutes	DVD, computer, LCD projector, and screen
4. Question time	Respond to questions	5 minutes	None

Note: Would include attachments with content details.

Critique of Lesson Plan 2

Objectives

The first two objectives are quite good in that they are measurable, fairly precise, and seemingly achievable. They could be even better if a qualifier of standard were added: "List four major food groups *according to . . .*" and "Describe the contents of a well-balanced meal *according to . . .*". This way the parameters and criteria of the objectives are specifically stated. Additionally, there is no clear indicator of evidence to prove the objective has been met. There are a few problems with objective 3. First, the verb *appreciate* is too vague; it should be followed by a verb that quantifies the objective. For example:

> Participants will appreciate the relationship between nutrition and health by listing on the whiteboard five positive effects that a sound diet can have on health, according to the workshop.

Also, the third objective is actually two objectives within one. This is not an uncommon problem with individuals who are inexperienced in objectives design. We have already discussed the difficulty with using ambivalent terms like *appreciate*, but now the facilitator has added another objective related to committing to an improvement in diet. Such a commitment is not a bad objective if a qualifier is added:

> Participants will make a commitment to improve their diets *by voluntarily joining a relevant support group.*

However, this objective cannot simply be tacked on to the end of another; it must be given its own importance. It is quite possible that participants will be able to list five positive effects of a good diet and yet will refuse to join a support group. In this case, has the instructor succeeded or failed to achieve the objective? Keep objectives simple, and beware of linking two objectives together by use of the word *and.*

Introduction

The intended introduction is an excellent attention getter and is a practical and effective way for the facilitator to both gain the audience's attention and lead into the subject matter of the workshop. Unfortunately, the presentation plan shows no evidence of any follow-up of this introduction in the development section. Warm-up exercises in the classroom and introductions in the community presentation are usually effective when they are innovative and capture the attention of the participants, but they have to be connected to the development section of the lesson/presentation so that their relevance and connection to the main topic become obvious. In this specific instance, the facilitator planned an extremely innovative introduction by bringing actual meals to the workshop to enable a practical comparison. After being rank-ordered, the meals could have been incorporated into the discussion of the major food groups and the preparation of nutritious meals. This inclusion would have added a real-life feel to the workshop, and the presentation would have tied together more effectively.

Development

The biggest weakness of this presentation plan is the passivity of the learning process. The participants are simply not actively involved in the workshop, and concerns about boredom and distraction must be considered. If the facilitator is an outstanding speaker who can hold the attention of audiences, then these concerns might be minimized. The question-and-answer period is the only part of the plan that calls for group participation, and even this method affords only a low level of participation.

The facilitator intends to show a 25-minute DVD. In contrast to the school setting (cited in Plan 1), where the discipline issue could be problematic, the concern with this target population could well be fatigue. Will the DVD be riveting enough to even keep the audience awake, especially after several minutes of lecturing preceding the DVD? Health education media are often dull and boring and should be used only if they impart important information, are relevant to the audience, and are at least minimally interesting. A more fundamental question might be, is a 25-minute DVD too long to use in a 1-hour workshop? Many experienced presenters might feel that unless the DVD is of exceptional importance, it is in fact too long to be used in such a brief workshop. A more effective approach might be to view only parts of the DVD so that at least some of the value of the media could be utilized.

Allowing 5 minutes to answer questions is almost certainly not enough, particularly in light of so much information being disseminated without any substantial discussion. The DVD would undoubtedly raise issues and concerns, and allowing only 5 minutes for responding to questions is simply poor planning.

Conclusion

There is no conclusion! The facilitator has allowed no time for it, nor for any type of evaluation. In an attempt to perhaps reinforce the material covered in the workshop, the facilitator plans to distribute pamphlets. Distributing pamphlets is common practice and can be an effective means to achieve several goals. This process, however, should not replace the summary or conclusion of a presentation and obviously plays no part in evaluation. In addition to some type of evaluation (however informal), dealing with what the audience has learned and how the facilitator has performed, the facilitator should also be concerned about the effectiveness of the DVD and whether or not using nearly half the workshop time showing it is worthwhile. Obtaining participant feedback on the DVD is one way to achieve this end.

Both of these presentation plans have some obvious problems. They are good examples of how crucial thoughtful planning is to the success of any presentation. Think about the type of class or workshop you would like to be involved in as a participant; conversely, remember some of the characteristics of the most boring and ineffective classes or presentations you have sat through. Do not perpetuate poor presentation methods! Thorough planning and method consideration can minimize your chances of boring someone else to death.

Exercise 2: Now You Try! Using your newfound knowledge of lesson/presentation planning, consider the following scenarios and develop an appropriate lesson/presentation plan for each. Remember to include achievable objectives and a variety of methods.

1. You are teaching the first of a four-session unit on cigarette smoking to a class of 25 seventh graders of mixed ability. The class period is 50 minutes long.
2. You are conducting a single, once-only workshop on hypertension for a group of 20 older adults (ages 50 to 65). The group is racially diverse and includes both men and women. The workshop lasts for 1 hour and 15 minutes.
3. You are teaching the final session of a three-session unit on sexuality and communication, including the subject of date rape, to a group of 20 tenth-grade high school students. The class period is 50 minutes long.
4. You are completing a two-session workshop on bicycle and traffic safety for a group of 18 ten-year-old children from a local youth group. Each session is 1 hour long, and all the children have brought their own bicycles with them.

For more information and tools related to this chapter visit http://healtheducation.jbpub.com/strategies.

CASE STUDIES REVISITED

Case Study Revisited: Michael   Appropriate planning allows the instructor to manage the educational environment, ensuring that the objectives are addressed. Michael's lack of variety, direction, and poor allocation of time resulted in a dreary presentation. His attitude that school and community health educators need to develop different sets of skills is all too common among many health education students. Regardless of what we call the "entity," the planning and delivery is virtually the same for both school and community health educators. When Michael stands up in front of a community group for an hour-long presentation and then declares that he does not teach, one has to wonder what he has been doing! (See page 198.)

Case Study Revisited: Shane   Shane and Mary have made numerous errors in planning. Shane has failed to construct an appropriate lesson plan with clear objectives, methods, and content. Mary has made several inappropriate decisions regarding content and format. Shane failed to make the school standards clear to his substitute for the day. The regular teacher at the high school should also assume some of the blame since she failed to share the school standards with the substitute. Generally, the regular teacher is held accountable for the presentation of any guest speaker, and that means she must communicate the standards of the school and school district to any speaker. (See page 201.)

SUMMARY

1. Lesson/presentation plans are vital to ensure coverage of important objectives in a purposeful manner.

2. Lesson/presentation plans and unit plans are important to ensure fidelity to the intention of the program developers.

3. A backup plan should be developed for components of a lesson plan that require the cooperation of the target group.

4. Evaluation is important for the improvement of any lesson or unit plan.

5. Unit plans are very useful for programs with more than 5 hours of contact time and are much more than a collection of lesson plans.

6. It is important to avoid the sin of reinventing the wheel. There are many good resources for purchase or to be shared via the Internet.

REFERENCES AND RESOURCES

Ames, E. E., Trucano, L. A., Wan, J. C., & Harris, M. II. (1992). *Designing School Health Curricula; Planning for Good Health.* Dubuque, IA: W.C. Brown.

Arends, R. I. (1991). *Learning to Teach.* New York: McGraw-Hill.

Bates, I. J., & Wider, A. E. (1984). *Introduction to Health Education.* Palo Alto, CA: Mayfield.

Bedworth, A. E., & Bedworth, D. A. (1992). *The Profession and Practice of Health Education.* Dubuque, IA: W.C. Brown.

Bender, S. J., Neutens, J. J., Skonie-Hardin, S., & Sorochan, W. D. (1997). *Teaching Health Science: Elementary and Middle School* (4th ed.). Boston: Jones and Bartlett.

Bloom, B. S. (Ed.). (1984). *Taxonomy of Educational Objectives (Book 1, Cognitive Domain).* White Plains, NY: Longman.

Breckon, D. J., Harvey, J. R., & Lancaster, R. B. (1994). *Community Health Education: Settings, Roles and Skills for the 21st Century* (3rd ed.). Gaithersburg, MD: Aspen.

Carroll, L. (1946). *Alice in Wonderland and Through the Looking Glass.* New York: Grosset and Dunlap.

Galli, N. (1978). *Foundations and Principles of Health Education.* New York: Wiley.

Goodlad, J. I. (1984). *A Place Called School: Prospects for the Future.* New York: McGraw-Hill.

Greenberg, J. S. (1988). *Health Education: Learner-Centered Instructional Strategies.* Dubuque, IA: W.C. Brown.

Greene, W. H., & Simons-Morton, B. G. (1984). *Introduction to Health Education.* New York: Macmillan.

Hellison, D. (1978). *Beyond Balls and Bats: Alienated (and Other) Youth in the Gym.* Washington, DC: AAHPER Publications.

Hoff, R. (1988). *I Can See You Naked.* New York: Andrews and McMeel.

Joyce, B., & Weil, M. (1986). *Models of Teaching.* Englewood Cliffs, NJ: Prentice Hall.

Kellough, R., & Kellough, N. (2007). *Secondary School Teaching: A Guide to Methods and Resources* (3rd ed.). Upper Saddle River, NJ: Pearson.

Lazes, P. M., Kaplan, L. H., & Gordon, K. A. (1987). *The Handbook of Health Education.* Rockville, MD: Aspen.

Mayshark, C., & Foster, R. (1966). *Methods in Health Education.* St. Louis: C.V. Mosby.

McKenzie, J. F., Pinger, R. R., & Kotecki, J. E. (1999). *An Introduction to Community Health* (3rd ed.). Boston: Jones and Bartlett.

Meeks, L., Heit, P., & Page, R. (1996). *Comprehensive School Health Education* (2nd ed.). Backlick, OH: Meeks Heit.

National Health Education Standards. (2007). (2nd ed.). American Cancer Society. Retrieved June 24, 2009, from http://www.cancer.org/docroof/PED/content/PED_13_2x_National_Health_Ed_Standards.asp/sitearea=PED

Pike, R. W. (2003). *Creative Training Techniques Handbook* (3rd ed.). Amherst, MA: HRD Press.

Read, D. A. (1997). *Health Education: A Cognitive-Behavioral Approach.* Boston: Jones and Bartlett.

Rubinson, L., & Alles, W. F. (1984). *Health Education: Foundations for the Future.* Prospect Heights, IL: Waveland.

Scott, G. D., & Carlo, M. W. (1979). *On Becoming a Health Educator.* Dubuque, IA: W.C. Brown.

U.S. Department of Health, Education, and Welfare. (1979). *Healthy People: The Surgeon General's Report on Health Promotion and Disease* (Publication 79-55071). Washington, DC: U.S. Public Health Service.

U.S. Department of Health and Human Services. (1980). *Promoting Health Preventing Disease: Objectives for the Nation.* Washington, DC: U.S. Public Health Service.

Wilgoose, C. E. (1972). *Health Teaching in Secondary Schools.* Philadelphia: W.B. Saunders.

Personal Computers and the Internet

Entry-Level and Advanced 1 Health Educator Competencies Addressed in This Chapter

Responsibility I:	Assess Individual and Community Needs for Health Education
Competency A:	Access existing health-related data.

Responsibility II:	Plan Health Education Strategies, Interventions, and Programs
Competency G:	Assess factors that affect implementation.

Responsibility III:	Implement Health Education Strategies, Interventions, and Programs
Competency A:	Initiate plan of action.
Competency B:	Demonstrate a variety of skills in delivering strategies, interventions, and programs.
Competency C:	Use a variety of methods to implement strategies, interventions, and programs.

Responsibility VI:	Serve as a Health Education Resource Person
Competency A:	Use health-related information resources.
Competency C:	Select resource materials for dissemination.

Responsibility VII:	Communicate and Advocate for Health and Health Education
Competency B:	Apply a variety of communication methods and techniques.

Note: The competencies listed above, which are addressed in this chapter, are considered to be both entry-level and Advanced 1 competencies by the National Commission for Health Education Credentialing, Inc. They are taken from *A Framework for the Development of*

Method Selection in Health Education

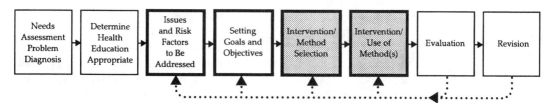

Heavy-bordered boxes indicate subjects addressed in this text; shaded boxes indicate subjects(s) of current chapter.

Competency Based Curricula for Entry Level Health Educators by the National Task Force for the Preparation and Practice of Health Education, 1985; *A Competency-Based Framework for Graduate Level Health Educators,* by the National Task Force for the Preparation and Practice of Health Education, 1999; and *A Competency-Based Framework for Health Educators—The Competencies Update Project (CUP)*, 2006.

OBJECTIVES   After studying this chapter the reader will be able to:

- Describe the development and importance of technology in health education.
- List the uses of a personal computer in the health education profession.
- Describe the components and process of evaluating websites.
- Correctly cite a source of information retrieved from a website.
- Describe the components and process of properly using chat rooms.
- Describe the uses of distance education in health education.
- Locate the email addresses of health educators using the Health Education Directory Internet Resource (HEDIR).

KEY ISSUES

Internet access	Distance learning
Evaluating websites	Virtual reality
Citing web sources	Chat rooms
Netiquette	Forums
PCs and health education	Blogs

The above listing of commonplace terms now used daily is perhaps evidence of the most explosive technological advances of the 20th century—almost limitless access to information through the use of personal computers and the Internet. Not long ago, searching for information about any subject usually involved a trip to a local library and a walk through the dusty stacks of books, hoping that the volume in question had not already been borrowed by another inquisitive patron. Although libraries today still fulfill an important role as providers of the printed word, even these institutions have altered their focus to utilize Internet access. According to a 2007 national survey of U.S. libraries, at least 99.1% of libraries provide online services to the public (Bertot, McClure, & Jaeger, 2007). Universally, vast numbers of individuals seeking information of all types turn, as a matter of course, to their personal computers and literally search the world for answers to their questions. The explosion of personal computer usage in the United States is an indicator of habits changed forever. In the mid-1980s only about 8% of Americans had a personal computer in their home, but by 2004 that number had increased to nearly 65% (International Telecommunications Union [ITU], 2006). It is estimated that there are over a billion personal computers in use around the world. In addition to personal computer ownership, computer experts estimate that approximately one-third of Internet users log on using either a laptop, handheld personal digital assistant (PDA), or smart phone using WIFI broadband or other cell phone networks (Horrigan, 2007). Perhaps most important for health educators is the statistic that nearly 53.5% of those individuals accessing the Web are seeking information related to health issues (Diaz et al., 2002).

Caveat Emptor

Although the Internet gives us the opportunity to access a wealth of current, accurate, state-of-the-art data, we can also be confronted with just the opposite . . . outdated, inaccurate, biased, controversial, and often unfounded information. Anyone who has access to the Internet can develop a website, and although many people assume information published on the Web to be accurate, the mere existence of a site means nothing with regard to legitimacy or objectivity. Many websites provide information that is vague as to its source or authorship. Some sites are blatantly biased; others appear to be legitimate but carry subtly prejudicial messages.

The Internet is a multibillion-dollar marketing tool, so users should be aware of the potential association between information and commercially marketed products. What makes the Internet unique with regard to legitimacy of information is that there is no screening device between the site developer and the user. Research or academic libraries, for example, have developed mechanisms whereby journals, books, and other resources have already been evaluated for inclusion in the library as legitimate resources. When you search for information on any given topic in such a library, any index or database that you access has been developed by a scholarly organization with an eye to maintaining strict standards of accuracy and legitimacy. No such screening device exists on the Internet; therefore, the user is exposed to an incredible diversity of material, often ranging from the sublime to the ridiculous. Clearly this is a case of *caveat emptor*, or buyer beware!

Objective: After reviewing the case study, the reader will explain how the principle of *caveat emptor* applies to Robyn's experience using Internet information.

Case Study: Robyn   Robyn has been asked to facilitate a prenatal workshop for a community group of expectant mothers. Robyn has been extremely busy lately, feeling overwhelmed with the numerous projects with which she has been involved. As the evening of the workshop date arrives, she has not yet pulled together materials for her presentation. Racing against time, Robyn decides to perform a rapid Internet search for relevant resources. Her search results in a myriad of sites, of which she selects a few that look the most promising and interesting. Hastily making photocopies of the information, Robyn heads to her workshop. The session begins well, with introductions, an explanation of the purpose of the workshop and the dissemination of the first Internet-generated handout— a discussion about diet during pregnancy. Robyn's growing confidence is abruptly punctured as an astonished and increasingly irate participant loudly notes that the author of the handout was a doctor who had lost his license to practice medicine for promoting his own diet plan that was judged to be unsafe and, in two instances, potentially fatal. Robyn, obviously shocked, stammers an apology and quickly moves on to another handout, fervently hoping that lightning won't strike twice! (See Case Studies Revisited page 247.)

Questions to consider:

1. What steps could Robyn have taken to avoid this problem?
2. Whose responsibility is it to assess the credibility of an Internet source?

The Feds Strike Back!

The Federal Trade Commission (FTC), the government watchdog organization responsible for monitoring, among other things, false claims developed by manufacturers and distributors of health and medical products, has created an innovative learning device. Instead of issuing boring, ineffective warnings about being fooled by unscrupulous "snake oil salesmen," the FTC has joined the game. In 1999 the FTC developed several bogus Web sites supposedly selling miracle cures and treatments like NordiCalite (weight loss), ArthritiCure (arthritis treatment), and Virility Plus (impotence) (see Figure 6-1). The screens describe the miraculous effects of the products and urge the consumer to purchase them immediately. When the consumer clicks on to the last screen to obtain the payment information, a screen explains that the Web site was developed by the FTC and is selling a nonexistent product. The site user is advised that many hundreds of Web sites exist that collect money without sending a product, sell products that have no medicinal or health value, and are being supported by false or exaggerated claims. This is an extremely innovative way to use the Internet to educate consumers about the dangers of purchasing from an unknown website.

According to *The Washington Post* (1999), the FTC visited about 800 sites over a 2-year period that contained questionable medical or health claims. The owners of these sites were sent an email warning that they were potentially violating federal law. When these same sites were rechecked some months later, approximately 62% were unchanged. Moreover, although the FTC charged 91 Internet sites with fraudulent advertising in a 4-year period, the number of new sites proliferates on a daily basis. This would seem to suggest that creating more educated and sophisticated consumers might be a more productive and effective route than legal action. The FTC advises consumers to beware of marketing that includes the following techniques (Meadows, 2006):

- Claiming the product will quickly cure a variety of ailments
- Using words such as "scientific breakthrough," "secret ingredient," or "ancient remedy"

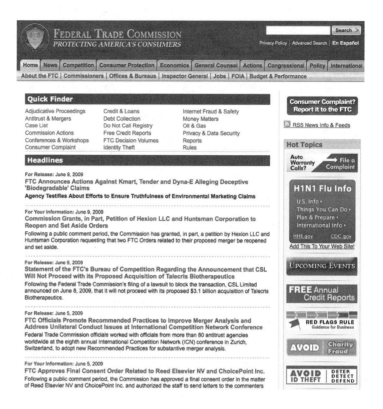

Figure 6-1
The Federal Trade
Commission Website

- Using impressive-sounding "medicalese" such as "thermogenesis" or "hunger stimulation point"
- Claiming the government, scientists, or the medical profession have conspired to suppress the product
- Including undocumented case histories or testimonials citing miraculous results
- Advertising the product as available from only one source or in limited supply
- Promise of no-risk or money-back guarantees

Evaluating Internet Sites

Assessing the credibility of an Internet site is an incredibly important concern given that millions of people are using the Web on a daily basis, and a high proportion of these users are seeking health-related information. Without some type of barometer, how do we evaluate the legitimacy and accuracy of information obtained from the Internet, and what types of issues should users consider? A list of such criteria was developed by Betsy Richmond (2000) of the McIntyre Library at the University of Wisconsin-Eau Claire; it is shown in Table 6-1.

Table 6-1 Ten Cs for Evaluating Internet Resources

Criteria	Explanation
1. Content	What is the intent of the content? Are the title and author identified? Is the document "juried"? Is the content "popular" or "scholarly," satiric or serious? What is the date of the document or article? Is the edition current? Do you have the latest version? (Is this important?) How do you know?
2. Credibility	Is the author identifiable and reliable? Is the content credible? Authoritative? Should it be? What is the purpose of the information, that is, is it serious, satiric, or humorous? Is the URL extension .edu, .com, .gov, or .org? What does this tell you about the "publisher"?
3. Critical thinking	How can you apply critical thinking skills, including previous knowledge and experience, to evaluate Internet resources? Can you identify the author, publisher, edition, and so on as you would with a "traditionally" published resource? What criteria do you use to evaluate Internet resources?
4. Copyright	Even if the copyright notice does not appear prominently, the material falls under the copyright conventions. Fair use applies to short, cited excerpts, usually as an example for commentary or research. Materials are in the public domain if this is explicitly stated. Internet users, as users of print media, must respect copyright.
5. Citation	Internet resources should be cited to identify sources used, both to give credit to the author and to provide the reader with avenues for further research. Standard style manuals (print and online) provide examples of how to cite Internet documents.
6. Continuity	Will the Internet site be maintained and updated? Is it now and will it continue to be free? Can you rely on this source over time to provide up-to-date information? Some good .edu sites have moved to .com, with possible cost implications. Other sites offer partial free use and charge fees for continued in-depth use.
7. Censorship	Is your discussion list "moderated"? What does this mean? Does your search engine or index look for all words, or are some words excluded? Is this censorship? Does your institution, based on its mission, parent organization, or space limitations, apply some restrictions to Internet use? Consider censorship and privacy issues when using the Internet. If you are working with young people, you need to apply some censorship.
8. Connectivity	If more than one user will need to access a site, consider each user's access and "functionality." How do users connect to the Internet, and what kind of connection does the assigned resource require? Does access to the resource require additional software, such as Adobe Reader or a media player?
9. Comparability	Does the Internet resource have an identified comparable print or CD-ROM data set or source? Does the Internet site contain comparable and complete information? (For example, some newspapers have partial but not full text information on the Internet.) Do you need to compare data or statistics over time? Can you identify sources for comparable earlier or later data? Comparability of data may or may not be important, depending on your project.
10. Context	What is the context for your research? Can you find "anything" on your topic—that is, commentary, opinion, narrative, statistics—and your quest will be satisfied? Are you looking for current or historical information? Definitions? Research studies or articles? How does Internet information fit in the overall information context of your subject? Before you start searching, define the research context and research needs and decide what sources might be best to successfully fill information needs without data overload.

Source: Richmond, B. (2000). *10 Cs for Evaluating Internet Resources.* Eau Claire, WI: University of Wisconsin, McIntyre Library (richmoeb@uwec.edu). Reprinted with permission.

| **NOTEWORTHY** | **Internet Example: Just Who *Is* Telling the Truth?** |

Access the Internet and go to http://healtheducation.jbpub.com/strategies. Follow the links to read *Ten Simple, Compelling Claims to Frame Arguments Against Drug Legalization* and *A Response to DEA Statements*.

You will find two entirely opposite views, with point-by-point rebuttals of established government arguments related to the issue of drug legalization. Which statements are true? How can the viewpoints be so different? Surely, a government (.gov) website is more credible than a private organization (.org) site? Check out the statements, and you be the judge. How could you best utilize information of this type that is seemingly so contradictory?

Another way to approach a critical evaluation of Internet sites is to examine how scholars evaluate print media and apply the same criteria to electronic information. Aleteia Greenwood (2008) developed six basic categories of such criteria: author and source, accuracy, currency, objectivity, coverage, and purpose. Greenwood's categories include a checklist of questions to help determine whether an electronic page is suitable. With Greenwood's permission, we will now present these (adapted) criteria:

1. **Author and source:** It is important to ask questions of authorship and source because often we are taught to believe that what we read in a magazine or book or on the Web is true. But this is not necessarily the case. If you cannot find an author or an organization connected to a website, be very, very suspicious. If no one is willing to stand behind the creation of the page, why should you believe what is written there? Even if you can find an organization or author, you still need to be cautious and make sure that the organization and/or author are who they say they are. This may include further research on a particular author or organization. Consider the following questions:
   - Is there an author of the work? If so, is the author clearly identified?
   - Are the author's credentials for writing on this topic stated?
   - Is the author affiliated with a credible organization?
   - Does the site or page represent a group, organization, institution, corporation, or government body?
   - Is there a link back to the organization's page or a way to contact the organization or the author to verify the credibility of the site (address, phone number, email address)?
   - Is it clear who is responsible for the creation and/or maintenance of the site or page?
   Authorship is perhaps the major criterion used in evaluating information. Is the author well-known in the field? Is the author a name that is recognized? If not, Kirk (1996) recommends you consider if:

- The author mentioned is referenced by an authority you trust.
- You arrived at the source (linked to it) from a trusted source.
- There is biographical information about the author—including the author's position, institutional affiliation, address, or a provided information link.

2. **Accuracy:** Unlike the world of traditional print where information undergoes a process of peer review, publications on the Web are not required to pass such rigorous review and revision processes. As a result, not all webpages are reliable. Documents can easily be copied and falsified or copied with omissions and errors—intentional or accidental. When using web resources, strive to review scholarly documents and peer-reviewed e-journals. These types of publications typically follow the review process of traditional print. When evaluating accuracy, consider the following:
   - Is this page part of an edited or peer-reviewed publication?
   - Can factual information be verified through footnotes or bibliographies to other credible sources?
   - Based on what you already know about the subject, or have checked from other sources, does this information seem credible?
   - Is it clear who has the responsibility for the accuracy of the information presented?
   - If statistical data are presented in graphs or charts, are they labeled clearly?

3. **Currency:** Some information is timeless; however, updating data is extremely important for many subjects, particularly the sciences where information may change quickly and drastically. One should evaluate the regularity with which the data are updated. The date showing the currency of a site is usually near the bottom of the page. If links to other webpages are not current, this is a fairly good sign that the site is not well-maintained. Evaluate the currency by considering the following:
   - When was the document originally created?
   - When was the site or page last updated, revised, or edited?
   - Are there any indications that the material is updated frequently or consistently to ensure currency of the content?
   - If there are links to other webpages, are they current?

4. **Objectivity:** Consider who is providing the information, because authors and publishers are rarely neutral. If advertisements are present, consider the possibility of a relationship between the content of the page and the advertising. Could there be a conflict of interest? Check other sources to verify the information. Look closely at how information is presented. Are opinions clearly stated, or is the information vague? It is acceptable for a page to present a biased opinion, but you—as the consumer of the information—should know what that opinion is. It should be clear, not hidden. Other questions to consider related to objectivity include:
   - Is the page free of advertising? If the page does contain advertising, are the ads clearly separated from the content?

- Does the page display a particular bias or perspective, or is the information presented factually, without bias?
- Is the view of the subject clear and straightforward?
- Does it use inflammatory or provocative language?

5. **Coverage:** Consider the completeness of the document. If there is any indication that the page is still under construction, it may be better not to use it, because aspects of the page and the information on it may change by the time it is finished. If you are looking at a webpage for which there is a print equivalent, check to see if the entire work is on the webpage. If it is a portion of the work, make sure that quotes have not been taken out of context or that information has not been misrepresented. Evaluate completeness by asking:
   - Is there any indication that the page is complete, or is it still under construction?
   - If there is a print equivalent to the webpage, is there clear indication of whether the entire work or only a portion is available on the Web?

6. **Purpose:** Consider why the webpage has been posted. If the primary purpose of the website is to sell a product, a more credible source should be considered. Perhaps the purpose of the electronic resources is to empower others with knowledge, skills, or to influence a person's attitude about a topic. One should consider how comprehensive the information provided is and remember to look at the page critically. If a page has a narrow focus, try to make sure that relevant information has not been left out. Consider the purpose by asking the following questions:
   - What is the primary purpose of the page? To sell a product? To make a political point? To have fun? To parody a person, organization, or idea?
   - Is the page or site a comprehensive resource, or does it focus on a narrow range of information?
   - What is the emphasis of the presentation: technical, scholarly, clinical, popular, elementary?

NOTEWORTHY   **Seal of Approval**

Several organizations are trying to help with the evaluation of Internet sites. One notable example is the HONcode developed by the Health On the Net Foundation, which was established in 1996 after an international conference in Geneva on the medical use of the Internet. The code was developed to direct proper use of the Internet in sharing health information. A "seal" of approval was adopted for sites that comply with the standards. Although there are a significant number of adopters, even a brief look at Internet sources demonstrates only a small percentage of sites adhere to these rules. Visit their website at http://www.hon.ch.

Correctly Citing Web Sources

The Internet has become a major source of information and resources for many individuals who need to research specific topics. Although the library has historically been the first research "port of call" for most people, the speed, efficiency, and global nature of the Internet has revolutionized the way research is conducted. When using the Internet you are obligated to reference materials cited just as you would for any other source (see Figure 6-2). It is unethical and usually a violation of copyright law to use the work of another without proper citation. Professional researchers, scholars, and students are familiar with citing references from printed information such as journal articles, government publications, and books. However, citing information taken directly from websites sometimes is a relatively challenging endeavor, and although it is similar in nature to traditional referencing, there are a few noticeable differences. When citing a website or other address you should provide the usual information, as well as the date the site was accessed. Refer to the newest version of the style manual you are using for your paper or publication.

One of the most commonly used styles of references is that of the American Psychological Association (APA). The following are examples developed using the guidelines provided in the APA's *Publication Manual* (2001).

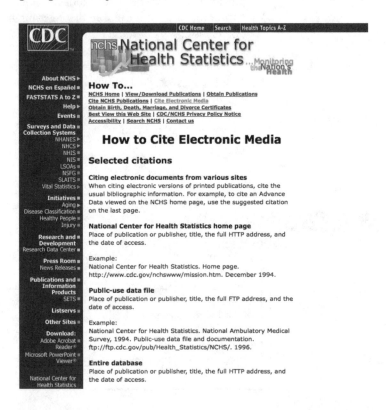

Figure 6-2
Electronic Resources
Need to Be Cited

- **Journal article:**
  McNeill, E., & Eddy, J. (2005). Planning ADE: Implications from literature on student perspectives. *International Electronic Journal of Health Education, 8,* 70–79. Retrieved September 16, 2008, from http://www.aahperd.org/iejhe/template.cfm?template=2005/mcneill.html
- **Newspaper article:**
  Yardley, J. (2008, September 15). Chinese baby formula scandal widens as 2nd death is announced. *New York Times.* Retrieved September 16, 2008, from http://www.nytimes.com
- **Abstract:**
  Andriole, D., Whelan, A. J., & Jeffe, D. B. (2008). Characteristics and career intentions for the emerging MD/PhD workforce. *Journal of the American Medical Association, 300*(10), 1165–1173. Abstract retrieved September 1, 2008, from MEDLINE (PubMed) database.
- **Action alert posted by APA's Public Policy Office:**
  American Psychological Association. (2006, June 27). APA public policy action alert: Political tensions impact grant awards [Announcement posted on the World Wide Web]. Washington, DC: Author. Retrieved September 25, 2007, from http://www.apa.org/ppo/istook.html
- **World Wide Web pages:**
  National Institutes of Health. (n.d.). Retrieved August 23, 2008, from http://www.nih.gov/index.html

There are a variety of interactive web tools designed to assist researchers in their efforts to credit sources appropriately. Many of these sites offer free access to software that can generate your citations in a designated format. Psych Web, operated by Dr. Russ Dewey, has an APA-style crib sheet that shows how to reference online resources:

Dewey, R. (2004). APA publication manual crib sheet. Retrieved August 15, 2008, from http://www.psychwww.com/resource/apacrib.htm

Public Domain in Health Education

A plethora of intellectual property is available to health educators from **public domain** sources. Information posted on most government websites is not owned or controlled by a specific entity; thus, it is considered in the public domain. Public domain information may be freely distributed and copied, but it is recommended that the source of the information be given appropriate acknowledgment. Keep in mind that you may discover materials such as illustrations, photographs, or other information resources on a public domain site that are contributed or licensed by private individuals, companies, or organizations; thus, they may be protected by U.S. and foreign copyright laws (National Library of Medicine [NLM], 2008).

When researching health-related data, it is a good practice to begin your search with sources that are recognized across the profession as credible sources. These include the sites of organizations such as:

- **National Institutes of Health (NIH):** http://www.nih.gov
- **Centers for Disease Control and Prevention (CDC):** http://www.cdc.gov
- **World Health Organization (WHO):** http://www.who.int/en

Additionally, you can explore sites that work in partnership to provide resources. For example, Partners in Information Access for the Public Health Workforce (http://phpartners.org/about.html) is a collaboration of U.S. government agencies, public health organizations, and health sciences libraries that provides access to selected public health resources on the Internet (NLM, 2008).

Technology in Health Education

Given that such revolutionary access to global information now exists, it is important to consider how this technology can be effectively incorporated as a tool of health educators. Certainly all health educators should have at least a rudimentary knowledge of computer usage, because most entry-level positions require such fundamental skills. Tasks that health educators might be expected to perform using this newer technology are as follows:

Using Handheld Devices (PDAs/ Smartphones)
- Texting
- Exchanging information between devices

Using Personal Computers
- Basic word processing functions, using programs such as Microsoft Word, that might range from simple reports to more complex activities such as newsletter or brochure development
- Data collection and recording with some type of spreadsheet software like Excel or SPSS
- Presentation preparation that might include charts, graphs, and presentation software such as PowerPoint (see Chapter 7)
- Utilizing health-related software, such as health risk appraisals or informational **CD-ROM** or **DVD**

Using the Internet
- Researching a topic to obtain the latest data
- Searching the Internet for websites that might provide differing viewpoints
- Searching specific websites for archival data
- Researching the application of methods by topic
- Reading or contributing to electronic professional journals. Many of these journals are good-quality, peer-reviewed publications that appear in an electronic format. In addition, many traditional health education journals are also accessible via the Internet (e.g., *American Journal of Health Behavior*).

Communicating via the Internet

This could be as basic as:

- Simple email messages
- Talking in a chat room
- Posting or reading messages on blogs, forums, or social networking sites

or something more elaborate like:

- Distance learning
- Videoconferencing
- Podcasting

The use of computer technology has certainly created exciting learning opportunities for classroom teachers, opening up new worlds to explore in addition to enhancing the more traditional modes of learning. Peck and Dorricot (1994) offer 10 reasons why classroom teachers should use technology in the classroom, presented in Table 6-2 with Steve Dorman's (1998) adaptation to the discipline of health education.

Table 6-2 Technology in the Classroom

Justification	Application to Health Education
#1 Students learn and develop at different rates.	One tenet of health education holds that the educator must consider the individual health and learning needs of the student. Use of technology in the classroom can facilitate this goal by evaluating and assessing the health needs of the user and starting the educational activity at an appropriate level for the learner. For example, many computer-based games and learning programs are able to assess the level of competence, record the playing history, and start the user at the appropriate level of the program.
#2 Graduates must be proficient at accessing, evaluating, and communicating information.	Living in the Information Age necessitates developing skills to access and evaluate health information. The average consumer is bombarded with information. Technology makes health information ever present. However, much of the information on the Internet, for example, is not evaluated and may be subject to error. Consumers must be able to access and evaluate the quality of information. Health educators, too, must be proficient in assessing, evaluating, and communicating health information as prescribed by the competencies of the entry-level educator.
#3 Technology can foster an increase in the quantity and quality of students' thinking and writing.	Technology opens avenues for study and exploration about health that until now would have required visiting a university campus or a major health center. The advanced information available allows the health education student to access an abundance of sources such as the Centers for Disease Control and Prevention (CDC), National Institutes of Health (NIH), and World Health Organization (WHO), which can stimulate advanced thinking about health issues and allow the student to develop more advanced solutions to health issues. Access to forums and listservs allows health education students to express themselves and to critique the expressions of others. HEDIR, the student HEDIR, and HLTHPROM are webforums that stimulate discussions and writings about health education related topics.
#4 Graduates must solve complex problems.	Technology allows students to explore complex health problems that would be difficult to simulate in a classroom without technology. For example, SimHealth, a computer game developed by the Markle Foundation, enables students to explore the impact of changes in government, health manpower, funding, taxation, and

(continues)

Table 6-2 Technology in the Classroom *(continued)*

Justification	Application to Health Education
	politics on the health of a local community. The average individual may take years to understand these complex relationships, yet this game presents them in a way that allows the user to grasp the dynamic impact they can have on health.
#5 Technology can nurture artistic expression.	Health-related graphic images such as those on the Visible Human Body Project give students access to visuals that previously were available only in the medical arena. These illustrations not only provide vital information about human anatomy, but also reveal the beauty of the human body in a way not seen before. In addition, with powerful software programs such as Freehand, Director Multimedia Studio, and 3D Choreographer, artistically inclined students can use technology to develop health-related computer activities, animations, and videos as class projects.
#6 Graduates must be globally aware and able to use resources that exist outside the school.	The Internet allows students inexpensive and instant access to health information around the world. Whether it is information about developments in biomedicine from the NIH, facts about disease transmission and epidemiology from the CDC, or late-breaking news on treatment and cures from the National Library of Medicine, the Internet allows the user access to this information found outside the walls of the school.
#7 Technology creates opportunities for students to do meaningful work.	Technology provides the conduit for individuals in the health and helping professions to contact difficult-to-reach populations. Many would listen to a mass communication message on television or other media, yet would not attend a public education lecture on the same topic. Health students can use technology to assemble highly creative venues for health information, which may indeed influence health behaviors. For example, students may be involved in video production, development of a computer-assisted instruction module on a health-related topic, or assembly of a dynamic set of webpages about a health issue.
#8 All students need access to high-level and high-interest courses.	Although the teacher should not rely on technology to supplant other stimulating forms of instruction or use technological application as a placating device for bored learners, technology can provide thought-provoking and stimulating avenues of study. CD-ROMs and DVDs, for example, provide the health education student with access to thousands of pictures of health-related issues and disorders.
#9 Students must feel comfortable with the tools of the Information Age.	The Information Age requires students to feel comfortable and proficient in accessing information about health by using technology. Students must feel capable and have a high level of comfort when interfacing with computers and technology formats to access health and other information.
#10 Schools must increase their productivity and efficiency.	Technology may help schools and teachers become more productive and efficient in health instruction. For example, electronic grading devices may give teachers more time to spend with students. Currently, several computer-based grade book programs are available for free downloading to an individual's computer. Local school-based electronic bulletin boards and email enable teachers to communicate easily with parents. CD-ROM technology allows teachers to implement learning stations in the health classroom, where students may engage in discovery learning at a pace on their level. Learners can be exposed to the basic facts about health by using technology, allowing the teacher to assist students with more complex tasks.

Source: Dorman, S. (1998). 10 reasons to use technology in the classroom. *Journal of School Health, 68*(1), 38–39. Reprinted with permission. American School Health Association, Kent, Ohio.

NOTEWORTHY   ## Health . . . the Internet . . . and Profit

Former surgeon general C. Everett Koop, famous for his then-radical position on HIV education and crusading attitude against the tobacco industry, became an Internet millionaire. Shares in the company that Dr. Koop founded were offered for public sale on Tuesday June 8, 1999, and the former surgeon general's share acquired a value of $56 million! Dr. Koop is well known to most health educators. (Washington Post, 1999).

It seems apparent that technology applications are considered standard practice in the training of educators. The National Council for Accreditation of Teacher Education (NCATE) accreditation standards pertaining to technology preparation require teacher training programs to demonstrate a commitment to preparing candidates who are able to use educational technology to help all students learn (Beasley & Wang, 2001). This standard requires programs preparing school-based health educators to show how information technology is integrated throughout the curriculum including instruction, field experiences, and assessments (Dorman, 2001). These standards impact the way school health teachers are prepared, and in turn influence the preparation of community health educators as well.

Distance Learning and Health Education

Distance learning, or *distance education,* is a term that has been with us for many years, employed whenever educators work with students over some distance. Early examples were homework help via "ham" radio in Australia and states with isolated communities like those found in Wyoming and Alaska. Later, regular phone lines were used, sometimes one-on-one and at other times at designated centers, sometimes in groups with a speaker phone. Educational television programming was often part of the package.

For many years the state of Wisconsin operated an audio network. This two-way audio network on a wide range of topics allowed groups to use teleconference equipment or to interact using a phone. There were approximately 30,000 participants as of April 22, 1999.

The addition of the computer and the Internet has opened up new and exciting avenues for meeting communication needs in health education through distance education, continuing education, and professional development. Advances in technology have spurred the evolution of off-site learning from correspondence courses to interactive video and virtual learning via distance education (Mattheos, Jonnson, Schittek, & Attstrom, 2000). Generally when we refer to distance education today we are discussing Internet use, using any combination of tools and sometimes involving an entire course or

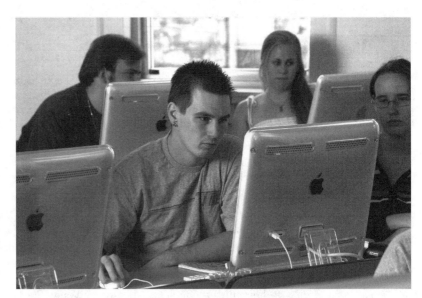

The abundance of personal computers and the Internet have made distance education a popular medium.

workshop. Many departments of health education and programs in public health are offering such courses or workshops today. Often they supplement traditional classroom courses with activities that require use of the Internet or offer Internet sites as sources of information.

Initially, technological problems limited the extensive use of the Internet for distance education by health educators—namely, slow speed of transmission, poor visual reception, bandwidth limitations on standard phone line capabilities, and high cost of quality hardware. All of these limitations have been overcome in most areas of the United States. Faster phone lines are available, and cable and other access points to homes are improving technical quality.

These limitations have been diminished with the enhancement of Internet speed, bandwidth capabilities, and increased accessibility of hardware devices. Sophisticated software such as Course Management Systems (CMS), Virtual Learning Environments (VLM), or Learning Management Systems (LMS) enable the student to become an active participant in the learning process by using capabilities like online chats, forums, testing, and submitting online text assignments. Along with the software, the course instructor can add a variety of tools (media) such as video lectures, Flash animations, podcasts, and videoconferencing to enhance the distance education student's experience. The addition of these tools and capabilities enables the student to take responsibility for the learning process and to determine the depth and breadth of exploration (McNeill & Eddy, 2005).

The growing demand for distance education is apparent. Student enrollments are escalating as students are shopping for education that meets their needs (Scott, Howell, Williams, & Lindsay, 2003). According to McNeill and Eddy (2005), multiple factors contribute to the increased interest in distance education. These include:

- **Convenience:** Students have the ability to access courses from remote locations and to complete course requirements during nontraditional hours.
- **Cost:** Although many distance education courses appear to be more expensive when compared to the cost per course hour at a traditional university, the savings in time and ancillary costs often offset the difference in expenses. The elimination of traditional supplemental costs related to room and board, travel, parking, and extracurricular expenses can very well make distance education a more economical solution for many students.
- **Flexible learning:** Not only does the distance education student have the ability to work when he or she wants, but he or she also has control over the pace of learning. The advantage of being able to set one's own pace without having to wait for the "rest of the class" to reach the same level of mastery saves the learner time that could be better used improving areas of weakness or exploring related topics of interest.
- **Expanded opportunities:** Opportunities to enroll in courses both nationally and internationally enhance the learner's exposure to a more diverse educational experience. The distance education student has the ability to gain insight from leaders in the profession in the comfort of his or her own surroundings.

As the interest in instructional technology continues to escalate, it is not surprising that universities are attempting to reach new student markets by enhancing the quality of distance instruction. Successful distance education programs are clearly linked to the quality of instructional applications and the extent to which the courses and programs meet the unique problems, needs, and capacity of the target audience (McNeill & Eddy, 2005). Although there are many advantages associated with distance education, it is important to be conscious of designing courses with pedagogical perspectives in mind. The U.S. Department of Education, Office of Post Secondary Education (2006) has identified common indicators of quality in distance education programs. These indicators include the following characteristics:

- A clear mission that includes a strong rationale for the distance education program that correlates to the mission of the institution.
- Centralized development of curriculum and instruction by a content expert including:
  - Defined course scope and objectives
  - Guidelines of course development and review of instructional materials established
  - Inclusion of active learning techniques, such as the use of personal risk assessments and methods that utilize diverse ways of learning (e.g., discussion boards, chat rooms)
  - Inclusion of program evaluation and assessment

- Faculty support services including training, access to specialized resources, and technical support designed to implement a distance education course.
- Attempts to plan for sustainability by incorporating student, academic, and faculty services as integrated components of the program. These plans might include:
  - Student support services to accommodate special needs of the distance learner, like a technical support line
  - Strategic technology plans to ensure quality, institutional support, and resources
- Incorporated techniques for evaluation and assessment.

In addition to the aforementioned indicators, two other commonly cited recommendations for developing quality distance education programs are providing opportunities for student–teacher interactions and providing prompt feedback (Chaney, Eddy, Dorman, Glessner, Green, & Lara-Alecio, 2007).

Internet Media

A by-product of the explosive growth in technology is the development of new jargon related to technology applications. Each type of medium, all of which may be used in distance education, provides a unique opportunity to retrieve or distribute information. The following sections attempt to describe various forms of commonly used media and highlight their unique features.

Web Lectures　Lectures are oral presentations designed to enlighten individuals about a particular topic. A web lecture is unique in that it performs this same function using the computer screen. Web lectures can be taped prior to or as they are being delivered and then made available for future viewing.

Podcasts　Consumers today have become accustomed to getting what they want when they want it. A podcast allows consumers to directly download or stream content from digital media formats at their convenience. A unique feature of a podcast is that it has the ability to be syndicated, subscribed to, and downloaded automatically to mobile devices such as an iPod, iPhone, or MP3 player. A student enrolled in a distance education course can download a podcast of a recorded lesson, which allows the student to listen to the lecture during the commute home from work or school.

Flash Animation　By using Adobe Flash, individuals have the ability to create animated films or Flash cartoons—what are commonly known as Flash animation. Once created, the Flash animations can be embedded on the distance education website. Flash animation methods are commonly used on video sharing websites like YouTube. Many video sharing sites are open source, allowing users to upload, view, and share video clips at no cost.

Videoconferencing   Videoconferencing has been with us for some time. Typically rooms are set up to handle a group of people who are linked to other sites that are similarly set up. The result is a sort of town meeting atmosphere where you can see and talk with others. Such sites are common at universities, community colleges, businesses, and many hotels. In addition, vendors often set up a site on a temporary basis for a special topic. Videoconferencing has become a common mode of operation to cut down on the costs and time required for travel.

A new twist on videoconferencing has come with the lowering of costs for hardware. Microphones and small digital cameras can now be purchased for as little as $15 each that will allow see-you-see-me conversations at any workstation so equipped (see Figure 6-3). Compatible software is required and, of course, an Internet provider. This holds true if it involves the next state or a distant country. The quality varies greatly depending on the speed of connection and the quality of the camera and other hardware.

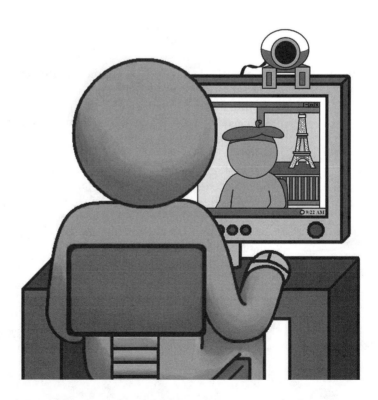

Figure 6-3
Videoconferencing

Virtual Reality in Health Education: Immersive Education

People, by nature, like games. Games enable players to safely try new ideas and experience new scenarios that are often not available in real life. Technological advancements have put a new spin on the ability of educators to use games as a method to reinvent the excitement of learning through the use of virtual reality. Virtual reality (VR) digitally encapsulates multiple media sources such as books, slides, pictures, audio, and video to create a hypothetical three-dimensional world on the computer (Balan & Swift, n.d.). The field of health education has embraced the idea of game-based learning and training systems via digital and virtual reality applications. According to an article in *Futurist*, the economic impact of serious games—games designed to educate not just entertain—is more than $150 million, with approximately 20% of these games dedicated to health-related content (Tucker, 2008). It is apparent that VR has the potential to significantly impact and improve health education and health promotion efforts.

Virtual reality can work for educators as a tool in assisting students to become immersed in a learning environment. An award-winning example of this type of technological application is immersive education, a learning *platform* that combines interactive 3D graphics, commercial game and simulation technology, virtual reality, voice chat (Voice over IP/VoIP), webcams, and rich digital media with collaborative online course environments and classrooms (Alhadeff, 2008). In immersive education, the term platform refers to any virtual world—simulator or 3D environment—that may be used for teaching or training purposes. Participants create avatars (characters) to visit the virtual worlds, allowing them to have a sense of "being there" when exploring the various scenarios. Imagine, if you will, your avatar being the first responder at the scene of an earthquake, bombing, or sarin gas attack in Beijing (Tucker, 2008). Consider also the ability of your avatar to experience life as a red blood cell flowing through disease damaged blood vessels of the body and chambers of the heart. A virtual island might be used to have your avatar participate in a virtual seminar where selections for insurance coverage are made based on your individual profile. These types of activities would be too costly and impractical to undertake in the physical world; however, these opportunities are available over the Internet (Alhadeff, 2008). The ability to weave health education concepts into the fabric of everyday life—especially in an interesting and challenging game format—has the potential to make a serious impact on the health of our society.

Many universities are now employing such technologies as an extension of their online courses. One of the clear advantages is the different way students communicate with one another. Their avatars can meet and converse much more like a real life group meeting. The participating campuses have set up sites that usually look much like their real campus buildings for group and class meetings. Some virtual campuses include rain and snow to reflect their current campus weather conditions. In most cases the controller has the weather set as ideal, which is an advantage for outdoor activities. The ability to set the weather as appropriate is something we have always wanted to do.

East Carolina University has an entire campus set up in "Second Life," one of the popular virtual environments, and is offering classes including several to high school students to prepare them for entering the less safe campus environment. One of the authors has an avatar for meeting with students.

Chat Rooms Most people are aware of chat rooms on the Internet. Such locations allow people to "talk" simultaneously on the Internet, often anonymously. You enter a "room" of people with similar interests and are free to "lurk" or participate as you choose. Many people find such opportunities enjoyable and stimulating. There are chat rooms available for almost any topic. As health educators, we need to be aware of the many chat rooms that are available for health information or social support. Individuals with special interests run some of these rooms, and others are operated by vendors such as America Online (AOL) as part of the package they sell to consumers. As with other Internet sites, *caveat emptor* applies: "Let the buyer beware." Strong cautions are in order about ever accepting any medical advice from such sources. Clearly, competent medical practitioners are not going to give a medical diagnosis over the Internet. Many vendors find such sites a good way to sell their books or other products.

Despite these cautions, it should be recognized that chat rooms can provide valuable social support to patients and family members. This can be especially true if one is in an isolated area or has a condition that is uncommon in the local community. Chat room access can be an important aid for someone caring for a patient with a serious and demanding illness or even trying to improve their personal health. For example, smoking cessation chat rooms have proved popular and helpful to many. Chat rooms are easily accessible through most vendors and generally have posted schedules of meeting times. Health issues are common subjects for chat rooms. Many health organizations run chat rooms. Examples are Narcotics Anonymous, Alcoholics Anonymous, and Sex & Love Addicts Anonymous. Figure 6-4 shows an example of an invitation to join a chat room discussion.

Monday

Narcotics Anonymous Discussion

6:00-8:00 a.m. ET (11:00 a.m. GMT)

Host: AARF NkenaA and Friends

Keyword:A&R> A&R Chat Center: A&Rs Chat Center

Figure 6-4
Chat Room Invitation

Objective: After reviewing the case study, the reader will discuss two or more potential hazards associated with the recommendations suggested to Pat while in the chat room.

Case Study: Pat

Pat finds a chat room on cancer. He is an observer for a couple of hours and then asks for information about his colon cancer. Quickly he receives recommendations regarding treatment centers. He also gets a recommendation to stop his current chemotherapy and to begin "inversion therapy." He is referred to the impressive-looking webpage of a Dr. Jacob Samm. According to Dr. Samm, "inversion therapy" is proven to eliminate many cancers, including his form of cancer. The focus of the treatment is an apparatus that allows users to hang upside down at least twice a day. Pat really is unhappy with the side effects of his current therapy and decides that the new therapy would be worth a try for a few months. (See Case Studies Revisited page 247.)

Questions to consider:

1. What are some "red flag" statements presented in the chat room that should elicit the notion of caveat emptor (buyer beware) for Pat?
2. What are the obvious dangers of Pat's use of the Internet?

Example: Positive Use of Chat Rooms

Theresa lives in an isolated area of Nebraska and has been caring for her grandmother who has been diagnosed with Alzheimer's disease. Day after day of working on her farm and looking after her grandmother has her tired and concerned that she is thinking ill of this woman she loves. She wonders if she is turning into an evil person because she has feelings that she thinks of as selfish—for example, wondering why she must be the one to constantly care for this woman. She attends a workshop on care of Alzheimer's patients run by a health educator who suggests that she join a chat room of like caregivers. After joining the chat room, she is surprised and relieved to hear many other caregivers express similar feelings. She finds the chat room helps her greatly with tips on helping her grandmother and on improving her self-esteem. She eventually even becomes one of the contributors.

Forums

Sites where you can post questions and later come back to read the replies, or where you post a note and ask people to respond to you directly, are called *forums*. Internet forums, formerly known as bulletin boards, are also referred to as web forums, newsgroups, message boards, or discussion groups. They are often topic specific, and many deal with health issues. Forums are set up much like chat rooms except that they are asynchronous, allowing you to add and review comments whenever you wish.

A pioneer in the use of technology by health educators is Michael Pejsach. He created the Health Education Electronic Forum (HEEF) before most health educators were ready to use it. Dr. Pejsach did much to raise awareness of health educators to the technology possibilities, but little use was made of the original service. His latest project is the Center for Excellence in Education about Health and can be found at www.healthbehavior .com. All health educators should review his new site.

Blogs   Similar to a forum, a blog is a website used to provide commentaries, descriptions of events, or opinions about a given subject. Blogs, however, are typically maintained by an individual and can be thought of as a digital diary that allows others to post comments that are typically displayed in reverse-chronological order (Wikipedia, 2008). Adding comments to your own blog or to another person's blog is referred to as blogging and has become a fairly common practice. According to Oomen-Early and Burke (2007), the use of blogs may serve as a powerful teaching resource for health education and a conduit to encourage individuals to take social and political action. Integrating blogging methods into classes has been shown to increase student motivation, critical thinking, class interaction, and student course satisfaction (Beldarrian, 2006; Halavais & Hernandez, 2004; Oomen-Early & Burke, 2007; Williams & Jacobs, 2004).

Social Networking   Social networking venues allow users to build personal "spaces" on a webpage, creating a user-submitted network of friends, personal profiles, blogs, groups, photos, music, and videos (Wikipedia, 2008b). Two examples of more popular social networking sites are Facebook and MySpace; however, in the field of health education, researchers and practitioners often will subscribe to the Health Education Directory, or HEDIR (pronounced heater).

The HEDIR was created in 1992 by Mark Kittleson, 2008 American Association of Health Education (AAHE) scholar, to help the health education profession incorporate technology, hence the acronym HEDIR. As stated on its website, the purpose of the HEDIR is to provide an electronic directory of health educators throughout the world where one can search by name, state, or professional interests and to provide an electronic communications system for news of interest to professionals and students on the listserv in the field of health education (Kittleson, 2008). Dr. Kittleson's site (http://hedir.org/) is a must-see for any health educator because it includes many useful features, including:

- A directory of health educators
- A directory of health educators by state and country
- A listserv (HEDIR) for practicing health educators
- Job openings
- . Archived messages from the listserv
- An electronic journal for health educators
- A chat room for health educators

Health educators also are encouraged to join the HEDIR group on Linked In, located at http://www.linkedin.com.

Finding Colleagues

Although the HEDIR is clearly a dominant source in health for locating colleagues, the Internet has expanded our ability to locate colleagues and people of similar interests. Most search engines now have databases of phone numbers, email addresses, and postal addresses. Most are a collection of available phone directories and assorted email directories. Simply enter the name and any other information you have on the individual into the search engine and it will provide a list of possible matches. It is fun to look for a long-lost friend or colleague. You may need to use several different search engines to find the latest information. One of the authors recently looked up his own address and found that most directories listed where he had lived and worked 2 years ago. Only by using a fourth search engine did he find the correct information. See Figure 6-5 for an Internet activity.

For more information and tools related to this chapter visit http://healtheducation.jbpub.com/strategies.

Find each site on the Internet and enter the URL (complete address). Good hunting!

SITE/ADDRESS	URL/ADDRESS
Twitter page of Mark Kittleson (health educator)	_____
MMWR	_____
Robin Sawyer academic vita (health educator)	_____
New York University professional resources—job postings in community health education	_____
Maryland Dept. of Health Education	_____
NCHEC–National Commission for Health Education Credentialing, Inc.	_____
The Youth Risk Behavior Surveillance System (YRBSS)	_____
HEDIR Directory for North Carolina	_____
ECU Department of Health Education and Promotion	_____
Society of Research Administration SRA's Grantsweb	_____
Go Ask Alice–Rohypnol	_____
Ann Rose's Ultimate Birth Control Links: Provide a proper APA citation of some located information here:	_____
_____	_____
_____	_____
Glen Gilbert's research interest (health educator)	_____
Elisa McNeill's philosophy of education	_____

Figure 6-5
Health Internet
Scavenger Hunt

NOTEWORTHY   Netiquette

A set of societal standards for Internet use exists. These guiding principles represent what is considered to be appropriate etiquette, or **netiquette**, for any type of electronic communication. Oscar Sodani (2003) suggests users practice netiquette by adhering to the following practices:

1. **Communicate clearly and politely.** Be aware that the absence of nonverbal cues can sometimes change the way a message is perceived.
2. **Be brief.** Time is a precious commodity for all. Strive to make your point while keeping your communications reasonably short.
3. **Keep to the topic.** If you are communicating in a chat room, newsgroup, or forum that is dedicated to the topic of AIDS awareness, it is not a good idea to start a conversation about the gold medal count of the last Olympics. People who are participating in the discussion are there for a reason.
4. **DON'T SCREAM.** WHEN YOU TYPE A MESSAGE IN ALL CAPITAL LETTERS, IT LOOKS LIKE YOU ARE SCREAMING. IN ADDITION, IT IS MUCH HARDER TO READ. Type everything in lowercase letters or mixed case if you want your communiqués to be read and accepted.
5. **Avoid flame wars.** Messages written to irritate the recipient are referred to as a **flame**. Flames often contain offensive material and are not considered appropriate electronic dialogue. The term is also used as a verb: If I send nasty emails to a colleague, then I have flamed him. It is a faux pas to electronically flame others. Keep in mind that the most effective way to end a flame is to ignore it. It is hard to fight with someone who does not fight back.
6. **Think before you type.** Unless your message is encrypted, it is not secure; thus it may be read by unintended recipients. Be certain what you type today is safe to be read later.
7. **Provide the subject.** The subject line helps the recipient to filter and to prioritize electronic correspondences. A brief, yet descriptive, subject line can alert the individual to items of high interest.
8. **Lurk before you post.** Before posting messages, take time to review the guidelines and explore what is currently posted. This practice is known as lurking. It is possible that the comment or question you might want to ask has already been asked and is available in the discussion archives or available in a FAQ (frequently asked questions) section.

EXERCISES

1. Select any health topic and perform *two* searches using different search engines (e.g., Yahoo!, Google, AltaVista, Bing). See how different the results of your search are, based on the first 20 sites listed by each search engine.

2. Using the evaluation criteria described in this chapter, access and evaluate five websites of your choice.

3. Select a health topic that might be deemed by some people to be controversial. Conduct a search on this topic, and try to identify two sites that offer opposite viewpoints. In your opinion, which site appears to be the most credible, and why?

4. Access an electronic health-related journal, and then read and critique in writing any article that you choose from the journal.

5. Access an electronic journal article. Compare and contrast its layout style to that of a traditional paper article.

6. Select a health topic of interest, and use the Internet to see if you can obtain the most recent incidence or prevalence data for that particular topic. What is the source for your data, and would you consider it reliable?

7. Locate the email addresses and websites of the authors of the textbook.

8. Locate chat rooms for prostate cancer and breast cancer.

9. Find the website for HEDIR, and determine what role students can play in it.

10. Examine the distance education offerings of your campus. Find a health education course similar to this one on the Internet. What do you see as the strengths and weaknesses of such courses?

11. Complete the Health Internet Scavenger Hunt found in Figure 6-5.

CASE STUDIES REVISITED

Case Study Revisited: Robyn

Robyn clearly felt overextended and preoccupied as she prepared materials for her workshop. This may have just been a bad day for her, or it may have been indicative of a chronic problem with leaving things until the last moment. Robyn's dilemma cannot be blamed on the Internet; however, this case provides an excellent example of the dangers of collecting information from a website without evaluating the source. Following the evaluative steps discussed in this chapter cannot guarantee that information gleaned from the Web will always be absolutely correct, but had Robyn performed even a cursory eval-uation of the websites, she might have avoided what must have been total humiliation and loss of face. The mere existence of a website is in no way indicative of legitimacy . . . check the source! (See page 223.)

Case Study Revisited: Pat

A phrase such as "proven to eliminate" and the unorthodox approach to treatment appears to be easily recognizable as questionable, yet in Pat's desperate attempt to find relief he may be vulnerable to the charms of a modern day "snake oil" salesman.

After a month of "inversion therapy," Pat is not feeling well. He returns to his physician, who says the cancer has progressed far more than expected. Probing, she learns of Pat's self-treatment. She encourages him to go back to his chemotherapy and warns him of the dangers of self-treatment. The physician also discusses the proper use of the Internet and even encourages such use and sharing of information. She also says Pat can use "inversion therapy" if he wants to as long as it does no harm but explains that she is ethically bound to inform him that she knows of no study that supports the claims of the treatment. She seems relieved when he says he will stay with chemotherapy and drop the "inversion therapy." Later Pat learns that Dr. Samm has a Ph.D. in geology and makes "inversion therapy" equipment in his basement. (See page 242.)

SUMMARY

1. The information explosion that occurred mostly in the 1990s has created an "age of information," and health educators need to be proficient and comfortable using this new medium to their best advantage.

2. The Internet offers a wealth of information sources that represent a great opportunity for all users. However, unlike written resources, most materials placed on the Internet are virtually unregulated in any way, and users need to develop evaluative skills to protect themselves from erroneous, misleading, and biased information.

3. Through the use of technology, teachers, presenters, and workshop facilitators have an outstanding opportunity to expand the world of their students/participants. Health educational professionals need to become familiar with as many facets of this technology as possible.

4. When using the Internet for research purposes, health educators should be able to effectively assess the legitimacy of the information and correctly cite the source of information.

REFERENCES AND RESOURCES

Alhadeff, E. (2008). When serious games meet immersive education—part 2. Retrieved December 10, 2008, from http://elianealhadeff.blogspot.com/2008/01/when-serious-games-meet-immersive_26.html

American Psychological Association. (2001). *Publication Manual of the American Psychological Association* (5th ed.). Washington, DC: Author.

American Psychological Association. (2008). Electronic media and URLs. Retrieved September 12, 2008, from http://www.apastyle.org/elecmedia.html

Balan, V., & Swift, M. J. (n.d.). Design of virtual reality systems for education: A cognitive approach. Retrieved December 10, 2008, from http://web-dev-csc.gre.ac.uk/conference/conf40/presentations/balan.ppt#258,14,DEFINITION

Beasley, W., & Wang, L. C. (2001). Implementing ISTE/NCATE technology standards in teacher preparation: One college's experience. *Information Technology in Childhood Education Annual*, pp. 33–44.

Beldarrain, Y. (2006). Distance education trends: Integrating new technologies to foster student interaction and collaboration. *Distance Education*, 27; 139–153.

Bertot, J. C., McClure, C. R., & Jaeger, P. T. (2008). The impacts of free public internet access on public library patrons and communities. *Library Quarterly*, 78(3); 285–301.

Chaney, B. H., Eddy, J. M., Dorman, S. M., Glessner, L. L., Green, B. L., & Lara-Alecio, R. (2007, October). A primer on quality indicators of distance education. Health Promotion Practice, doi:10.1177/1524839906298498.

Dewey, R. (2004). APA style resource. [Publication manual crib sheet]. Retrieved August 15, 2008, from http://www.psychwww.com/resource/apacrib.htm

Diaz, J. A., Griffith, R. A., Ng, J. J., Reinert, S. E., Friedmann, P. D., & Moulton, A. W. (2002). Patients' use of the Internet for medical information. *Journal of General Internal Medicine, 17*(3), 180–185.

Dorman, S. (2001, February). Are teachers using computers for instruction? *Journal of School Health, 71*(2), 83. Retrieved August 28, 2008, from Academic Search Complete database.

Dorman, S. M. (1998). 10 reasons to use technology in the classroom. *Journal of School Health, 68*(1), 38–39.

Dorman, S. M. (1999). Technology briefs: Cookies—Tricks or treats? *Journal of School Health, 69*(2), 82.

Federal Citizen Information Center. Retrieved September 23, 2000, from http://www.pueblo.gsa.gov

Federal Trade Commission. (1999). Beware false marketing techniques. Retrieved July 1, 1999, from http://www.ftc.gov

Gilbert, G. G., Sawyer, R., & Mardon, B. F. (1997). Using the Internet in health and physical education in Maryland. *Maryland Journal of Health, Physical Education, Recreation and Dance.*

Greenwood, A. (2008). Criteria for evaluating internet resources. University of British Columbia. Retrieved August 14, 2008, from http://www.library.ubc.ca/home/evaluating/Easyprint.html

Halavais, A., & Hernandez, P. (2004, December). Blogs, threaded discussions accentuate constructivist teaching. *Online Classroom,* 1–5.

Horrigan, J. (2007). Wireless Internet access. Pew Internet and American Life Project. December 2006. Survey. Retrieved August 13, 2008, from http://www.pewinternet.org/~/media//Files/Reports/2007/PIP_Wireless.Use.pdf.pdf

International Telecommunication Union. (2006). *World Telecommunication Indicators 2005.* Geneva: ITU. Retrieved August 17, 2009, from http://www.itu.int/ITU-D/ict/publications/world/world.html

Kirk, E. E. (1996). Evaluating information found on the Internet. Retrieved on June 16, 2009, from: http://milton.mse.jhu.edu:8001/research/education/net.htm/

Kittleson, M. (2008). HEDIR policies and procedures. Retrieved August 30, 2008, from http://www.kittle.siu.edu/hedir/about.html#purpose

Mattheos, N., Jonnson, J., Schittek, M., & Attstrom, R. (2000). Technology and media for distance learning in academic health education. *Journal of Dentistry.* Retrieved June 20, 2009, from http://www1.elsevier.com/homepage/sab/jdentet/contents/mattheos/mattheos.html

McNeill, E., & Eddy, J. (2005). Planning ADE: Implications from the literature on student perspectives. *International Electronic Journal of Health Education, 8*; 70–79. Retrieved September 16, 2008, from http://www.aahperd.org/iejhe/template.cfm?template=2005/mcneill.html

Meadows, M. (2006). Cracking down on health fraud. Federal Trade Commission. *FDA Consumer Magazine, 40*(6). Retrieved August 13, 2008, from http://www.fda.gov/ForConsumers/ConsumerUpdates/default.htm

National Library of Medicine. (2008). NLM copyright information. Retrieved August 20, 2008, from http://www.nlm.nih.gov/copyright.html

Oomen-Early, J., & Burke, S. (2007, December). Entering the blogosphere: Blogs as teaching and learning tools in health education. *International Electronic Journal of Health Education, 10,* 186–196. Retrieved August 31, 2008, from http://www.aahperd.org.iejhe/2007/07_J_Oomen.pdf

Peck, K. L., & Dorricot, D. (1994). Why use technology? *Education Leader, 51*(7), 11–14.

Richmond, B. (2000). 10 Cs for evaluating Internet resources. Retrieved August 14, 2008, from http://www.uwec.edu/review/work/library/research/guides/tenCs.pdf

Scott, L., Howell, S. L., Williams, P. B., & Lindsay, N. K. (2003). Thirty-two trends affecting distance education: An informed foundation for strategic planning. *Online Journal of Distance Learning Administration, 4*(3). Retrieved August 30, 2008, from http://www.westga.edu/~distance/ojdla/fall63/howell63.html

Sodani, O. (2003). Internet etiquette (netiquette). Retrieved September 2, 2008, from http://www.help2go.com/Tutorials/Internet_Basics/Internet_Etiquette_(Netiquette).html

Tucker, P. (2008, September). Virtual health. *Futurist, 42*(5), 60–61. Retrieved December 11, 2008, from Professional Development Collection database.

U.S. Department of Education, Office of Postsecondary Education. (2006, March). Evidence of quality in distance education programs drawn from interviews with the accreditation community. Retrieved August 30, 2008, from http://www.ysu.edu/accreditation/Resources/Accreditation-Evidence-of-Quality-in-DE-Programs.pdf

Washington Post. (1999). Web site makes Koop an IPO millionaire. Business section, p. 1.

Wikipedia. (2008a). Blog. Retrieved August 31, 2008, from http://en.wikipedia.org/w/index.php?title=Blog&oldid=234419569

Wikipedia. (2008b). MySpace. Retrieved August 31, 2008, from http://en.wikipedia.org/w/index.php?title=MySpace&oldid=235179571

Williams, J., & Jacobs, J. (2004). Exploring the use of blogs as learning spaces in the higher education sector. *AJET, 20*(2); 232–247.

Use of Media in Health Education: Literacy, Selection, Marketing, Development, and Equipment

Entry-Level and Advanced 1 Health Educator Competencies Addressed in This Chapter

Responsibility III: Implement Health Education Strategies, Interventions, and Programs
  Competency A: Initiate a plan of action.
  Competency C: Use a variety of methods to implement strategies, interventions, and programs.

Responsibility VI: Serve as a Health Education Resource Person
  Competency A: Use health-related information resources.
  Competency C: Select resource materials for dissemination.

Responsibility VII: Communicate and Advocate for Health and Health Education
  Competency B: Apply a variety of communication methods and techniques.

> Note: The competencies listed above, which are addressed in this chapter, are considered to be both entry-level and Advanced 1 competencies by the National Commission for Health Education Credentialing, Inc. They are taken from *A Framework for the Development of Competency Based Curricula for Entry Level Health Educators* by the National Task Force for the Preparation and Practice of Health Education, 1985; *A Competency-Based Framework for Graduate Level Health Educators,* by the National Task Force for the Preparation and Practice of Health Education, 1999; and *A Competency-Based Framework for Health Educators—The Competencies Update Project (CUP),* 2006.

Method Selection in Health Education

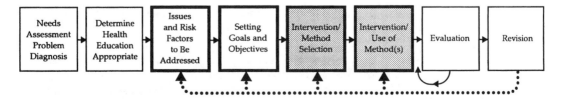

Heavy-bordered boxes indicate subjects addressed in this text; shaded boxes indicate subjects(s) of current chapter.

OBJECTIVES   After studying the chapter the reader will be able to:

- Justify the need for media literacy.
- Explain the criteria for selection.
- Describe the major steps involved in media development.
- Develop a personal checklist for media evaluation.
- Describe the major advantages and disadvantages of using each media method and its required equipment.
- Present a rationale for using a particular form of media, including how that medium complements the overall learning objectives.

KEY ISSUES   Media literacy
Selecting and evaluating media
Media development
Equipment dinosaurs
Major types of media equipment:

- DVDs
- Document cameras
- Interactive whiteboards
- Presentation software
- Audience response systems
- Personal computers

Media Literacy

The powerful nature of the media and its influences on young people's lives is well documented. It has been suggested that media could be considered as a "super peer" in the lives of young people (Ziegler, 2007). With the continuous exposure to messages from advertisements, television programs, movies, song lyrics, and video games, one cannot deny the potential for media sources to influence today's youth. According to Rideout, Roberts, and Foehr (2005), children ages 3–12 spend what is considered hours equivalent to a full-time job with overtime (44+ hours per week) engaged in some form of media, averaging 6.3 hours per day. The average person in the United States spends 4 hours a day watching television (Herr, 2001).

Although television's primary purpose is to entertain, it has the ability to convey messages about serious health issues. In an effort to understand the potential of educational (edutainment) entertainment, the Kaiser Family Foundation supports research to explore the use of edutainment to promote health.

In one study, conducted by Victoria Rideout (2008), the writers of a prime-time soap opera–style medical program, *Grey's Anatomy*, embedded health messages related to HIV into one of its episodes. Viewers were pre- and post-surveyed to identify changes in knowledge related to the content of the embedded massage. Rideout concluded:

> This study documents the enormous potential of popular entertainment television to serve as a health educator—even on a show that has a "soap-opera"-like feel and a comedic bent. A very large proportion of viewers absorbed the information that was provided in *Grey's Anatomy*, and many of them had retained that knowledge six weeks later. (p. 8)

Media has become such an intricate part of society—it is no longer considered to be just a part of our culture, it is considered a culture on its own (Ziegler, 2007). With the explosive growth in the number and types of devices that provide instant access to media sources, it is unlikely that the "media culture" is a temporary phenomenon.

The concept of media literacy emerged during the 1980s and continues to receive much attention. Media literacy is based on the premise that much of what people see and believe is derived from contact with various forms of media, which would not represent a problem if what the media provided was consistently accurate, honest, unbiased, and neutral information. In reality, financial profits tend to drive the agenda of many privately owned media organizations; thus, the neutrality of the message may get lost in the desire to attract audiences. Consequently, the messages rendered by media sources ". . . can be confusing or disruptive to individuals looking to the media for direction, purpose and meaning" (Silverblatt, 2004). Many writers and researchers have suggested that media is more interested in ratings and sales than in presenting an undistorted reality (Considine, 1990; Melamed, 1989; Silverblatt, 2004); therefore, in order to protect individuals from falling prey to the vagaries of media messages, media education should become a necessary part of existing educational programs (Dorman, 2000; Ziegler, 2007). The public's reliance on the media, coupled with their inability to effectively scrutinize its content, can be problematic without the ability or desire to filter its content—which is the point of teaching media literacy.

Early definitions of media literacy were based on the idea of helping young people develop an informed and critical understanding of the nature of mass media, the techniques utilized by various media, and how these techniques influence each individual's perceived reality (Ontario Ministry of Education, 1989). As the interest in media literacy grew, basic definitions broadened to include all populations. Currently, media literacy is considered as having the competencies to access, analyze, evaluate, and communicate information in both print and electronic venues (Aufderheide, 1993; Considine, 1995; Galician, 2004; Ziegler, 2007). According to the Center for Media Literacy (CML, 2004), media literacy is a four-step process of informed inquiry that includes:

- **Awareness:** Exploring a variety of media sources by accessing information from multiple sources
- **Analysis:** Exploring how messages are assembled while identifying, comparing, and contrasting the content from various sources
- **Reflection:** Evaluating the implicit and explicit messages from one's own philosophy
- **Reaction:** Using media devices to participate in the exchange of ideas by expressing or creating messages using media devices

Clearly, if the mass media plays some type of role, either intentionally or unwittingly, in distributing material that somehow contributes to the negative

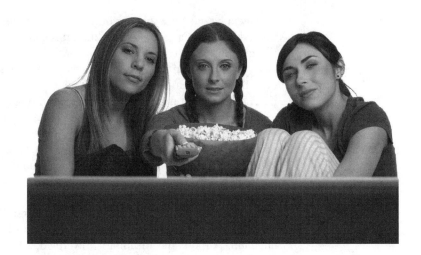

The media, especially television, is one of the biggest educators in today's society.

health status of the public, then a logical preventive measure would be to better educate the public on how to be more critically aware of received messages. Expecting the producers of mass media to take a more open and perhaps honest approach to programming is unrealistic in that the driving force of private media is a sound profit margin. Given this stark reality, media literacy becomes an important concept to consider in the realm of health education. A greater understanding of how mass media can shape people's perceptions can only help to make individuals more critical and selective when receiving health-related messages. These same analytical skills are also fundamental in the evaluation of health information and the development of health literacy (see Chapter 8).

Resources   An abundance of available information exists regarding media literacy, and much of it can be found on the Internet. Here are three websites that provide some excellent resources in addition to a wealth of links to other related sites:

- **The Media Literacy OnLine Project:** This website, maintained by the University of Oregon, has a wealth of information on this topic in addition to a large number of links to related websites. (http://interact.uoregon.edu/medialit/mlr/home)
- **Center for Media Education:** This is the home page for a national, nonprofit organization "dedicated to improving the quality of the electronic media." Information on research, advocacy, policy making, and public education. (http://www.densondesign.com/CME.html)
- **Center for Media Literacy:** This nonprofit organization, established in 1989, develops and distributes educational materials and programs that "promote critical thinking about the media." This website has a large amount of resources on this topic including books, videotapes, and teaching

materials and also provides a free email bulletin, a discussion group, and a calendar of events describing upcoming conferences and training. (http://www.medialit.org)

Selecting and Evaluating Media

The selection of visual media forms is crucially important, particularly in health education. All too often, audiovisual materials are used for the wrong reasons. For example:

- Because the item (videotape or DVD) has *always* been used for a certain topic.
- To fill a blank space on the schedule.
- Because a particular item is the only one available.
- Because an item is the only one that can be afforded.
- Because the topic is applicable, even though the level of the material is inappropriate.

Although these reasons for using audiovisual materials may seem obviously inappropriate, they occur frequently. The use of visual media is routine; unfortunately, there is limited research on the criteria to evaluate its quality.

There have been some early attempts to somehow objectively evaluate media, particularly in the area of drug education. The Audiovisual Group of the Addiction Research Foundation (ARF) provided a rating of films based on the following nine criteria (Fejer et al., 1972):

1. The scientific accuracy of information presented
2. Its merits as a teaching aid
3. Whether or not it was contemporary
4. The clarity of the message
5. Whether or not it could influence attitudes
6. Its believability
7. Its technical merits
8. Whether or not it maintained interest
9. Whether or not it was applicable to individuals from different social strata

Although this early effort at least provided some basic guidelines for audiovisual material selection, the ambiguities of its components are obvious. It is not within the scope of this text to document further specific audiovisual research in health education, but a review of the literature clearly denotes a paucity of meaningful evaluation . . . a sad commentary, particularly in the light of how frequently such materials are used today.

To aid the health educator in choosing the most appropriate media materials, a helpful evaluation checklist has been designed (see Figure 7-1).

```
┌─────────────────────────────────────────────────────────────┐
│                                                             │
│                 MEDIA EVALUATION CHECKLIST                  │
│  ─────────────────────────────────────────────────────────  │
│                                                             │
│    Media Objectives                                  ____   │
│                                                             │
│    Level of Media                                    ____   │
│                                                             │
│    Language                                          ____   │
│                                                             │
│    Content                                           ____   │
│                                                             │
│    Culture/Ethnicity                                 ____   │
│                                                             │
│    Time/Duration of Media                            ____   │
│                                                             │
│    Cost                                              ____   │
│                                                             │
│    Interest Level                                    ____   │
│                                                             │
│    Production Qualities                              ____   │
│                                                             │
│    Evaluation of Media                               ____   │
│                                                             │
│    Availability                                      ____   │
│                                                             │
│    Format                                            ____   │
│                                                             │
│    Approved Material                                 ____   │
│                                                             │
│    Others                                                   │
│                                                             │
│    ───────────────────────────────────────────────────     │
│                                                             │
│    ───────────────────────────────────────────────────     │
│                                                             │
└─────────────────────────────────────────────────────────────┘
```

Figure 7-1
Choosing Appropriate
Media

This checklist is by no means exhaustive, and additional categories could be added, but those included here are some basic principles to consider when selecting media materials. Let us examine each of these in detail, bearing in mind that the order of the items implies no ranking. For a more comprehensive and complicated media rating system, health educators should examine a scale called "An Analysis Checklist for Audiovisuals" developed by Martin and Stainbrook (1986). Another valuable resource available from the Food and Nutrition Information Center of the USDA's National Agricultural Library is a publication summarizing a collection of resources on the topic of health literacy, tools for developing/evaluating materials, and sources of easy-to-read nutrition materials (Widen, Pellechia, & Schneider, 2007). Although much of the content is tied to nutrition, the principles of development and evaluation of media are fundamental and easily applied to other health-related topics.

Media Objectives   Will the materials used fulfill or facilitate achieving the objective(s) of the presentation? All too often materials are chosen because they are topic appropriate, and yet they may do little to achieve objectives. For example, in AIDS education, films depicting factual information about the disease or showing interviews of people with AIDS have traditionally been shown in school and community settings in an attempt to elicit attitude and sexual behavior change. Using cognitive information may well improve knowledge levels, but such an approach does little to influence attitude or behavior. If attitude change is an objective—perhaps in this case, in dealing with AIDS education, the objective might be to increase perceived susceptibility to HIV—then the film selected should be affective in nature and not didactic. If a simple increase in knowledge is the objective, then the factual film is appropriate. Clearly, an awareness of specific objectives is crucial to media selection.

One condition that has exacerbated this problem is that until relatively recently the vast majority of available media materials has been of the factual variety, thus perpetuating the axiom of "if that's all there is, then we'll have to use it!" On many occasions using nothing is more appropriate than using ineffective, inappropriate materials! Since factual information can be addressed through many different methods, using media to address affective or other more difficult objectives can often be a useful strategy.

Level   Is the level of the material suitable for the audience? It is important to consider the learning styles and levels of the audience when considering media materials. If the material is either too complex and difficult or too simplistic, the audience may become, respectively, frustrated or uninterested. Again, the availability of level-appropriate materials might be limited, so the health educator must make a decision as to the material's potential utility. As stated earlier, inappropriate materials may well do more harm than good.

Language   Is the language used in the materials appropriate for the audience? This question can be posed on two levels: Is the language used offensive in any way, and possibly inappropriate, particularly in school settings? Perhaps more important, is the language intelligible to the audience? For example, can you use a film in English in a predominantly Hispanic setting? There are no easy answers to these questions, and solutions may be different in each case. For example, if the only film available on a certain topic is in English, showing such a film to an Asian or Hispanic group is not necessarily out of the question. The group's level of English may be quite sufficient to understand the meaning of the film. Health educators should consider both the language capabilities of the group, and the language complexity of the media materials.

Content   Is the content of the materials accurate and up to date? Here is where the "we've always used this film!" doctrine can be dangerous. Many health issues change so quickly that as new information succeeds the old, media materials can become outdated and, even worse, inaccurate in relatively short periods of time. The high cost of some materials makes updating media libraries a difficult task, and, again, the health educator may be faced with the decision of not using media materials rather than risking the dissemination of inaccurate information. It is perhaps useful to note that affective materials less concerned with cognitive information probably have a longer "shelf life" than their more factual counterparts.

Culture/Ethnicity   Are the media materials culturally sensitive? That is, are they appropriate for a specific audience? This question is probably one of the most difficult to address in a satisfactory manner. In an ideal situation the health educator would be able to choose media materials that are both topic specific and completely culturally appropriate. For example, when considering a drug education film, the health educator should ideally be able to choose from affective to factual films, with alternative versions for each different ethnic group, whether black, Hispanic, Asian, white, and so on. But wouldn't we then also have to have even more versions, not only for race but for socioeconomic status? It would certainly seem insensitive to assume that individuals within races are all the same! To that end, achieving this Utopia would necessitate the development of literally hundreds of new media materials, each culturally specific and appropriate. Given the cost of media development, this situation will never exist, and the health educator is again left with making some type of compromise. The search for media materials that will satisfy the needs of *every* group is both futile and unreasonable. The health educator must make every effort to obtain materials that are as inclusive as possible and will not patently offend groups or individuals. A decision that no useful or appropriate materials are available to be used in certain contexts would not be unusual.

Time/Duration of Media   Just how long does it take to show specific materials? Is it reasonable to take up the entire 50-minute classroom period to show a film? In the community setting while facilitating a 90-minute workshop, what length of DVD would be reasonable to show? Is it reasonable to show a film in two parts because the film is too long to complete in one session? Again, each situation must be evaluated individually, with both the context of the presentation and the objectives of using specific media materials being of paramount importance in making a decision. What should be avoided is the selection of media materials because they happen to fit the presentation time frame. If some materials are deemed to be valuable but too lengthy, perhaps with careful preparation crucial pieces can be substituted for the whole. Another thing to remember is the attention span of the audience. Adult learners find it difficult to concentrate for more than 20 minutes (Protective Services Training Institute, 2004). Generally a 10- to 15-minute window of time is optimal for maintaining focus in adult audiences.

Cost   No matter how useful some educational materials may be, there will always be the question of cost. As with anything related to consumerism, you tend to get what you pay for. High-quality, well-produced, interesting, educationally sound media materials are usually expensive. As production costs continue to rise, the price of the finished media products also increases. The average cost of a high-quality 20-minute DVD will range from $150 to $400. With ever diminishing budgets in both the school and community settings, media selection must be made very carefully, and made with an eye to longevity and maximized usefulness of the materials. It is perhaps sad to note that with all the important factors incorporated in media selection in an effort to maximize the educational experience, the single greatest factor determining the final decision may well be the issue of cost.

Interest Level   How interesting are the materials? Will students in the classroom find the materials so dull that they mentally absent themselves from the experience, making the time and expense of using such materials futile? Will the community health smoking-cessation group find the DVD "talking head" to be so technical and boring that they begin to question continuing their involvement in the program? Perhaps the single most common criticism of health education materials has been their dull, lifeless, uninspiring format. No matter how important and useful the health information may be, if individuals have "tuned out," then the whole experience has achieved nothing. One useful tip when seeking media materials is to look for something the audience can *closely* relate to. For example, some of the best health education films for middle and high school audiences have been media sources from the Public Broadcasting System series *PBS Kids*. But would this material be applicable to college students, or would they dismiss the information as irrelevant because of the age difference? Is it effective to show a predominantly young, heterosexual, non-drug-using college population a film depicting middle-aged drug abusers or homosexual men describing how they contracted AIDS? The ability of the audience to see themselves in the scenario promotes interest in the outcome and enables the audience to explore their own feelings or perspectives about the scenario. As participant interest increases it is ". . . likely to result in greater student engagement, higher levels of intrinsic motivation, higher student productivity, greater student autonomy, increased achievement, and an improved sense of self-competence" (Cox, 2008, p. 53). Health education materials have certainly improved over the past few years, but in selecting such products, health educators should never underestimate the importance of interest levels in making their final decision.

Production Quality   How good are the production levels of health education materials? Historically, health education materials have been of poor quality. Over a decade ago, health education leaders were complaining about the appalling quality of educational materials. These materials were being produced to combat the much more sophisticated and glossy materials originating on Madison Avenue to promote unhealthy products. The criticism of the health education productions was that they tended to be boring, preachy, and unimaginative and that by making such films, health educators were wasting the most powerful medium of all. Today's youth in particular has become accustomed to the high-tech, high-quality level of media typically found in contemporary television. To present health education materials in a form any less sophisticated is to risk a total loss of credibility and usefulness. High-quality, interesting health education materials are now becoming more common, but as mentioned earlier, they come at a significant cost. Health educators may well be faced with deciding between using materials of poor quality, or using nothing at all . . . and it would not be unreasonable to choose the latter.

Evaluation   One factor to consider is, have the materials under review ever been evaluated in any way? It would probably be safe to say that the vast majority of media materials have never been evaluated. DVDs may have been reviewed by other health educators, but often these reviews are very subjective and are prey to the vagaries of personal opinion. Little or no quantitative evaluation exists that examines the effects of specific forms of media (Sawyer & Beck, 1991). Most evaluation tends to center around the effects of specific programs or courses of study, giving scant attention to the individual component of media. With such little objective data available, the health educator should take great care to always preview new materials prior to use, and if necessary seek additional opinions from colleagues.

Availability   In selecting educational materials, the health educator needs to be concerned with the issue of availability. Do companies provide preview copies of materials? How long can you keep the materials? Is renting expensive products an option? If so, how much notice is needed for reservations? If you want to purchase something, how long will it take to receive the material? Although these questions appear to be fairly obvious concerns, the importance of planning ahead and gaining all possible relevant information cannot be overemphasized. If, for example, a film is a crucial part of a presentation, then the presenter should begin planning to obtain the film well in advance of the presentation. All types of complications are possible, and the simple process of determining the availability of materials can prevent many problems.

Format   Format is a particular concern in the area of videotape and computer usage. As will be discussed later, videotape is now used much less frequently than DVD. To that end, many productions are no longer available on VHS, or have become prohibitively expensive. Health educators need to establish what type of equipment is available before ordering. Ordering software for computer usage also presents some choices. Some software is still not compatible with other types, so if educators see software programs that they want to order, they must make sure that the program is available in the correct format.

Approval   Being able to use specific media materials in an educational setting may well be determined not by the individual health educator but by outside agencies. For example, in most public school settings any materials used in the classroom must be preapproved by a board or committee in the school system. This is particularly common when teaching "sensitive" topics such as human sexuality. A school health educator would obviously be well advised to ensure that materials he or she intends to use are "approved." Individual teachers may not always agree with a committee's opinions on which materials are acceptable, yet ignoring this approval process invites professional sanctions. The community health educator is less likely to confront such formal approval procedures. Nevertheless, the educator should take every precaution to ensure that he or she selects materials that will be deemed appropriate by the community. Consultation with professional peers and community leaders would certainly reduce the possibility of embarrassment.

Objective: After reviewing the case study, the reader will recommend two strategies Amy could implement to ensure the selection of useful media products.

Case Study: Amy   Amy has some end-of-the-year funds in her budget and decides to spend the money on some educational DVDs that look very good in the catalogue. Later she is disappointed when her staff gives the media resources poor reviews and most refuse to use them. It appears that Amy has wasted valuable resources. What steps could Amy have taken to prevent this situation? (See Case Studies Revisited page 281.)

Questions to consider:

1. What are some ways Amy could involve her staff when making her media selections?
2. What are the advantages and disadvantages of previewing the material prior to purchase? Do you believe the advantages outweigh the disadvantages? Explain your position.

Media Development

One of the major problems of applying rigorous evaluation standards to media materials is that given the limitations of many of the products currently available, the health educator may be unable to find anything suitable. Some individuals may be able to compromise and use the materials despite their obvious limitations. Others may decide that the price of compromise is too high, and the media materials are simply not used. Finally, some individuals may decide in the absence of useful materials that they will develop their own.

Historically, health education materials have been designed by media production companies, not health educators, and health educators have used them because the subject matter has been health-related . . . a sort of marriage of convenience. This situation has often resulted in high-quality production levels but less effective health education messages than desired. Conversely, many of the productions designed by health educators have adhered more closely to principles of health education but because of low production qualities were viewed as boring, amateurish, and ineffectual. The development of high-quality, credible health education materials that can compete with glossy and sophisticated commercial productions is of paramount importance. Health educators know better than anyone else the types of materials that would be effective. Unfortunately, their lack of technical expertise makes them reluctant to embark on media development. Although the development of new, exciting, high-quality materials is not easy, the process is well within the grasp of many educators. Some important points to consider when contemplating media development follow:

1. Objectives
2. Present resources
3. Format
4. Expertise
5. Cost
6. Financing
7. Marketing
8. Production quality
9. Evaluation

Once again, this list is not exhaustive, but it provides some useful fundamental questions that you, the health educator, should consider. Let us examine each in detail.

Objectives   What do you specifically want to accomplish? The development of specific objectives or learning outcomes is the first crucial step in material development. From which domains are the objectives derived: cognitive, affective, or psychomotor? Do the objectives include components from more than one domain? Before even deciding what type of media to produce, think through and commit to paper no more than three behavioral objectives. A common mistake is expecting to be able to accomplish multiple objectives from one production . . . an incredibly difficult task irrespective of the elaborate nature of the materials. You may well find yourself needing to concentrate on and limit yourself to only one major objective.

Present Resources   Does a vehicle already exist that will meet your desired objective(s)? Before embarking on what is usually a very time-consuming and often expensive venture, you need to be absolutely certain that such materials have not already been developed. This is of particular importance if you intend to market your materials in an effort to recoup production costs.

Format   What will be the most effective format for the new materials—PowerPoint presentation, billboard, poster, DVD? Unfortunately, the most effective format is not necessarily the most practical. For example, a DVD might be considered the most effective manner to lessen the fears of adolescents before experiencing their first pelvic examination. However, the production of a good-quality DVD can be quite involved and very expensive. The health educator might decide that the development of a high-quality set of PowerPoint slides accompanied by a well-written script would be a more practical strategy. The sequence of brainstorming here is important. Begin by thinking through *the* most effective format, regardless of cost and impracticality, and do not compromise until you have explored every possibility to develop your first choice. Talk to others in your field or individuals who have expertise in media development—you may be surprised at what is possible!

Expertise   Do you have the knowledge and level of expertise necessary to develop your own materials? For most of us in health education the answer to this question will be a resounding "No!" . . . and that's all right. You may be an expert in health education, but probably your skills and knowledge concerning the intricacies of media production are limited. Finding individuals who are skilled in production is an absolutely vital component in the successful development of quality materials. Such individuals exist in many settings, not only the expensive, professional film production company but also the university where talented students are studying film and television, graphics, art, journalism, and other related fields. Develop your ideas for media materials, shape them into a preliminary proposal, and then seek out some individuals who can react to your ideas. Many individuals in the university setting would be delighted to be involved in media development. Some will be looking for payment, but not necessarily exorbitant payment. Students might be interested in course credit. Other individuals might simply be interested in the experience. The key point here is to pursue your ideas with enthusiasm. You won't know what is possible unless you try!

Cost   How much will the development and production of your materials cost? The answer is nearly always "too much!" In most cases the cost of production will be the critical determining factor in deciding on the media format. Once again, as a health educator, you might have little idea as to production costs, so the necessity of consulting the media professional becomes obvious. For example, if your initial objective is to produce a DVD, in order to obtain a fairly accurate estimate of cost, you would need to develop a rough script and outline. If money is no problem, a production company could do this for you, but a more likely scenario is to collaborate with someone who has an interest in this area. The DVD producer can then give you a fairly accurate estimate of cost, given your project requirements.

The sequence of events is fairly similar for all media formats—think through your ideas, focus on specific objectives, develop an outline and proposal, and then research cost. Obviously, selecting a less involved format of materials means that you can do more of the production yourself and be less concerned with cost. Once you feel that you have a fairly accurate estimate, the next step is to seek financing.

Financing   Can you access sufficient sources of funding to develop your materials? Now that you know what you would like to produce and how much it is going to cost, you need to work out if you can fund the materials. If you feel that your intended materials might fill a need shared by others, then with some persistent searching you may be able to find some financial help. Collaboration with several groups, organizations, or departments will certainly reduce individual burdens. Investigate the possibility of funding through grant writing. Many federal, state, and private organizations offer grants for health-related issues, and the development of educational materials is certainly a legitimate avenue. Again, consulting with individuals who are knowledgeable in obtaining grants would be very useful.

Also, approach private companies who manufacture products relevant to your topic. Although you would need to tread carefully in the area of sponsorship, the development of useful new educational materials can sometimes be facilitated by collaboration with the private sector. Media distributors who produce their own materials may be receptive to a proposal, leading to their producing the educational materials. Often the key to confronting the cost of media development is a combination of creativity and sheer persistence. Before you decide that the cost of developing your materials is too prohibitive, make sure that you have solicited every source!

Marketing   Do you intend to develop your materials for personal use, or would you consider marketing your product at the local or national level? One important point to consider is that if you are developing materials because a void exists in what is currently available, there is a good chance that other health educators are experiencing the same problem and may be interested in what you produce. This whole issue is integrally linked to obtaining initial funding. If you can provide a very strong proposal that includes evidence of a widespread universal need for your materials, the chance of winning some type of funding is greatly enhanced. If individuals or groups are likely to recoup their initial investment and even perhaps make a profit, they are far more likely to help finance a project than if they perceive their support as a donation. Health educators could certainly distribute their own materials, but without any real expertise in this area, their success would be limited.

Professional organizations could be helpful in this process, either in distributing the actual materials or in providing mailing lists of fellow professionals (at a cost!). Examples of such organizations are the American College Health Association (ACHA); American Alliance for Health, Physical Education, Recreation and Dance (AAHPERD); American School Health

Association (ASHA); and American Public Health Association (APHA). In addition to professional organizations, commercial media distribution companies are only too glad to distribute high quality products, but at a large cost to the developer. For example, commercial distributors of DVDs will customarily take 70–75% of the selling price of each disc sold, leaving the producer with a much lower 25–30% of the share. Although the rates might seem unreasonable, a good, aggressive distribution company can potentially sell many more DVDs than could the producer, thus compensating for offering a smaller share of the profits. As with sponsorship discussed in the previous section, association with commercial distribution companies should be thoroughly investigated, often with legal advice, before any commitment is made.

Finally, be advised that publishing companies that previously concentrated only on printed materials have begun to broaden their horizons. In the light of diminishing book sales these companies are becoming more progressive and are demonstrating a firm interest in alternative or supplementary educational materials, in particular DVDs, interactive DVDs, and computer software programs.

Production Quality   What level of production quality do you anticipate developing? A good part of this question will have already been answered by considering the factors of cost and marketing previously mentioned. These factors are inextricably linked and probably should be considered simultaneously. Obviously, if national marketing is anticipated, then production qualities must be of the highest order. This in turn will ensure that production costs are fairly high. On the other hand, there is absolutely nothing wrong with setting your sights lower, keeping production costs to a minimum, and confining the use of the materials to yourself and local colleagues.

Evaluation   Although the vast majority of media materials has not been exposed to rigorous outcome evaluation, many of the products currently available have at least been developed through some type of professional and/or student validation. When developing media materials it is often useful to involve the intended target audience in the production. Small focus groups to test various components of the materials can provide invaluable feedback, as can input by fellow professionals. Changes and alterations can easily be made along the way, whereas attempting to change completed materials can be expensive, time-consuming, and sometimes impossible.

Major Types of Media Equipment

Community health, school health, small groups, large groups, schoolchildren, or senior citizens—no matter what the setting or clientele, the health educator will usually use some form of audiovisual equipment or media. Devices aimed at optimizing the effectiveness of presentations are numerous, and

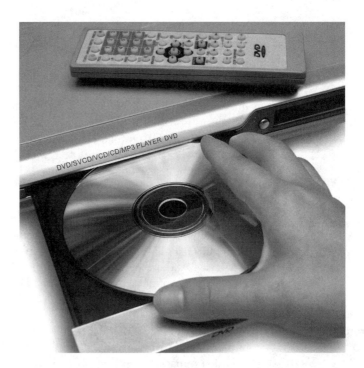

DVDs are a cheap and easy method to bring new information into your classroom.

the past decade has seen incredible technological advances, providing the presenter with some interesting choices. This section is intended to describe the available types of equipment and help the potential user grasp some of the advantages and disadvantages of each one.

The major types of media equipment include:

- DVDs
- Document cameras
- Interactive whiteboards
- Presentation software
- Audience response systems
- Personal computers

DVDs   The DVD has become the dominant format for data storage and the distribution of prerecorded content. Like most sources of media, video storage formats continue to evolve. The DVD (digital video disc or digital versatile disc) essentially replaced outdated formats such as laserdiscs, VHS (tapes), and CDs. The optical disc storage provided by a DVD continues to improve in quality with the addition of high definition and Blu-ray.

Advantages

1. Instructors have many options of how to use a DVD. For example, the disc can be stopped and then restarted at any point the instructor selects. This allows the instructor to efficiently skip to desired segments of the content contained on the disc.

2. Quite often, DVDs are designed to encourage frequent pauses to allow for discussion. This is particularly useful for reinforcing cognitive information and permitting processing of affective ideas. It is also a major advantage for instructors dealing with groups who have short attention spans!

3. Perhaps the greatest advantage of the DVD is its interactive nature. This allows learning to be less of a spectator sport and more of a mutual endeavor. Groups can interact with the program in a community or classroom setting, or programs can be utilized that focus on the individual. The individual focus is particularly useful when dealing with sensitive, personal issues such as human sexuality and drug abuse.

4. Increasingly, DVDs are being produced with two soundtracks, one in English and another in a second language, usually Spanish.

5. Because this technology is relatively new, the programs that exist tend to be more current than some of the other forms of instructional materials. Additionally, the ability to digitize archived content enables the user to include pieces of data that have historical relevance.

6. The sound and picture quality of the DVD are outstanding.

7. DVDs can be played on many laptop computers and used in conjunction with the most recent video projectors, which are both small and relatively portable.

Disadvantages

1. The enhancement of features provided by the DVD often requires more advanced and sometimes costly systems, such as Blu-ray players, to display the content.

2. Scratches to the DVD can result in diminished ability to view or hear the content. Care must be taken to avoid scratching the disc.

Document Cameras   Think of a document camera as the hybrid of its predecessors, the opaque and overhead projectors. The document camera—commonly known as a video visualizer/presenter—is a modern replacement for the stand-alone overhead transparency projector, a device first developed to train soldiers during World War II (Crystal, 2008).

An illuminated platform serves as a display base for a mounted camera. The camera lens is pointed at the material placed upon the platform, which is then projected onto a TV monitor or ceiling projector using an S-Video cable. The document camera is superior to its predecessors in that almost anything can be enlarged and displayed under its lens. In addition to the ability to project transparencies using the base light, it can also display paper printouts, pages from a book, photographs, and three-dimensional (3D) objects without losing the ability to see the colors of the original document (Frisk, 2008). The camera can even display live images. For example, an educator might use the document camera to display a breast model while performing the steps of a breast self-exam. The students would be able to view the teacher's movements in actual time, allowing the participants to follow along step-by-step. The zooming feature allows the educator to isolate

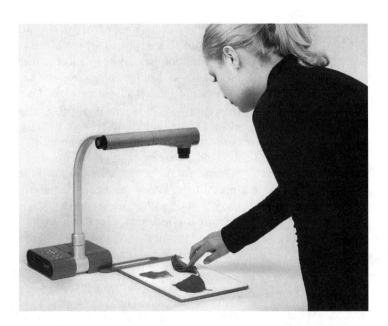

Three-dimensional objects are easily displayed using a document camera.

specific parts of the displayed object. An additional feature is the ability to allow students to display their artifacts without changing the integrity of the product. Although there are some disadvantages of using document cameras, according to Frisk, the advantages are significantly greater. Its advantages and disadvantages follow:

Advantages

1. The technology is easy to use with a short learning curve limited to adjusting the zooming features.
2. It enables the educator to display fragile or 3D objects without fear of damage.
3. It does not require a computer or networking.
4. It eliminates the need to transfer materials into other formats such as transparencies, thus reducing preparation time and additional costs.

Disadvantages

1. Like most technology, the cost of the equipment can be quite expensive, far greater than the cost of a stand-alone transparency projector. However, as this medium becomes more commonly used, the cost of purchase is likely to decrease.
2. The camera requires a projection unit or TV to display the image.
3. When displaying handwritten materials, illegible handwriting may interfere with the effectiveness of the technology.

**Interactive
Whiteboards**

An interactive whiteboard is basically a giant touch screen computer. When the board is connected to a computer and digital projector, the software enables the computer applications to respond to touch commands from the whiteboard. This feature minimizes the amount of time spent returning to the computer to change applications. An additional feature is the ability to write notes using "digital ink," which can be saved and be reproduced at a later time. The ability to have multiple applications available at the touch of a finger allows the instructor to move smoothly among methods of delivering content. A health educator presenting a lecture on chronic obstructive pulmonary disease (COPD), for example, could transition, with a touch of the screen, to a media clip showing how to use an inhaler. Following the media clip, the instructor might use the digital pen to record brainstormed ideas about eliminating barriers to using inhalers, and then print or email the entire presentation to the participants later. Advantages and disadvantages of interactive whiteboard use are as follows:

Advantages

1. The interactive boards accommodate many learning styles, are appropriate for a wide range of age groups, and can accommodate participants with limited motor skills (Bell, 2002).
2. The ability to create, save, post, and share lessons allows the educator to create a library of resources.
3. They potentially expand the amount and variety of content that can be delivered in an educational session. The whiteboard interfaces well with the document camera.
4. They also have the potential to engage participants by having them touch or draw on the board.
5. Numerous interactive templates and activities are readily available on the Internet.
6. The digital markers can be used to underline, circle, or highlight information, allowing the educator to add emphasis to key concepts.
7. It is user friendly, but it does take practice to adjust to the sensitivity of the board and the response of the digital ink pens.

Disadvantages

1. The expense and necessary electronic ancillaries make interactive boards expensive.
2. Setup and maintenance of the equipment can be complicated, because the board must be calibrated to ensure that the display is congruent with the position of the virtual digital ink.
3. Lighting of the room can impact the clarity of the projected image. The boards need to be mounted or placed in locations within the room where light is limited.
4. The size of the board and its required ancillaries limit its portability.

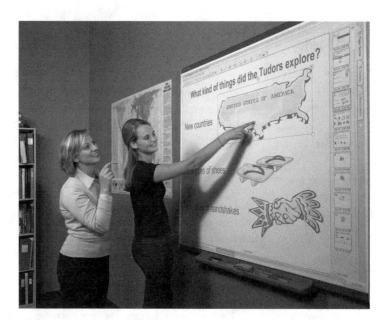

Interactive whiteboards provide another opportunity to actively engage participantss in the learning process.

Presentation Software

Imagine a really slick, colorful, sophisticated, personalized, easily operated set of overhead transparencies and you will have the sense of what presentation software can provide. To continue the media analogy, presentation software is to the overhead what the DVD is to the videotape . . . more sophisticated, professional, and definitely more impressive. There are different types of available presentation software, but Microsoft's PowerPoint is by far the most used and has become the accepted standard. PowerPoint allows the user to basically custom create a set of slides or transparencies for use in a presentation. The program provides a set of templates with many different features, including subtle backgrounds, interesting title styles, and organizational choices. The ideal use of such a program is to store the presentation materials on a disc or hard drive, then connect a computer to a video/computer projector to display the materials with the click of a mouse. If a computer/projector setup is not available, with the use of a color printer, PowerPoint materials can be displayed on a document camera or can be used to develop overhead transparencies. Simply print the materials directly onto transparencies. Although your presentation may not look quite as polished as the computer/projector version, you will still have a set of very professional-looking resources. Advantages and disadvantages of presentation software are as follows:

Advantages

1. Presentation software allows the instructor to custom develop his or her own materials, thereby tailoring presentations specifically to the instructor's goals, rather than merely adapting less suitable material.

2. Using the computer/projector or document camera, the instructor will be able to easily show materials to small or large groups.
3. Materials developed with presentation software such as PowerPoint look very professional.
4. Written material and tables can be displayed on a large screen, making visibility for the audience very easy.
5. The order of presentation can be readily changed, and previous slides can be revisited with little difficulty.
6. Presentation slides can be made from just about anything, so information from books, magazine advertisements, newspaper headlines, and so forth can all be used in a very creative manner. Additionally, there are many commercially prepared slide programs available.
7. The computer/projector setup is becoming more feasible as both the price and size of computers and projectors become smaller.
8. Presentations can be stored on portable flash drives, allowing the presenter to carry a pocket-sized version of the presentation.
9. Presentation files can be sent to others electronically via the Internet.

Disadvantages

1. The instructor will need to use some type of screen or find a very white wall to use either a computer or a document camera.
2. Use of either form of projector necessitates semi-darkness. This has the potential for lessening the speaker/audience bond—and in the classroom setting can initiate disruption.
3. Although laptop computers are readily available and projectors are becoming more portable, the inconvenience of transporting expensive and sometimes awkward equipment should still be considered a disadvantage.
4. Again, although the cost of computer equipment has steadily fallen into the relatively affordable range, the initial outlay for both hardware and software could, in some cases, be prohibitive.
5. The development of PowerPoint presentations necessitates access to both a computer and available software, in addition to a reasonable amount of computer expertise.
6. Because PowerPoint presentations take some time and effort to create, this could be a great barrier for many individuals.
7. PowerPoint presentations have the potential of being very boring. With the lights necessarily being lowered, the potential exists for behavior problems in a classroom setting and lack of interest/attention in a community setting.

Audience Response Systems

"Toss me my remote" seems like an unusual phrase to hear in an educational setting, yet it is one you might hear more often as "clickers" become as commonplace as pencils in a classroom. An audience response system or "clicker" is a handheld transmitting device that uses wireless technology to beam audience responses to a receiver attached to a computer. Clickers can be used for a variety of applications such as administering in-class quizzes, voting on debate issues, surveying game show audiences, or even polling registered voters. The audience response system can instantly display the results, tally them, and present them in elaborate spreadsheets using eye-catching graphics like spaceships or *Jeopardy!*-style boards (Hu, 2008). Participant responses are linked to the clicker being used by a serial number, thus the anonymity of the participant is well protected. The ability of the clicker's computer program to monitor participation rates and track the percentages of accurate responses provides instant feedback and gratification for both the instructor and participant (Hu, 2008). The educator has the ability to embed questions into presentation software, allowing the question to appear during the lecture and thereby challenging all the audience members to actively participate by responding to the question. "Student response systems can be used in situations where students are required to apply prior knowledge or use higher-level, critical thinking skills to predict an outcome" (Chapman & Conner, 2006, p. 1). For example, after reviewing the health profiles of three individuals (A, B, and C), students can be asked to predict which one is at greatest risk for a stroke. The data collected from the use of clickers could be of great value when providing evidence of formative assessment, especially in a community health setting. Draper and Brown (2004) have identified the following advantages and disadvantages of using audience responses:

Advantages

1. The lectures become more interactive and interesting because participants are able to contribute without embarrassing themselves.
2. The ability to respond and see the responses of others provides feedback on individual performance in relationship to other individuals.
3. Techniques can provide feedback on student comprehension and help to identify content that needs greater clarification.
4. The technology is relatively inexpensive. A price range for a typical clicker is about $15 to $25, in addition to a registration fee to the service provider. Classroom sets are available to instructors for about $800 to $1,000, which includes the registration fee.

Disadvantages

1. Setting up of handsets and incorporating the technology into a lesson can be time consuming.
2. Overuse of questions can distract from learning. It is recommended that no more than five or six questions be asked within a typical 50-minute educational session.
3. They can facilitate low-level cognition if questions are poorly designed and limited to assessing the comprehension level of thought.
4. Intentional mis-voting can skew the accuracy of the displayed data.
5. The clicker devices are battery operated, thus dead batteries can inhibit the use of the technology.

Personal Computers   Personal computer (PC) technology has become a legitimate health education instructional tool in both the school and community settings. Computer applications are diverse, including small-group or individualized usage and spanning a full range of interest areas from health assessments to health education games and puzzles to statistical analysis. The most significant advantage of using personal computers is the ability to individualize instruction. By using a PC, one can input data specific to his or her health condition; then one can access reliable information that is tailored to his or her demographic. The ability to interact with the computer empowers the person to analyze his or her wellness concerns and exert control over health choices (Steinbronn & Merideth, 2003). (For more complete information on the computer, see Chapter 6.)

Advantages and disadvantages of personal computers are as follows:

Advantages

1. Computers offer an incredibly diverse set of possibilities for use in health education, ranging from complicated statistical analysis to simplified elementary school–level health education games.
2. Computers can be fun to use and of particular value in the classroom as a motivational tool.
3. Computers can allow individual usage that permits working on personal programs where privacy might be a concern.

Disadvantages

1. The format of one computer per person is ideal but not always feasible. Although greatly reduced in price (compared to a few years ago), computers are still relatively expensive, and therefore, accessibility can be limited. Having three or four individuals crowded around one terminal can become frustrating and lower the effectiveness of the method.
2. Computer equipment can vary greatly from one machine or piece of software to the next. Some individuals may be expert on one type of machine yet total novices on another type. Learning can be difficult with such differing levels of skill and experience.
3. Some health educators rely on the technology to accomplish health education instead of viewing it as an additional tool in their repertoire.

The Dinosaur Section

The rapid pace of technological change inevitably consigns some of the older forms of media to the proverbial scrap heap. However, in the rare likelihood that some hapless health educator finds him- or herself confronted by such dinosaurs, we have not completely obliterated from this text the existence of these "not so new" forms of media!

Table 7-1 summarizes the evolution of these proverbial dinosaurs. Figure 7-2 serves to remind us that failure to keep up with the advances in technology can reflect poorly upon the health educator's efforts.

Table 7-1 Evolution of Media Equipment

Dinosaur Device	Replaced By
Chalkboard and chalk	Whiteboard and dry erase markers
Overhead projector	Document camera
Slide projector	Document camera Presentation software
Film	DVD movies
Filmstrips	Electronic video clips (see Chapter 6) DVD short takes

Objective: After reviewing the case study, the reader will identify three or more indicators that suggest the medium being used is outdated and, consequently, is a contributor to the participant's disinterest.

Case Study: Jason   The room was hot and dark. Jason was trying to count the number of dust motes as they slowly passed in front of the projector's rays of light. At a subconscious level, he could hear the narrator's voice droning on interminably about the effects of alcohol on the liver, but even a pictorial switch from talking head to a grossly abused and swollen liver was insufficient to disturb Jason's reverie. Sure, he saw the offending organ, glistening on the marble slab . . . sure, he could hear the narrator listing the dangers of an intemperate lifestyle . . . but Jason wasn't actually in the room. The warmth and darkness had transported him to a far more interesting place . . . his imagination. The football game this weekend . . . the party at Scott's place . . . catching that new movie . . . much more interesting than the talking head who had just returned to the screen. The visual switch was enough to make

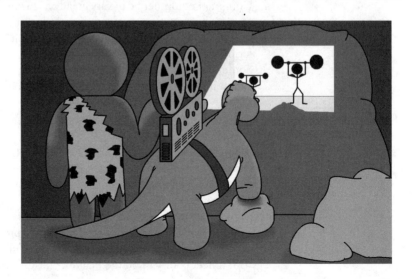

Figure 7-2
Are You Guilty of
Not Evolving with
Technology?

Jason briefly wonder why all talking heads wore white coats and horn-rimmed glasses, and sported haircuts from the 1960s . . . not that it really mattered; it was back to the party for him! Boy, the party was crowded—was everyone in the room counting dust motes and partying? . . . an alarming prospect! (See Case Studies Revisited page 282.)

Questions to consider:

1. What are some indicators that suggest the medium being used is out-dated?
2. How might the use of outdated media devices impact the effectiveness of health education efforts?

Preparing Visual Materials

Eight specific problems to avoid when preparing visual materials with presentation software follow (Figures 7-3 and 7-4 illustrate a poor use of graphics and good use, respectively, which can either confuse or help the viewer understand your message):

1. Beware of using a tiny font size. Many presenters simply copy their notes onto a transparency for use with groups, thus importing a size 12 font that may look fine on a printed page but proves unrecognizable from the back of a large room! Always increase font size to at least 16 or 18, particularly when using smaller fonts like Times.
2. If you ever hear yourself saying, "You probably can't read this, but . . ." you probably shouldn't be projecting the text. If people can't read what you have provided, you either need to redo the document, making it legible, or think of another method of presentation without the fairly useless visual.
3. The rainbow effect is undesirable. Some presenters equate lots of color with high-quality visuals, but instead of being impressive, overly colorful materials are distracting and difficult to read. The rule of thumb is to keep things simple and clear. Color can be very effective . . . just don't overdo it!
4. Busy, busy, busy . . . some transparencies have way too much material on them and are so crammed with information that they become overwhelming and ultimately confusing. Rather than trying to put literally everything on the screen, limit the type of material you put on any slide to core issues and essentials, adding to and expanding information from your narrative. Most people are easily bored and do not want to look at the same transparency for very long, so have more, shorter transparencies rather than fewer, complex images.
5. More busy, busy, busy . . . in addition to too much material, some presenters tend to confuse the inclusion of a logo or background image common

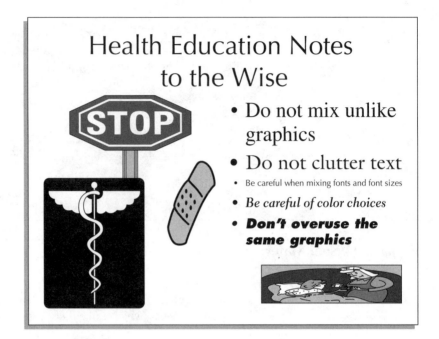

Figure 7-3
Disorganized Clutter

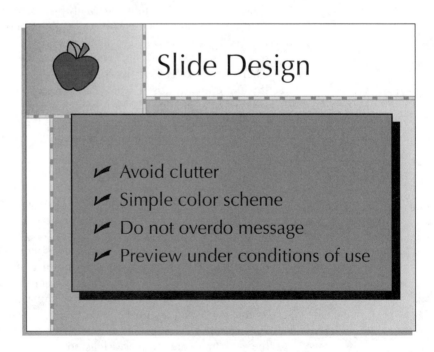

Figure 7-4
Organized Design

to all the transparencies with sophistication and quality. Logos or icons can prove to be very distracting and detract from the message. Keep things simple and clear.

6. Avoid using too many font changes. Some transparencies look like a ransom note — as if the presenter couldn't decide which font to use, so decided to use them all! Unless you need to change font types to make a specific point, be consistent with the appearance of the transparency, again to avoid detracting from the material itself. Strive to limit yourself to two typefaces to minimize visual confusion. AVOID USING ALL CAPS; it is harder for the eye to differentiate between the letters when they are all the same size.

7. Organize your information with boxes, borders, and areas of contrasting color. This allows the participant to visually take in the content in smaller segments, making it easier to retain.

8. Keep it simple. The visual aids that you develop should be just that, aids to complement your presentation, not a colorful extravaganza to advertise the fact that you've just got a new computer! Develop and use only what will enhance your presentation, and avoid bombarding the audience with too much material that ultimately may swallow up the point of your presentation. Always test your materials in the actual room of delivery (if possible). Otherwise, find a similar room with similar lighting to test the presentation. Be certain to stand in the back of the room.

Marketing Interventions

Effective interventions don't happen by chance; they require hours of advanced planning and preparation. The majority of the work of a health educator is done long before the presentation of the program. It is not enough to create dynamic programs; one must also be effective in enticing participants to attend. How dreadful it would be to spend countless hours creating a dynamic intervention that no one or very few attended. For this reason, it is critical to at least consider some fundamental aspects of marketing.

According to the Centers for Disease Control and Prevention (CDC, 2006), health marketing is the creating, communicating, and delivering of health information and interventions using customer-centered and science-based strategies to protect and promote the health of diverse populations. Effective health marketing ensures that a product is tailored to meet customer needs, realistically priced, conveniently delivered, and effectively promoted to the target population (Lovelock & Wirtz, 2004). There are four fundamental elements that should be present when developing a marketing plan; these four elements are referred to as the "four Ps" in the marketing mix (CDC, 2006):

- **Product:** The item being promoted and the benefits of the item to the targeted consumer
- **Price:** The monetary and nonmonetary costs of the item
- **Place:** Where or how the product can be obtained
- **Promotion:** The mechanisms used to publicize and advertise the product

These elements are important to consider as health educators develop interventions and strategies to deliver them. The quality of a product is irrelevant if consumers cannot obtain it.

Objective: Using the example in the case study, the reader will be able to identify the activities that represent each of the "Four Ps."

Case Study: Lauren   Lauren works as the health educator on the campus of a major university. During a staff meeting, the director of health services reports that there has been a dramatic increase in the number of clients they are seeing in the sick clinic. The one thing most of these clients have in common is the use of the open access computer labs (OACLs) on campus. Lauren is charged to design an intervention to control the spread of infectious disease in the computer labs. After many hours of research and planning, she develops a 1-day educational seminar targeting the student workers in the OACL. In this seminar, student workers will be trained to promote sanitary practices such as the proper use of hand sanitizers and the skills related to sanitizing computer stations between clients. The student workers will not only act as a catalyst in reducing the spread of disease, but also decrease their individual risk for contracting an infectious disease.

Lauren secures financial backing from the university's Department of Environmental Health and Safety. Their support enables Lauren to offer the training as a free service to the student workers and provide incentives for those who attend. She schedules the workshop during the days allotted for mandatory training and hosts the program at the central computer lab on campus. The workers will be able to choose between Lauren's workshop and their normally scheduled in-service training.

Using the roster provided by computer services, Lauren sends a flyer describing the program and its benefits for attendees via email to the inboxes of each student worker. The email includes a link enabling the workers to register for the workshop electronically. Workers are encouraged to sign up quickly for the limited number of spaces available. The electronic sign-up allows Lauren to send additional reminders to registered participants and recruitment emails to those who have not registered yet. Five days prior to the scheduled workshop, Lauren is almost at capacity for the training. It appears that her marketing plan was a success. (See Case Studies Revisited page 282.)

Questions to consider:

1. What would you consider to be the product, price, place, and promotion of Lauren's intervention?
2. What elements of Lauren's plan do you believe contributed most to the success of her marketing?
3. Lauren chose to make the program available to the participants free of charge. In your opinion, is this the best approach? How might charging a fee for the program impact the participation rate?

Preparing Promotional Materials

In an ideal world, health educators would have the ability to hire advertising firms to develop slick promotional campaigns; however, budget limitations often dictate this becoming the responsibility of the community health educator. A fundamental concept is to market where your target population is likely to be found. If promoting proper use of infant car seats, it would be illogical to post flyers at the community senior center. It makes much more sense to post these flyers in the windows of the local toy store or distribute program information via the community pediatric clinic.

Consider a variety of venues to deliver your message, including newspaper advertisements, pamphlets, flyers, webpages, emails, and bulletin boards or billboards. Today, an event T-shirt is often given as an incentive, which serves as a walking advertisement for anything and everything. Movie theater, television, and radio advertisements are more expensive options to reach an expanded target audience. One free resource available to community interest groups is the public service announcement (PSA). Broadcast companies are required by the Federal Communications Commission (FCC) to donate a percentage of their air time to playing PSAs. Theoretically, this appears to be an ideal venue for advertising programs; however, the lack of regulations about the placement of the PSA within the programming schedule leads to less than optimal airtime placement. "Overall, the data suggest that despite the seemingly large amount of airtime and media dollars donated to PSAs by television stations, the advertisements are reaching a very limited number of people" (Lancaster & Lancaster, 2002). When using broadcast media, it might be worth considering the use of PSAs in conjunction with other promotional efforts.

The following tips are suggestions to help you develop promotional materials that will stand out and ideally have a positive impact on your advertisement efforts:

1. Be consistent in your marketing message. Repeat the same ideas, color schemes, logos, and basic information on all your materials. Repetition is an effective technique to helping potential consumers remember the dynamics of your product.
2. Strive to draw the attention of the consumer by using a catchy title or a colorful/striking logo or photograph. Buzz words or phrases often entice the reader to take a look at or listen to the advertisement. Some common buzz words/phrases might include:
   - Easy
   - Discover
   - The secret to
   - Unlock
   - Insider
   - How to
   - Free
   - Now you can

Be careful not to make unrealistic claims that might cause the consumer to discredit your product based on the advertisement. The use of the buzz word "proven" is problematic, for example, because it is very difficult to prove anything. There may be a strong correlation between your product and its ability to achieve its goals, but it is improbable that the product will have perfect results every time.

When developing a logo, remember the cliché, "simple is elegant." One simple large image is better than many small images. The validity of the concept can be clearly seen in the ability of a multi-million-dollar business to get the average consumer to associate a large, golden, arching M with its chain of hamburger restaurants.

3. Promote the benefits of participation to the target audience. What will your participants gain from using your product? Consider using testimonials that focus on the benefits. Entice the consumer by listing and promoting the incentives that are included with the product. For example: "You can present the tear-off coupon at the bottom of this flyer to receive a free T-shirt upon arrival." Use words that promote individual gain like "you" and "your" instead of words like, "we," "us," "I," or "our."

4. Provide the necessary information on how to obtain the product or more information about the product. This might include dates, times, locations, web addresses, and the name, email address, and phone number for a contact person.

5. In addition to the same guidelines suggested earlier in this chapter on preparing visual presentations, be certain to have an outsider proofread your materials prior to printing. This includes dialing the listed phone numbers, connecting to the webpages using the provided web address, and emailing the person listed as the point of contact. It is a sickening feeling to know that you just printed 1,000 flyers with the name of your program spelled incorrectly.

The promotion of a product can be very costly, so three key ideas to remember with your promotion campaign are:

- **Kiss it!:** Keep it simple, sweetie.
- **Proof it!:** Proofread everything.
- **Budget it!:** Select promotional materials that will enable you to get the most exposure for the least monetary and nonmonetary expense.

For more information and tools related to this chapter visit
http://healtheducation.jbpub.com/strategies.

EXERCISES

1. You are a high school health teacher and have just been told by a friend about a new DVD on HIV/AIDS. You are scheduled to teach a unit on AIDS in a few weeks and would potentially like to use the DVD. Carefully describe all the steps you would take to achieve this goal.

2. You are a school or community health educator who has received a $1,000 grant to purchase media materials related to heart health. Make a detailed budget list of the materials you will purchase. (Do not make up a fictitious list! Do some research and consult some audiovisual catalogues, libraries, bookstores, health professionals, etc.). You must reference all items, for example, the name of the DVD distributor, address, cost, and so on. You may be surprised how little you get for $1,000!

3. You are a school or community health educator who is interested in media materials. Thinking of your particular area of interest or expertise (if you do not have one, just select a health topic), what sort of media materials could be developed that would really enhance education in this area? Where do you consider the gaps to be in available media when related to your area of particular interest? Do some initial research to ensure that the materials do not already exist, and then write a descriptive outline of *your* proposed new media materials. Be creative! Do not worry about budget or lack of previous experience. What do you think would really enhance your teaching or presentations? What type of media would you develop? What would be your goals and objectives? What type of approach would you use? Give it a try!

4. Select two videotapes or DVDs from the same subject area, and, utilizing Figure 7-1 (or, if you prefer, a similar instrument), evaluate the videotapes/DVDs. Include in your evaluation what you would consider the goals and objectives of each videotape/DVD and whether or not you would use either of them in your work.

5. Collect two or three samples of flyers displayed in your community. Determine which of your examples meet the criteria described for creating effective marketing materials. Design a flyer based on the principles discussed in the text to promote the "anti-bullying program" you have created for the children at the community youth center.

6. Using the National Institutes of Health website (http://www.nih.gov), identify a grant that could be used to support the production of media for your topic selected in exercise 3.

CASE STUDIES REVISITED

Case Study Revisited: Amy   Amy should probably have consulted her staff initially to see whether they had seen the DVDs that she was about to order and also to ask them if they had any suggestions. Also, to purchase a DVD without previewing it is a very risky if not foolhardy practice. Most media companies will allow the customer to preview prior to purchase. Amy would have been wise to do just that, in addition to asking her staff members to preview the materials with her to obtain some additional input. (See page 261.)

Case Study Revisited: Jason

This case presents an alarming prospect indeed, but unfortunately an all too common one. As modern technology has become more sophisticated and available, the use of educational media has increased in both the school and community settings. This increased usage, however, has not always proved beneficial to program participants. Too often the materials used are outdated, of poor technical quality, too heavily laden with facts, inappropriate for the audience, or, perhaps the greatest sin of all, they are often excruciatingly boring! Modern-day individuals like Jason, who have been nurtured on extremely high production-quality shows on television (like MTV) and in movie theaters have developed the uncanny ability of being able to identify poor quality in health education media within a matter of seconds. The classic clues on a media source might include an extremely dated soundtrack, characters wearing flared pants and giving the "peace" sign, no sign of any automobiles built since 1978, and the talking head in the form of a physician wearing the ubiquitous white coat and pointing to a list of written information. Any or all of these attributes are guaranteed to encourage Jason and his peers to leave their bodies in search of greater stimulation! (See page 274.)

Case Study Revisited: Lauren

Lauren has done several things right in her marketing plan. Her intervention addresses a need and targets a specific clientele, allowing Lauren to tailor her marketing efforts. When considering the 4 Ps, Lauren appears to have included all the necessary elements:

- **Product:** The training workshop benefits the target population by reducing their individual risk for disease while increasing the environmental quality of their work environment.
- **Price:** Lauren has addressed the monetary barriers by identifying a sponsor to underwrite the initiative while minimizing the non-monetary costs by offering the program when the student workers would normally be in training. Additionally, she increases the likelihood that the workers will choose her workshop over their typical in-service by offering incentives for attending.
- **Place:** Lauren has selected a central location that is easily accessible by the target population.
- **Promotion:** Considering the target population, Lauren's choice to use electronic means to publicize the workshop makes sense. Her ability to monitor sign-up within her promotional materials is an effective use of resources. Her choice to promote the limited availability of spaces may have been directly related to the early participant sign-up.

Lauren's choice to underwrite the participant cost was likely a good one in this situation. When participants are placed in a forced compliance situation, as is the case with a mandatory attendance policy, they often begrudge having to attend. Eliminating participant costs can serve to minimize the negative emotions related to the mandatory compliance. Free, however, is not always best. It is human nature to be skeptical of the quality of a product when it is free. It is sometimes advantageous to charge a minimal fee for participation. When participants pay, they tend to place more value on the product because there is a vested interest. (See page 278.)

SUMMARY

1. Media literacy is a field that advocates the critical analysis of mass media messages to enable the individual to more accurately distinguish between reality and the media's version of the truth.

2. The use of media materials in health education has become extremely common. Unfortunately, much of the material produced in earlier years is of poor production quality and low interest and generally does little to enhance health education programming.

3. Media selection is a multifaceted process that should be based on a combination of sound principles described in this chapter.

4. Selecting media materials should be based on more than cost, availability, and personal preference. Selection should be based on the goal of achieving behavioral objectives formulated before the review process.

5. The decision to use no media material rather than something of dubious quality will usually be the right decision. Poor-quality, outdated, or boring materials will usually have a detrimental effect on the presentation.

6. Media materials should be viewed as vehicles to enhance learning, not products that stand alone. Processing materials is an essential part of using educational resources.

7. New media development should always be considered an option when existing materials are deemed to be insufficient. The production of media should be based on the sound principles of development discussed in this chapter.

8. A recent trend in media materials is a move away from the fact-filled production to a more affective, process-oriented approach.

9. There is an obvious need for health educators to use materials that match the quality of shows produced by commercial agencies that often promote unhealthy lifestyles.

10. Health educators need to be aware of the advantages and disadvantages of the various forms of media.

11. Health educators would be well advised to develop a basic operating knowledge of media equipment.

REFERENCES AND RESOURCES

Agency for Healthcare Research and Quality. (2008). Background on AHRQ. Retrieved December 18, 2008, from http://www.ahrq.gov/about/budgtix.htm #background

Aufderheide, P. (1993). Media literacy: A report of the national leadership conference on media literacy. ERIC Document Reproduction Service No. ED 365 294.

Bell, M. A. (2002). Why use an interactive whiteboard? A baker's dozen reasons! teachers.net. Retrieved December 12, 2008, from http://teachers.net/gazette/JAN02/mabell.html

Campeau, P. L. (1974). Selective review of the results of research on the use of audiovisual media to teach adults. *Audio-Visual Communications Review, 22,* 5–40.

Center for Media Literacy. (2007). The heart of media literacy is informed inquiry. Retrieved on June 20, 2009, from http://www.medialit.org/about_CML.html

Centers for Disease Control and Prevention. (2006). Health marketing basics. Retrieved December 16, 2008, from http://www.cdc.gov/healthmarketing/basics.htm

Chapman, S., & Connor, P. (2006). "Clickers" aka classroom response systems. The Institute for Learning and Teaching. Retrieved December 12, 2008, from http://tilt.colostate.edu/mti/tips/tip.cfm?tipid=46

Considine, D. (1995). An introduction to media literacy: The what, why and how to's. *Journal of Media Literacy, 41*(2). Retrieved December 18, 2008, from http://www.ced.appstate.edu/departments/ci/programs/edmedia/medialit/article.html

Considine, D. M. (1990). Can we get there from here? *Educational Technology, 30*(12), 27–32.

Cox, S. G. (2008). Differentiated instruction in the elementary classroom. *Education Digest, 73*(9), 52–54.

Crystal, G. (2008). What is an overhead projector? Wisegeek. Retrieved December 12, 2008, from http://www.wisegeek.com/what-is-an-overhead-projector.htm

Dorman, S. M. (2000). American Academy of Pediatrics sponsors media matters. *Journal of School Health, 70*(1), 33–34.

Draper, S. W., & Brown, M. I. (2004). Increasing interactivity in lectures using an electronic voting system. *Journal of Computer Assisted Learning, 20*, 81–94. Retrieved June 8, 2006, from http://www.psy.gla.ac.uk/~steve/ilig/papers/draperbrown.pdf

Fejer, D., Hawley, P., Kuchar, E., Lucitis, D., & Webster, C. (1972). *Assessing audiovisual aids for drug education: Preliminary study.* Toronto, Canada: Addiction Research Foundation of Ontario.

Frisk, J. (2008, October 1). The document camera: Advancing classroom visual technology. *Educators' eZine.* Retrieved December 11, 2008, from http://www.techlearning.com/showArticle.php?articleID=196605452

Galician, M. (2004). Introduction: High time for "disillusioning" ourselves and our media. *American Behavioral Scientist, 48*(1), 7–17.

Herr, N. (2001). The sourcebook for teaching science. Retrieved December 18, 2008, from http://www.csun.edu/~vceed002/health/docs/tv&health.html

Hu, W. (2008). Students click, and a quiz becomes a game. *New York Times.* Retrieved June 20, 2009, from http://www.nytimes.com/2008/01/28/education/28neck.html?pagewanted=all

Kahn, T. M., & Master, D. (1992). Multimedia literacy at Rowland: A good story well told. *Technological Horizons in Education Journal, 19*(7), 77–83.

Lancaster, A. R., & Lancaster, K. M. (2002). Reaching insomniacs with television PSAs: Poor placement of important messages. *Journal of Consumer Affairs, 36*, 150.

Lovelock, C., & Wirtz, J. (2004). *Services Marketing: People, Technology, Strategy.* Upper Saddle River, NJ: Prentice Hall

Martin, C., & Stainbrook, G. L. (1986). An analysis checklist for audiovisuals when used as educational resources. *Health Education, 17*(4), 31–33.

Media Literacy Project. (1999). Definition of media literacy. Retrieved June 3, 1999, from http://www.babson.edu/medialiteracyproject

Melamed, L. (1989). Sleuthing media "truths." *History and Social Science Teacher, 24*(4), 189–193.

Ontario Ministry of Education. (1989). *Media Literacy.* Ontario: Ministry of Education, p. 225.

Palmer, P. (1990, Jan/Feb). Critical thinking. *Change,* 14.

Protective Services Training Institute. (2004, December). Trainers corner. Retrieved December 19, 2008, from http://www.utexas.edu/research/cswr/psti/newsletter/trainerscorner/TC_12.php#Commissioner

Rideout, V. (2008, September). Television as a health educator: A case study of *Grey's Anatomy.* Kaiser Family Foundation. Retrieved December 19, 2008, from http://www.kff.org/entmedia/upload/7803.pdf

Rideout, V., Roberts, D., & Foehr, U. (2005). *Generation M: Media in the Lives of 8–18-year-olds.* Report for the Henry J. Kaiser Family Foundation. Menlo Park, CA: The Henry J. Kaiser Family Foundation.

Sawyer, R. G., & Beck, K. H. (1991). The effects of videotapes on the perceived susceptibility to HIV/AIDS among university freshmen. *Health Values, 15*(2), 31–40.

Silverblatt, A. (2004). Media as social institution. *American Behavioral Scientist, 48*(1), 35–41.

Sneed, D., Wulfmeyer, K. T., Van Ommeren, R., & Riffe, D. (1989). Media literacy ignored: A qualitative call for the introduction of media studies across the high school social science curriculum. Paper presented at the annual meeting of the Association for Education in Journalism and Mass Communication, Washington, DC.

Steinbronn, P. E., & Merideth, E. M. (2003). An outward design support system to increase self-efficacy in online teaching and learning. *Campus Wide Systems, 20*(1), 17–24

Widen, E., Pellechia, K. M., & Schneider, J. K. (2007). *Health Literacy Resource List for Educators.* Beltsville, MD: Food and Nutrition Information Center Agricultural Research Service, USDA. Retrieved December 19, 2008; from http://www.nal.usda.gov/fnic/pubs/bibs/edu/health_literacy.pdf?

Yates, B. L. (1999). Media literacy: A health education perspective. *Journal of Health Education, 30*(3), 180–184.

Ziegler, S. G. (2007). The (mis)education of generation M. *Learning, Media and Technology, 32*(1), 69–81.

Minority Health

Entry-Level and Advanced 1 Health Educator Competencies Addressed in This Chapter

Responsibility I: Assess Individual and Community Needs for Health Education
  Competency A: Access existing health-related data.
  Competency F: Infer needs for health education from obtained data.

Responsibility III: Implement Health Education Strategies, Interventions, and Programs
  Competency B: Demonstrate a variety of skills in delivering strategies, interventions, and programs.
  Competency C: Use a variety of methods to implement strategies, interventions, and programs.

Responsibility VII: Communicate and Advocate for Health and Health Education
  Competency A: Analyze and respond to current and future needs in health education.
  Competency D: Influence health policy to promote health.

> Note: The competencies listed above, which are addressed in this chapter, are considered to be both entry-level and Advanced I competencies by the National Commission for Health Education Credentialing, Inc. They are taken from *A Framework for the Development of Competency Based Curricula for Entry Level Health Educators* by the National Task Force for the Preparation and Practice of Health Education, 1985; *A Competency-Based Framework for Graduate Level Health Educators,* by the National Task Force for the Preparation and Practice of Health Education, 1999; and *A Competency-Based Framework for Health Educators—The Competencies Project (CUP),* 2006.

Method Selection in Health Education

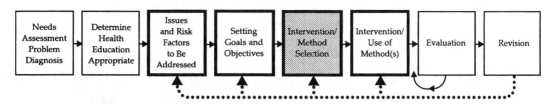

Needs Assessment Problem Diagnosis → Determine Health Education Appropriate → Issues and Risk Factors to Be Addressed → Setting Goals and Objectives → Intervention/ Method Selection → Intervention/ Use of Method(s) → Evaluation → Revision

Heavy-bordered boxes indicate subjects addressed in this text; shaded boxes indicate subjects(s) of current chapter.

After studying this chapter the reader should be able to:

- List some populations that might require the health educator to prepare material differently for presentation.
- Describe ethnic and racial disparities in selected areas of health.
- Describe the extent of research related to health and minority populations.
- Justify the need for the development of health literacy in minority populations.
- Explain the research concerns and difficulties in studying minority health.
- Describe the legacy of suspicion and concern among ethnic and racial minorities in the wake of the Tuskegee study.

KEY TOPICS

Race	Cultural competence
Ethnicity	Health knowledge levels
Culture	Sources of health information
Literacy levels	Political awareness
Language	Institutional review board
Health literacy	Community gatekeepers

Proportionately, most health educators today are both white and middle class. As opportunities for ethnic minorities increase, the discipline will become more multicultural and sensitive to the specific needs of others will be heightened. However, health educators currently practicing in the United States need to make great efforts to gain information about the individuals or groups with whom they will be working. Sometimes that information will make little difference to how a presentation is made, but in other situations radical change will be necessary. The key to successful teaching and presentations in any discipline is preparation, and learning about the lives of different populations is essential to preparation. This chapter presents suggestions for facilitating this learning process, but, as the reader will discover, for some minority populations little research has been performed to identify specific health needs; in these cases, documented methodologies for health education interventions are scarce.

Objective: After reviewing the case study, the reader will identify three or more potential cultural barriers that can interfere with the delivery of health education.

Case Study: Susan   Susan is a community health educator who has recently been planning and implementing presentations related to increasing the number of women receiving pelvic examinations. She has been asked to present a program to a women's group on the east side of the city. Having performed several of these presentations before, Susan gives little thought to preparation

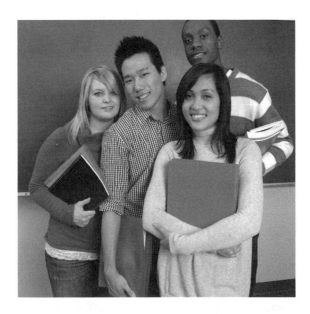

Health educators must consider ethnic diversity when planning programs and strategies.

and arrives with her materials at the appointed time and place. Susan quickly realizes that this will not be a "standard" presentation because the audience is predominantly Asian, with almost no grasp of English. The group leader graciously offers to translate, and the presentation moves laboriously along despite the translator obviously being troubled at having to translate graphic information related to sexuality. The presentation finally concludes with both audience and presenter feeling uncomfortable and dissatisfied. How could Susan have reduced the likelihood of this situation occurring? (See Case Studies Revisited page 318.)

Question to consider:

When planning for a presentation where language is a barrier, what recommendation would you make to improve the delivery of the content?

Changing Demographics in the United States

The United States has often been described as a "melting pot" in reference to the diverse ethnic backgrounds of its population. This country is indeed heterogeneous, and along with the richness and vitality that such diversity brings comes an intriguing complexity. Here are some important questions to consider:

- Are all ethnic groups affected in the same way by specific health problems?
- Do we even have data that will enable us to generalize about health problems of certain ethnic groups?

- Will an educational intervention that seems to be successful with one group work with another?
- Can only health educators who are themselves from an ethnic group work successfully with that particular group?
- Do ethnic groups trust "outside" sources of information?
- Is ethnicity the real "key" to planning health behavior interventions, or is socioeconomic status a more powerful factor?

These are important questions to consider, particularly in the light of the rapidly changing demographic face of America. According to the 2000 United States Census (2008), minorities represent roughly one-third of the U.S. population and are expected to become the majority in 2042. In the year 2039, the population of the nation is expected to reach the 400 million milestone. Projections suggest that by the year 2050 the nation will be 52% minority (U.S. Census Bureau, 2008). The graph in Figure 8-1 vividly demonstrates the projected population changes the United States will experience in the first half of the 21st century. Such a shift in populations will inevitably affect the healthcare system and, specifically, how health educators develop and implement successful programming with the ever increasing diversity of communities. The graph was developed by the Kaiser Family Foundation (2008b), based on U.S. Census Bureau, 2004, U.S. interim projections by age, sex, race, and Hispanic origin.

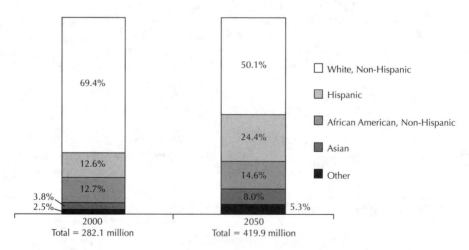

Notes: Data do not include residents of Puerto Rico, Guam, the U.S. Virgin Islands, or the Northern Marina Islands. íOther" category includes American Indian/Alaska Native, Native Hawaiian or Other Pacific Islander, and individuals reporting "Two or more races." African American, Asian, and Other categories jointly double-count 1% (2000) and 2% (2050) of the population that is of these races and Hispanic; thus, totals may not add to 100%.

Figure 8-1
Distribution of U.S. Population by Race/Ethnicity, 2000 and 2050

Source: Kaiser Slides, The Henry J. Kaiser Family Foundation. (2008, May). Based on U.S. Census Bureau (2004). U.S. Interim Projections by Age, Sex, Race, and Hispanic Origin. Available at http://www.census.gov/population/www/projections/popproj.html. Reprinted with permission. The Kaiser Family Foundation is a nonprofit private operating foundation, based in Menlo Park, California, dedicated to producing and communicating the best possible information, research, and analysis on health issues.

Should We Study Minority Health?

Although many health professionals believe studying minority health as a separate entity is a reasonable strategy, an opposing viewpoint certainly exists. Some researchers argue that separating health issues out by race, and examining race as a unique variable, encourages misinterpretation of the data and potentially increases racism. The argument continues that because race is not considered a scientifically valid biological concept, discrepancies in race data serve only to perpetuate racist stereotypes about biological differences and genetic inferiority (Leslie, 1990; Leonard, 2006; Osborne & Feit, 1992). However, other health professionals argue that we need more, not less, research on minority health and, to avoid encouraging racism, that we simply need to do a better job of performing the research (LaVeist, 2002).

One criticism of using race as a variable in health studies is that the term *race* is poorly defined. All too often, researchers assume that there is no variance within ethnicity, nationality, or culture, lumping individuals together because they speak the same language (Spanish–Hispanic) or because they originate from approximately the same part of the world (Asian). Two individuals, one from Mississippi and one from Haiti, may both be black, but they come from cultures worlds apart and may engage in completely different patterns of health behavior. Hispanic Americans originate from many different countries and continents, such as Mexico, Puerto Rico, South America, Central America, and Cuba, as indicated in Figure 8-2. Additionally, many Dominicans and some Puerto Ricans consider themselves racially black but ethnically Hispanic, while Hispanics from some Central American countries are racially Indian (Bowsworth, 2008; Nickens, 1995).

Similar ranges of diversity are also found in what is known as the "Asian" population. Such a blanket term actually tells us very little with regard to

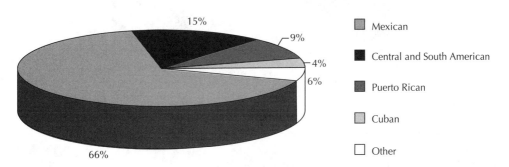

Figure 8-2
Hispanic Americans in the United States, 2006
Source: U.S. Census Bureau. (2007, October). Current population survey. Annual Social and Economic Supplement, Ethnicity and Ancestry Statistics Branch, Population Division. Retrieved on January 3, 2009, from http://www.census.gov/population/socdemo/ hispanic/cps2006/2006_tab1.2a.xls

specific ethnicity or culture in groups of individuals originating from countries such as China, Vietnam, Japan, Korea, or the Philippines. In addition, such broad categories result in missing many differences *within* groups or categories. For example, Americans of Vietnamese and Mexican origin tend to have low mean family incomes and low median age, whereas Japanese Americans and Cuban Americans have relatively high mean incomes and high median age (U.S. Census Bureau, 2007). In fact, one could argue further that although the white majority population in the United States today is also all categorized as one entity, the health behaviors of Irish, Italian, Swedish, and German Americans are not necessarily the same.

The authors of this text believe that health issues as they relate to minority populations should indeed be discussed, with the condition that such topics be viewed not through the narrow lens of race alone, but rather within a fuller context that more accurately reflects the complexity involved. There is a clear need to look beyond the obvious markers of race such as skin color or language and examine the additional factors of culture, country of origin, and socioeconomic status. For example, an obvious influence on health status is access to health insurance coverage, and as Figure 8-3 clearly shows,

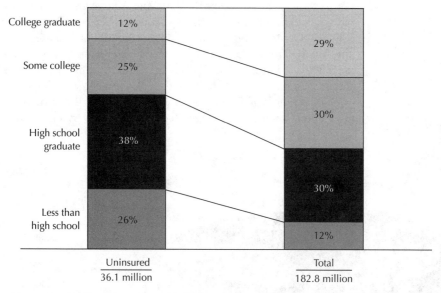

Notes: "Some college" category included respondents with an associate's degree. Adults includes all individuals aged 19 to 64. Data may not total 100% due to rounding.

Figure 8-3
Uninsured Adults vs. All Adults, by Education, 2007

Source: Kaiser Slides, The Henry J. Kaiser Family Foundation. (2007, October). Kaiser Commission on Medicaid and the Uninsured/Urban Institute Analysis of 2008 ASEC Supplement to the CPS. Reprinted with permission. The Kaiser Family Foundation is a nonprofit private operating foundation, based in Menlo Park, California, dedicated to producing and communicating the best possible information, research, and analysis on health issues.

access is by no means equal and is affected by, among other things, educational levels. As the level of education increases, so does access to higher-skilled jobs that are more likely to provide health coverage (Kaiser Family Foundation, 2008b). Additionally, there are numerous intervening factors that shape the connection of race and health outcomes, as illustrated in Figure 8-4. Health educators need to understand that looking at race or ethnicity as a single descriptor is too simplistic; additional factors should also be considered.

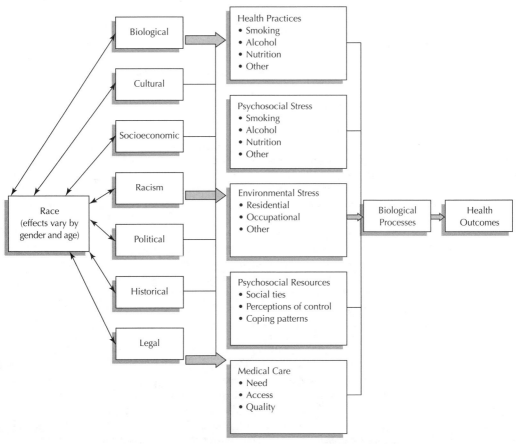

Figure 8-4
A Framework for Understanding the Relationship Between Race and Health

Racial and Ethnic Disparities in Health

Rather than develop an exhaustive list of health problems, laboriously broken down by ethnicity, the reader might be better served by examining a selected number of important contemporary health issues that provide telling examples of discrepancies by ethnicity. The following section describes six health problems that have been targeted by the federal government in an attempt to eliminate such discrepancies and is taken from the Office of Minority Health and Health Disparities (OMHD) (Centers for Disease Control and Prevention [CDC], 2007a).

The Initiative to Eliminate Racial and Ethnic Disparities in Health

Based on the nation's Healthy People (HP) 2010 goals, these six identified areas were selected from a list of 28 objectives because they represent multiple racial and ethnic groups at various life stages. At the time HP 2010 was developed, near-term goals were established for the year 2000 to help measure progress toward the 2010 goal. Revisions to the existing goals are currently underway. Policy makers are reviewing progress toward the objectives as they outline directives for the nation's future goals in the year 2020. Healthy People 2020 objectives are expected to be released in January 2010 along with guidelines for the new 10-year near-term goals. The Department of Health and Human Services (HHS) is leading the effort to eliminate disparities in health access and outcomes in the following areas:

Goal 1. Infant Mortality Rates

Infant mortality is often cited as a measure of a country's health status. The infant mortality rate—the rate at which babies less than 1 year of age die—has been decreasing over the past few decades. In 2000 it was at a record low of 6.9 deaths per 1,000 live births in the United States. This is significant progress when you consider that in 1960 the infant mortality rate was 26.0 per 1,000 live births. The United States, however, still ranks 28th in infant mortality compared to other Western industrialized nations, largely due to the disparities among the African American population (CDC, 2002).

Rates of infant mortality vary greatly between and within racial and ethnic groups (African American, American Indians, Alaska Natives, and Hispanics). The infant death rate among African Americans was 14.1 per 1,000 live births, more than double that of the national average (6.9 per 1,000 live births in 2000). Sudden infant death syndrome (SIDS), pre-term/low birth weight, complications associated with pregnancy, and respiratory distress are leading causes for elevated mortality rates. Although American Indians and Alaska Natives represent a small portion of the population, SIDS deaths are 2.3 times the rate for non-Hispanic white mothers (CDC, 2007a).

One well-established predictor of improved pregnancy outcome is involvement in prenatal care, particularly in the first trimester of pregnancy. The likelihood of delivering a very low birth weight (VLBW) baby (less than 3 lb 4 oz) is estimated to be 40% higher among women who receive late or no prenatal care compared to women entering prenatal care during the first trimester. Approximately 95% of VLBW babies are born early (less than 37 weeks) and the risk of death for VLBW babies is about 65 times that of infants who weigh at least 3 lb 4 oz. Rates of preterm birth among black women have remained rel-

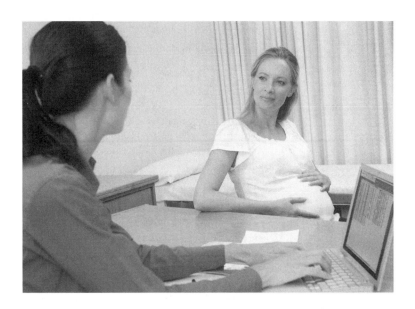

Prenatal care is an important factor in the effort to reduce infant mortality.

atively constant at 18% over the last few years and are higher than that of any other racial or ethnic group (Hamilton, Martin, & Sutton, 2003).

In 2002 the proportion of pregnant women in the United States receiving prenatal care in the first trimester was 83.8% (Hamilton et al., 2003) This proportion reflects a consistent improvement from the 1996 figure of 81.8% and the 1989 figure of 75.5%. However, the sad fact remains that one in five pregnant women, nearly three-quarters of a million women, did not receive timely prenatal care, and nearly 47,000 pregnant women received absolutely *no* prenatal care. There are substantial racial disparities in the receipt of prenatal care. Although 88.7% of white pregnant women received timely prenatal care in 2005, that proportion was only 76.5% for black and 77.6% for Hispanic pregnant women (U.S. Department of Health and Human Services [USDHHS], 2007).

When examining specific causes of infant deaths, racial and ethnic disparities seem to be particularly acute in preterm or premature birth (PTB) and SIDS. A much higher incidence of PTBs occurs among black mothers than among white mothers (17.7 versus 9.7), with nearly two-thirds of the deaths related to infant mortality being attributed to PTBs in African American women (Savage et al., 2007). SIDS, which accounts for approximately 10% of all first-year infant deaths, is also more common in minority populations.

Higher rates of infant mortality in minority groups are influenced by many factors, such as socioeconomic and demographic factors, medical conditions, and quality of and access to health care. The near-term goal is to reduce infant mortality in African Americans (the group with the greatest disparity in terms of infant death rates) by at least 22%, from the 1996 rate by the year 2000—or from 14.1 per 1,000 to 11.0 per 1,000 live births.

Near-Term Goal: Reduce infant mortality among African Americans by 22%.

Goal Progress: As of 2005, the infant mortality rate for African Americans was 13.6 per 1,000 live births, indicating the near-term goal has not been met (CDC, 2008a).

Goal 2. Cancer Screening and Management

Cancer is the second leading cause of death in the United States, resulting in more than 553,800 deaths each year. The chances of developing cancer in a lifetime are nearly 45% for men and nearly 41% for women. Although cancer deaths are on the decline, racial disparities exist in both mortality and incidence rates. For example, African Americans in the United States carry the greatest burden for all cancer types combined with a death rate 25% higher than that of whites (National Cancer Institute, 2008). Table 8-1 summarizes the incidence and death rates in the United States for all cancers by racial/ethnic group.

Major Mortality Discrepancies:

- African Americans have a cancer death rate about 35% higher in men and 18% higher in women than that of whites.
- The African American male cancer death rate is about 50% higher than it is for white men.
- The death rate for lung cancer is about 30% higher for African Americans than for whites.
- The prostate cancer mortality rate for African American men is 60% higher than that of white men.

Major Incidence Discrepancies:

- The incidence of lung cancer in African American men is about 40% higher than in white men.
- Native Hawaiian men have elevated rates of lung cancer compared with white men.
- Alaska Native men and women suffer disproportionately higher rates of cancers of the colon and rectum than do whites.
- Vietnamese women in the United States have a cervical cancer incidence rate more than five times greater than white women. Hispanic women also suffer elevated rates of cervical cancer.

Table 8-1 Incidence and Death Rates in the United States for All Cancers, by Racial/Ethnic Groups

	All Sites	
Racial/Ethnic Group	**Incidence**	**Death**
All	470.1	192.7
African American/Black	504.1	238.8
Asian/Pacific Islander	314.9	115.5
Hispanic/Latino	356.0	129.1
American Indian/Alaska Native	297.6	160.4
White	477.5	190.7

Statistics are for 2000–2004, age-adjusted to the 2000 U.S. standard million population, and represent the number of new cases of invasive cancer and deaths per year per 100,000 men and women.

Source: National Cancer Institute. (2008). Cancer disparities: Questions and answers. National Institutes of Health. Retrieved January 6, 2009, from http://www.cancer.gov/cancertopics/factsheet/cancer-health-disparities

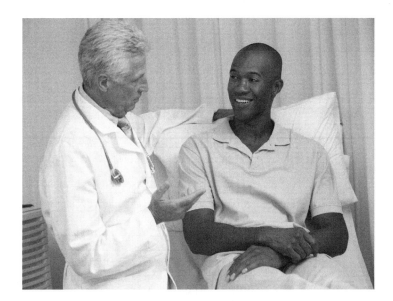

Equal access to health-care screening is essential to reduce cancer mortalities in minorities.

The incidence of certain forms of cancer could be greatly reduced through various types of prevention. For example, tobacco use is responsible for nearly one-third of all cancer deaths, while evidence suggests that diet and nutrition are probably associated with another 30–40% of cancer deaths. For the forms of cancer we do not know how to prevent, early detection can reduce the risk of death. Regular mammography screening and follow-up can reduce deaths from breast cancer by about 30% for women 50 years of age or older, while regular Pap tests for cervical cancer along with follow-up care can virtually eliminate the risk of developing this disease. Despite the gains in screening in the African American community, the mortality rate from breast cancer for black women is greater than that for white women. Some possible reasons for this might include irregular screening, limited follow-up opportunities, and lack of access to treatment services. Hispanic, American Indian, Alaska Native, and Asian and Pacific Islander women also experience similar barriers related to screening, access to treatment, and follow-up, often compounded by problems such as culture differences, language, and in some cases, negative provider attitudes.

This HHS initiative hopes to decrease the existing discrepancies in this category by eliminating these barriers to prevention and screening practices.

Cervical cancer: The goal for the year 2000 is to increase to at least 85% the proportion of all women age 18 or older who have received a Pap test within the preceding 3 years.

Goal Progress: As of 2006, there has been no change in the percentage of women obtaining Pap tests (USDHHS, CDC, & NIH, 2007).

Near-Term Goal: Increase to at least 60% those women of all racial or ethnic groups, age 50 or older, who have received a clinical breast exam and a mammogram within the preceding 2 years.

Goal Progress: As of 2006, the target for this objective has been met (USDHHS et al., 2007).

Goal 3. Cardiovascular Disease

Cardiovascular disease, primarily coronary heart disease and stroke, kills nearly as many Americans as all other diseases combined. The annual national economic impact of cardiovascular disease is estimated at $300 billion as measured in healthcare expenditures, medications, and lost productivity due to disability and death. The major modifiable risk factors for cardiovascular disease are high blood pressure, high blood cholesterol, cigarette smoking, excessive body weight, and lack of physical activity.

Major disparities exist among minority groups, with a disproportionate burden of death and disability from cardiovascular disease existing in minority and low-income populations.

- The age-adjusted death rate for coronary heart disease for the total population declined by 46% from 1997–1998; for African Americans, the overall decrease was only 33%.
- Compared to non-Hispanic white men, African American men were 30% more likely to die from heart disease in the year 2005.
- High blood pressure is 1.4 times more common in African Americans than in non-Hispanic whites.
- Obesity is 1.7 times greater in African American women and 1.2 times more likely in Mexican American women than in non-Hispanic white women.
- Non-Hispanic white men were 70% more likely to die from heart disease compared to Mexican American men in 2005.
- Compared to their white counterparts, African American adults are twice as likely to have a stroke.
- In general, American Indian/Alaska Native adults are 60% more likely to have a stroke than their white adult counterparts.

Not all racial minority groups, however, are at a disadvantage:

- Heart disease is less common in Asian/Pacific Islander adults, and they are less likely to die from heart disease compared to non-Hispanic white adults.
- Asian/Pacific Islander adults are less likely to die from or experience a stroke than white adults.
- In 2005, Hispanic men were 15% less likely to die from a stroke than non-Hispanic white men.
- Hispanics, in 2006, were 10% less likely to have heart disease compared to non-Hispanic whites.

Near-Term Goals:

- Reduce the heart disease mortality rate among African Americans by 25%.
- Reduce the stroke mortality rate among African Americans by 40%.

Goal Progress: As of 2006, progress was made toward both of these goals. In 2002 the coronary heart disease death rate dropped from 203 deaths per 100,000 population to 180 per 100,000 population, moving toward the target of 162 per 100,000 population. The decline in stroke-related deaths is attributed to a decrease in smoking behaviors, an increase in blood pressure and cholesterol level management, and an increase in physical activity and leisure time (USDHHS et al., 2007).

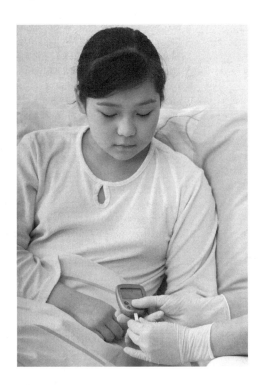

Diabetes is a serious health problem disproportionately affecting minorities.

Goal 4. Diabetes

Diabetes is the sixth leading cause of death in the United States and is a serious public health problem, affecting nearly 20.8 million Americans. A significant strain is placed upon the healthcare system as the number of persons with diabetes or diabetes-related complications continues to grow. It has been suggested that the existing healthcare system could be overwhelmed by the number of persons with diabetes mellitus (USDHHS et al., 2007). By 2050, the CDC projects the prevalence of diagnosed diabetes in the United States will increase 165%. The estimated direct and indirect costs of diabetes to the nation was estimated to be $174 billion in 2007.

- The prevalence of diabetes in African Americans is approximately 70% higher than in whites, and the prevalence in Hispanics is nearly double that of whites.
- African Americans and Hispanics born in the year 2000 have a 2 in 5 risk for diabetes.
- The prevalence rates among American Indians and Alaska Natives is more than twice that for the total population, and at least one tribe, the Pimas of Arizona, have the highest known prevalence of diabetes of any population in the world.
- Among people younger than 20, American Indians ages 10–19 have the highest prevalence of type 2 diabetes.

Cardiovascular disease is the leading cause of death among people with diabetes, killing almost 75% of all diabetics. Achieving mortality reduction among high-risk populations will require an effort to reduce cardiovascular risk factors among these groups. Individuals with diabetes not only face a reduced life span, but also the possibility of many acute and chronic complications, including end-stage renal disease (ESRD), blindness, and lower extremity amputations. All of these complications have the potential to be prevented:

- If uncontrolled hypertension among people with diabetes were reduced by half, about 25% of ESRD due to diabetes could be prevented.
- Diabetic retinopathy is the leading cause of new cases of blindness among people 20–74 years of age. Clinical trials have demonstrated that approximately 60% of diabetes-related blindness can be prevented with good blood glucose control or by early detection and laser photocoagulation treatment, which is widely available but underused.
- One half of all lower extremity amputations can be prevented through proper foot care and by reducing risk factors such as hyperglycemia (abnormally high blood sugar), cigarette smoking, and high blood pressure.

Preventive interventions should target high-risk groups. African Americans and American Indians, for example, are more likely than white populations to experience diabetes-related complications such as ESRD and amputations. Even among similarly insured populations, such as Medicare recipients, African Americans are more likely than whites to be hospitalized with septicemia, debridement, and amputations—signs of poor diabetic control. Although diabetes is a serious problem, recent studies have shown that careful control of blood glucose levels is a strategy that can be successful for preventing complications of diabetes. The challenge is to make proper diabetes management part of daily clinical and public health practice.

Near-Term Goal: Reduce the rate of ESRD from diabetes among African Americans and American Indians/Alaska Natives by 65%.

Goal Progress: The data on ESRD rates are not promising. In 2006, the rate increased by 2.5% (159 per million population) from what was considered a stabilized rate in 2001. This rate—significantly higher than the HP 2010 target of 90 per million—is reflective of the prevalence of diabetes in the general population. In 2006, rates of ESRD by race and ethnicity were three times greater in African Americans. Some improvement, however, has occurred in the Native American population. The rate of ESRD among Native Americans has decreased by 27.7% since 1995, suggesting that some progress had been made (U.S. Renal Data System, 2008).

Goal 5. HIV Infection/AIDS

In 1998, HIV infection/AIDS was the leading cause of death for all persons 25 to 44 years of age. Between 650,000 and 900,000 Americans were estimated to be living with HIV infection, while by June 1998, over 400,000 of the 665,357 adults and adolescents reported with AIDS in the United States had died from the disease (CDC, 1999). By the year 2003, over a million persons in the United States were living with HIV/AIDS and approximately 25% of them were unaware of their infection (Glynn & Rhodes, 2005). Although from 2003 through 2006 the estimated number of newly diagnosed HIV/AIDS cases increased among whites (8.2 per 100,000) and Asians/Pacific Islanders (6.7 per 100,000), the incidence rates were still clearly disproportionately elevated in the black (67.7 per 100,000) and Hispanic (25.5 per 100,000) populations (CDC, 2008b).

AIDS has clearly disproportionately affected minority populations.

- In 2002, racial and ethnic minorities accounted for almost 70% of the newly diagnosed cases of HIV/AIDS.
- In 2006, blacks accounted for 49% of all HIV/AIDS cases diagnosed (CDC, 2008b).
- Of the babies born with HIV, more than 90% belong to minority groups.
- Racial and ethnic minorities constitute about 26% of the total U.S. population, and yet they account for nearly 67% of all AIDS cases.
- While the epidemic is decreasing in some populations, the *number* of new AIDS cases among African Americans is now greater than the number of new AIDS cases among whites. Data from the 2000 census indicate that blacks make up approximately 13% of the U.S. population. Yet in 2005, an estimated 37,331 new cases were diagnosed in the United States with blacks, alarmingly, accounting for 18,121 (49%) in the 33 states with long-term, confidential name-based HIV reporting (CDC, 2007b).
- Women constitute roughly 25% of the population living with HIV/AIDS. Of the 126,964 women living with HIV/AIDS, black women are disproportionally over-represented. Of those afflicted, 64% were black, 19% were white, 15% were Hispanic, 1% were Asian or Pacific Islander, and less than 1% were American Indian or Alaska Native (CDC, 2007b).
- Although the number of AIDS diagnoses among men who have sex with men (MSM) has decreased dramatically since 1989, the number of AIDS diagnoses among African American men having same-gender sex has increased.

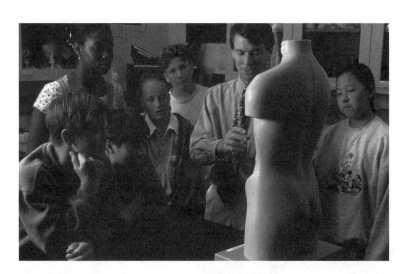

Innovative methods of education can help to reduce high-risk behaviors.

- New cases of AIDS where the identifiable route of transmission is injecting drug use are increasingly concentrated in minorities; of these cases almost 75% are among minority groups (56% African American and 20% Hispanic).
- American Indians are three times more likely to have AIDS than whites.

In addition to disproportionate rates of AIDS, minority groups have not kept pace with reduced death rates reported in majority populations. For example, in each racial/ethnic group, the rate decreased significantly from 1995 through 1998. Among non-Hispanic blacks, however, the percentage decrease in the rate was proportionally smaller (58%) than in the other radical/ethnic groups. The percentage decrease in the other groups ranged from 67% among American Indians/Alaska Natives to 76% among non-Hispanic whites (see Figure 8-5). Major contributing factors to this discrepancy include late identification of disease and lack of health insurance to pay for drug therapies and treatment that can cost between $20,000 and $25,000 per patient per year.

The stability in the mortality rate from 1999 to 2005 is an important sign of progress considering that the total number of people living with HIV is increasing. Inadequate recognition of risk—detection of infection and referral to follow-up care—is a major issue for high-risk populations. It is estimated that about one-third of persons who are at risk of HIV/AIDS have never been tested. More effective prevention strategies are needed that are acceptable to the target

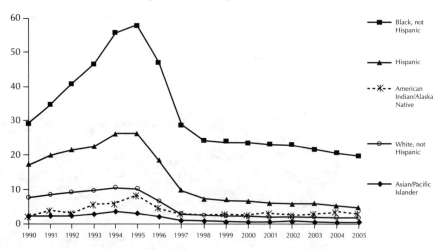

Trends in Age-Adjusted* Annual Rates of Death Due to HIV Disease, by Race/Ethnicity, United States, 1990–2005

Note: For comparison with data for 1999 and later years, data for 1980–1988 were modified to account for *ICD-10* rules instead of *ICD-9* rules.
*Standard: age distributution of 2000 US population

Figure 8-5
HIV Morbidity Rates by Ethnicity
Source: Centers for Disease Control and Prevention. (2008c). HIV mortality (through 2005). U.S. Department of Health and Human Services, Division of HIV/AIDS Prevention. Retrieved January 13, 2009, from http://cdc.gov/hiv/topics/surveillance/resources/slides/mortality/slides/mortality13.ppt

audience (i.e., they must be culturally and linguistically appropriate). Organizations serving at-risk populations need to develop, implement, evaluate, and fund programs that promote basic knowledge and skills such as knowing one's serostatus and being able to access counseling, testing, and referrals to medical services, including efficacious therapies. Such promotion will continue to guide the development and administration of federal initiatives to prevent HIV transmission and improve access to care for individuals living with HIV/AIDS.

Near-Term Goal: Make appropriate health services more available.

Goal Progress: Some progress has been made toward reaching the near-term target. Three of four measurable subobjectives are related to the proportion of HIV-infected adolescents and adults who receive testing, treatment, and prophylaxis consistent with current treatment guidelines. The data suggest that use of highly active antiretroviral therapy achieved 51% of the targeted change, use of any antiretroviral therapy demonstrated 33% of the targeted change, and *Mycobacterium avium* complex prophylaxis achieved 29% of the targeted change (USDHHS et al., 2007).

Goal 6. Child and Adult Immunization

The reduction in incidence of vaccine-preventable diseases is one of the most significant public health achievements of the past century. This success is best illustrated by the global suppression of smallpox. The major factor in this success is the development and widespread use of vaccines, which are among the safest and most effective preventive measures.

Childhood immunization rates are at an all-time high, with the most critical vaccine doses reflecting coverage rates of over 90%. The 1996 immunization targets for all five vaccines (measles, mumps, and rubella [MMR]; polio; diphtheria, tetanus, and pertussis [DPT]; *Haemophilus influenzae* type B [Hib]; and hepatitis B [Hep B] were exceeded. Although immunization rates have been lower in minority populations compared with the white population, minority rates have been increasing at a more rapid rate, thus significantly narrowing the gap. However, efforts must be made to achieve and maintain at least 90% coverage for all recommended vaccines in all populations. Particular areas of concern are pockets of need within each state and major city where numbers of under-immunized children reside. These areas are of great concern because, particularly in large, urban areas with traditionally underserved populations, there is a potential for outbreaks of vaccine-preventable diseases.

In addition to the very young, older adults are also at increased risk for many vaccine-preventable diseases. Approximately 90% of all influenza-associated deaths in the United States occur in people age 65 or older, the fastest growing age group of the population. Reduction of deaths in this age group has been hindered in part by relatively low vaccine utilization. Each year, an estimated 50,000 adults die of infections related to influenza, pneumococcal infections, and hepatitis B despite the availability of safe and effective vaccines to prevent these conditions and their complications. There is a disproportionate burden of these diseases in minority and underserved populations. Although vaccination levels against pneumococcal infections and influenza among people 65 years or over have increased slightly for African Americans and Hispanics, the coverage in these groups remains substantially below the general population and the year 2000 targets.

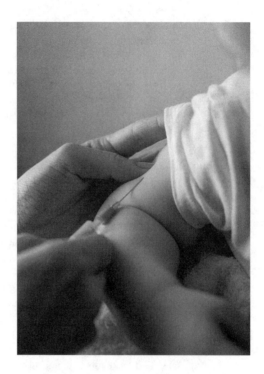

Immunization contin-
ues to be one of the
most effective methods
of controlling infectious
diseases.

Childhood Immunization:

Near-Term Goal: Achieve and maintain at least 90% coverage for all recommended childhood vaccines in all populations.

Goal Progress: This goal continues to meet the HP 2010 objectives. Evidence suggests that providing pneumococcal vaccine to children has contributed to a decrease in new cases of invasive pneumococcal disease in adults (CDC, 2005).

Adult Immunization:

In order to achieve this near-term goal, the 1994 influenza immunization rates among African Americans, Hispanics, and Asians and Pacific Islanders will need to nearly double, and among these same groups, the 1994 pneumococcal immunization rates will need to quadruple.

Near-Term Goal: Increase pneumococcal and influenza immunizations among all adults age 65 years or older to 60%.

Goal Progress: Immunization for influenza and pneumococcal disease of high-risk adults has exceeded its near-term target but still has room for improvement to reach the HP 2010 goal. Data from the 2006 and 2007 Behavorial Risk Factor Surveillance System (BRFSS) suggest that only 72.1% of adults over the age of 65 were vaccinated in the 2006–2007 season (CDC, 2005).

Health Literacy

Health outcomes for minority populations often differ from those of the majority population; such health disparities are a consequence of multiple factors, one of which is poor health literacy. **Health literacy** is "the degree to which individuals have the capacity to obtain, process, and understand basic health information and services needed to make appropriate health decisions" (USDHHS, 2000). Estimates indicate that approximately 9 out of 10 adults lack proficient health literacy skills (Agency for Healthcare Research and Quality [AHRQ], 2007). As one might expect, the absence of these requisite skills results in poorer health outcomes due to the difficulty or inability to manage one's health. Adverse effects of poor health literacy rates are associated with ". . . low health knowledge, increased incidence of chronic illness, higher risk of hospitalization, and less than optimal use of preventive health services" (AHRQ, 2007). Health literacy is not just about being able to locate and read health information—it is the ability to interpret and apply the information to improve one's quality of life. In addition to a basic understanding of health topics, the consumer must be able to provide an accurate health history, access healthcare services, practice numeric skills, follow directive documents, and communicate personal needs (see Figure 8-6). Health professionals often underestimate how overwhelming it can be to be diagnosed with a health complication.

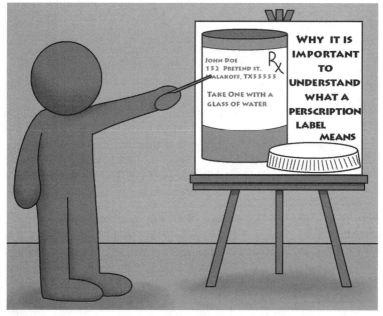

Figure 8-6
The Ability to Follow Directives

The development of health literacy skills is paramount to obtaining optimal outcomes. Imagine the shock a patient feels when he makes an appointment with the doctor to see about his extreme fatigue, frequent urination, and thirst and is surprisingly diagnosed with type 2 diabetes. Although the physician's diagnosis was likely explained in detail, the patient's lack of time to process the information, especially in an emotional state, may result in the inability to comprehend the content or to retain the information. The need for oral communication skills becomes evident as healthcare providers attempt to identify aspects of the patient's condition related to his or her health history and current lifestyle. A patient must be able to articulate his or her health concerns and describe his or her symptoms accurately. Often the provider and patient need skills to negotiate beyond cultural, language, and literacy barriers to effectively communicate (Smith et al., 2007).

As patients get inundated with new directives to self-manage their health care, the need for health literacy skills becomes more apparent. It is critical that the patient be knowledgeable about the disease process and the signs and symptoms of his or her condition so that he or she can report changes that indicate control or lack of control of the disease. Without this knowledge, he or she may not understand the relationship between lifestyle factors such as diet and exercise and various health outcomes (USDHHS, 2000). Mathematical (numeracy) skills also play an important role in disease management. To effectively manage blood glucose levels, the patient will need to calculate sugar levels, measure medication dosages, and interpret nutrition values from food labels. Numeracy skills will also be vital when estimating the cost of treatment—co-pays, insurance premiums, medications, and deductibles (Kelly, 2007). Skills related to visual literacy also become necessary when interpreting graphs or information presented in illustrated formats.

Finally, skills related to analyzing and evaluating become the foundation for allowing patients to make informed choices. The development of decision-making skills enables the consumer to analyze options by comparing and contrasting the negative and positive aspects of his or her options.

The development of health literacy has been identified as a cornerstone for the reduction of health disparities. Healthy People 2010 emphasizes two key areas for attaining measurable improvements: to develop materials for audiences with limited literacy and to target the development of the health literacy skills mentioned above (USDHHS, 2006).

Guidelines for Developing Materials for Health Literacy

The U.S. Department of Health and Human Services, Office of Disease Prevention and Health Promotion (n.d.) has developed a quick guide that provides strategies to improve the development of usable health information. Tables 8-2 through 8-4 provide three key questions to ask along with aspects to consider when designing and disseminating health information.

Improving health literacy, especially for minority populations, will be a step in the right direction toward minimizing health disparities. Application of improved communication techniques and implementation of suggested guidelines in developing materials offers a good possibility for success.

Table 8-2 Question #1 for Improving the Usability of Health Information

---

Question #1: Is the information appropriate for the users?

Identify the users.	• Identify the intended users based on epidemiology (who is affected?), demographics, behavior, culture, and attitude. • Be sure the materials and messages reflect the age, social and cultural diversity, language, and literacy skills of the intended users. • Consider the communication capacities of the intended users.
Evaluate user understanding before, during, and after introduction of information and services.	• Determine the target population's need for communication materials before they are designed. • Design a method to test the effectiveness of your communication materials.
Acknowledge cultural differences and practice respect.	• Ensure that health information is relevant to the intended users' social and cultural contexts. • Some aspects to consider include: 　• Accepted male/female roles 　• Value of traditional medicine over Western medicine 　• Favorite and forbidden foods 　• Manner of dress 　• Being aware of body language and concerns related to touching or proximity in various situations (National Cancer Institute, n.d.)

Table 8-3 Question #2 for Improving the Usability of Health Information

---

Question #2: Is this information easy to use?

Keep it simple.	• Limit the number of messages to four or fewer. • Use plain language in simple sentences that avoid jargon. • Focus on action; request the performance of a behavior.
Supplement instructions with pictures.	• Graphics should function to enhance the delivery of information—not just to decorate. • Add captions under pictures to clarify meaning. • Use images that are familiar and culturally relevant to the audience (Doak, Doak, & Root, 1996).
Make written communication easy to read.	• Select easy-to-read fonts of 12 points or greater. • Keep text plain, reserving bolding for key points. • Use bullets and white space to break up the text.
Improve usability of information on the Internet.	• Enhance text with video or audio files. • Include interactive features and personalized content. • Use uniform navigation. • Organize information to minimize searching and scrolling (USDHHS, 2005). • Give users the option to navigate from simple to complex information.

Table 8-4 Question #3 for Improving the Usability of Health Information

Question #3: Are you speaking clearly and listening carefully?	
Ask open-ended questions.	• Eliminate the use of questions that can be answered by simple one-word answers (i.e., yes or no). • Strive to use "what," "how," or "why" as part of the question.
Use a medically trained interpreter.	• Use interpreters who can provide examples in culturally relevant terms to enhance communication.
Check for understanding.	• Have the receiver of the information restate the content in his or her own words. • Restate, act out, or use graphics to clarify information when needed.
Get adequate training.	• Participate in plain language and cultural competency training.

Cultural Competency

Another fundamental concept aimed at improving health outcomes for traditionally underserved populations is that of **cultural competency**. This concept developed from the premise that not all individuals within the healthcare system are treated equally, particularly those with cultural mores outside the "mainstream." Cultural competency is intended to optimize the likelihood that individuals from all cultures, ethnicities, and races will receive appropriate and sensitive care. This is considered to be one of the main ingredients in closing the disparities gap in health care. In response to Public Law 101-527, the Office of Minority Health created the Center for Linguistic and Cultural Competence in Health Care (CLCCHC). The role of the center is to fulfill the law's mandate to support research, demonstrations, and evaluations and to test innovative models designed to ameliorate cultural and linguistic barriers to health care while promoting understanding of health risk factors and preventive measures. Through collaboration with federal agencies and other public and private entities, the CLCCHC strives to enhance the quality of the healthcare system to provide information and service to populations with limited English-speaking proficiency. In an effort to promote cultural and linguistic competency, a set of standards has been developed and organized around three key themes.

- **Theme 1:** Developing culturally competent care by:
  - Providing care that is respectful of and compatible with the client's cultural health beliefs, practices, and preferred language
  - Implementing strategies to recruit and retain a diverse staff that is representative of the demographic characteristics of its clientele
  - Providing training in culturally and linguistically sensitive service delivery

- **Theme 2:** Increasing language access services by:
  - Providing timely language assistance services (verbal offers and written notices) in the client's preferred language about his or her right to receive language assistance services
  - Ensuring the competencies of individuals providing language assistance
  - Ensuring patient-related signage and materials are easily understood by the clientele according to demographic characteristics
- **Theme 3:** Utilizing organizational supports by:
  - Establishing written policies related to providing culturally and linguistically appropriate services
  - Conducting training and incorporating evaluation techniques to maintain or improve strategies for cultural and linguistic competency
  - Integrating and updating demographic data into organizations' management information systems to be used in planning and implementation of services
  - Developing partnerships to facilitate community involvement
  - Establishing policies related to grievance resolution
  - Communicating public information, strategies, and progress related to building cultural and linguistic competency

The intent of these standards is evident—we should be taking the extra steps to ensure that all individuals are treated equally.

When planning interventions and interacting with people of other cultures, it is important to be cognizant of potential barriers. A common cultural barrier is verbal communication, but one must also consider the impact of nonverbal communication. Approximately 70% of the messages we send and receive are nonverbal. For example, in the Middle Eastern culture, intense eye contact communicates respect for the speaker if male; however, in U.S. culture intense eye contact can be misconstrued as a sign of hostility. Personal space is also an important consideration. A person from one subculture might touch or move closer to another as a friendly gesture, whereas someone from a different culture might consider such behavior invasive. Although people's comfort zones vary, spatial requirements tend to be similar among cultural groups. Latin Americans typically have a much tighter proximity zone that may cause some Europeans to feel as if their privacy were being invaded. Social organizations—such as family, kinships, tribes, and political, economic, and religious groups—are critical in the socialization of a culture. An understanding of the socialization of a culture can provide insight for the health educator. Understanding the close-knit familial relationships that are common in a Hispanic culture, for example, can yield a potential source for influencing behaviors through subjective norms.

A barrier that is commonly ignored when considering cultural values is time. As health educators, we often have an extreme sense of urgency in our desire to motivate behavior. Failing to consider cultural influences related to time—such as worship, fasting, or meal time—when setting goals for self-managed care can lead to frustration and noncompliance. Although these are only a few examples of barriers to consider, they help to emphasize the need to target interventions that are culturally sensitive.

Obviously, the development of effective cultural competence in the health professions could have a profound effect on potential or existing clients, particularly those who have felt marginalized by the system. Health care should acknowledge the client's health-related beliefs and cultural mores, as well as consider the community from which the person has come.

Case Study: Denise

Objective: After reviewing the case study, the reader will recommend two or more suggestions related to cultural competency that could improve Denise's ability to discover this target population perceived need for health services.

Denise, a community health educator, has been asked to speak with representatives from several local Hispanic women's groups to explore their perceived needs concerning preventive health services. Eager to be prepared for the encounter, Denise thoroughly researches health issues relevant to Mexican Americans. On learning that fluency in English among the women is very limited, she persuades a good friend visiting from Madrid to accompany her in the role of translator. Denise's confidence that she is well prepared is short-lived as the workshop begins. Denise had made the seriously wrong assumption that all Hispanic people are alike and come from the same culture. The women at the workshop represent group members from Mexico, South America, Central America, Cuba, and Puerto Rico. Although the women had some similar concerns, they were offended that Denise was making broad assumptions based on information that was foreign to their particular cultures. To make matters worse, Denise's interpreter friend was experiencing major difficulties understanding and being understood! This exploratory session was rather less than effective. (See Case Studies Revisited page 318.)

Questions to consider:

1. What type of impact did Denise's assumptions have on her workshop?
2. How could she avoid making that same mistake again?

Tuskegee—A Legacy of Doubt

One of the major issues discussed in this chapter is the difficulty experienced by health educators attempting to plan and effectively implement programs when viewed as an "outsider." Although most young health education students will probably be unaware of research begun in the 1930s, the Tuskegee Syphilis Study provides an excellent example of why a community, in this case the African American community, might exhibit a pervasive sense of distrust of public health agencies.

In the late 1920s the Public Health Service (PHS) was completing a study of the prevalence of syphilis in the black population in Mississippi. In order to expand syphilis research in the rural south, the PHS was awarded a grant from the Julius Rosenwald Foundation, a philanthropic organization located in Chicago. The research was to study the testing and treatment of syphilis in five rural counties in the south: Albemarle County, Virginia; Glynn County, Georgia; Pitt County, North Carolina; Macon County, Alabama; and Tipton County, Tennessee (Parran, 1937).

The Depression, beginning in 1929, played havoc with the research funding, and the treatment phase of the study was never completed. In Macon County, Alabama, the prevalence of syphilis had been reported as high as 35–40% of all age groups tested. It was this community in Alabama that was to serve as the proving ground for the effects of untreated syphilis. A PHS physician, T. Clark, stated simply, "The Alabama community offered an unparalleled opportunity for the study of the effect of untreated syphilis" (Jones, 1981).

One of the great ironies of this study was the astonishingly thorough and textbook approach taken by the PHS in implementing the program. Prestigious black institutions were persuaded to cooperate, several black churches added their credibility, and individual black community leaders ensured participation (Thomas & Quinn, 1991). The research continued, and little concern was voiced that anything questionable was taking place. However, in addition to not treating the infected individuals, the PHS team also chose not to provide any education about syphilis (Jones, 1981). No mention was made of the disease by name. It was simply referred to as "bad blood," a rural, southern term descriptive of many health problems at that time. Individuals were not told that the disease could be sexually transmitted, or that infants could be born infected (Thomas & Quinn, 1991).

America's involvement in World War II began in 1941. The PHS was so desperate to avoid losing their subjects to the war that they pressured the draft board to exclude these men from the draft. In 1943 the recently developed "miracle drug" penicillin was being widely used, including in the treatment of people infected with syphilis. This effective form of treatment was withheld from the men in the study. Clearly, treatment of the infected individuals would end the study and future research, something the PHS did not want to occur. The study and the withholding of treatment continued until 1972 when the *Washington Star*'s front-page exposé created enormous public outcry, finally stirring health officials into ending the study.

What are the implications of the Tuskegee study for health educators? What can we learn from this obviously inhumane and unethical research? Thomas and Quinn (1991) draw a powerful connection between the Tuskegee study and the current AIDS epidemic. The authors point out that the legacy of Tuskegee is a legitimate and understandable fear and distrust of the "health establishment." They cite the fears of some African Americans who believe that AIDS is an agent of white forces developed as a form of genocide. Mark Smith from Johns Hopkins University described the African American community as "already alienated from the health care system

. . . and somewhat cynical about the motives of those who arrive in their communities to help them" (National Commission on AIDS, 1990, p. 19). A health educator from Dallas, testifying before the National Commission on AIDS, commented, "So many African American people that I work with do not trust hospitals or any of the other community health care service providers because of that Tuskegee experiment. It is like . . . if they did it then, they will do it again" (National Commission on AIDS, 1990, p. 43).

The sentiments of distrust continue to be a barrier to reducing health disparities. In a study conducted by Braunstine, Sherber, Schulman, Ding, and Powe (2008), the researchers report that almost twice as many blacks as whites believe that their physicians secretly experiment on patients. "African American participants expressed markedly greater concerns about experiencing harm from participation in clinical trials and distrust toward medical researchers than white participants" (Braunstine et al., 2008, p. 1). They suggest that this distrust is correlated to the reluctance of African Americans to participate in clinical trials. Lack of participation in clinical trials handicaps minority populations because they are left out of important findings about treatments and new medications for disease (Braunstine et al., 2008). It seems apparent that the legacy of doubt left by Tuskegee is still a mitigating factor in reducing disparities.

As health educators, we must not underestimate the importance and power of past events. Over 35 years after the study ended, and over 75 years since it began, the effects of the Tuskegee study are still with us. It would be easy to dismiss as preposterous the notion that AIDS is a deliberate attempt at genocide. Yet, in the light of Tuskegee, is that type of fear so far-fetched? Thomas and Quinn (1991) make a forceful point when they describe the necessary ingredients for a successful community-based HIV education program that is ethnically acceptable and culturally sensitive: (1) the use of program staff indigenous to the community, (2) the use of incentives, and (3) the delivery of health services within the target community. The authors comment, though, that these were the exact methods used in the Tuskegee study and that health educators will have to work hard to ensure that these sound strategies are not diminished by their association with this fateful study.

Tuskegee Postscript

In a White House ceremony on May 16, 1997, nearly 65 years after the advent of the now notorious Tuskegee study, President William Clinton apologized for the 40-year government study. In 1997 there were only eight survivors of the Tuskegee experiment still alive, and five of them, accompanied by family members of some of the deceased, attended the ceremony. The president remarked,

> The legacy of the study at Tuskegee has reached far and deep, in ways that hurt our progress and divide our nation. We cannot be one America when a whole segment of our nation has no trust in America. What was done cannot be undone, but we can end the silence, we can stop turning our heads away,

NOTEWORTHY   **Tuskegee Revisited?**

President Clinton's words were prophetic in that in September 1997 the media and popular press had picked up a controversy surrounding the Centers for Disease Control and Prevention (CDC) and National Institutes of Health (NIH) sponsored drug treatment trials in Third World areas. One trial under scrutiny was a project that sought to test the efficacy of reduced dosage treatment of an AIDS drug, AZT, in a population of more than 12,000 HIV-positive pregnant women. The study design included one group that was to receive the full dose, another that was to receive a half dosage, and a control group that would receive a placebo. The purpose of the study was pragmatic in that most developing countries could not afford expensive medications such as AZT, and researchers were trying to see whether or not a lower, less expensive dose would still be effective. The withholding of an effective treatment regimen certainly reminded some ethicists of the Tuskegee situation. Writing in the *Washington Post*, William Raspberry described how Marcia Angell, the executive editor of the *New England Journal of Medicine*, had written an editorial fiercely criticizing such studies, calling them unethical and akin to the Tuskegee study (Raspberry, 1997). Dr. Angell asserted, "Some of the same arguments that were made in favor of the Tuskegee study many years ago are emerging in a new form in the AZT studies in the third world." Raspberry had also talked to two ethics professors about the issue, both of whom thought that the removal of the control group would eliminate any ethical problems.

Elizabeth Kiss of Duke University stated, "The inarguable point is that it is totally unethical to withhold a known effective treatment," while Arthur Kaplan of the University of Pennsylvania remarked that the Tuskegee comparison was rash. He stated, "Tuskegee was clearly in the inexcusable zone, because it didn't have the interest of the subjects at heart. The AIDS research, on the other hand, is undertaken by people who are seriously trying to do something to help poor people who otherwise might get no effective treatment at all." Responding to the criticism of the studies, Dr. Helene Gayle, director of the CDC's National Center for HIV, STD, and TB prevention, stated that the tests had not been carried out "behind closed doors" and noted that "this was done with a lot of discussion from the international community" (Stolberg, 1997).

Whether or not this latter day example of medical research could be construed as "another Tuskegee" is a matter for discussion. What is perhaps a positive legacy of Tuskegee is the fact that individuals are now more sensitized to the obvious unethical and inexcusable treatment of individuals in a government-sponsored research project, and future studies will be scrutinized far more carefully in the light of the shameful events that have become known simply as "the Tuskegee study."

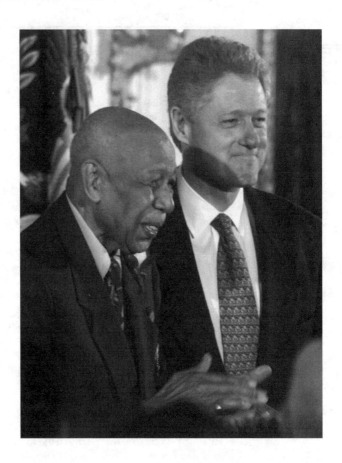

Sixty-five years after the
Tuskegee study began,
President William
Clinton apologized to
the survivors.

we can look at you, in the eye, and finally say, on behalf of the American people, what the United States government did was shameful, and I am sorry.
(White House, 1997)

President Clinton also announced that he was awarding a $200,000 grant
to Alabama's Tuskegee University to help build a center on bioethics and research and that he had directed Donna Shalala, secretary for the Department of Health and Human Services, to report back to him in 180 days with
recommendations for how to more effectively include minority populations
in healthcare research (Harris & Fletcher, 1997). In 2004, the last living sur-
vivor of the Tuskegee Syphilis Study, Ernest Hendon, died at the age of 96 in
his home state of Alabama.

Institutional Review Boards

One of the more positive consequences of the Tuskegee legacy was the development of regulatory agencies, known as the institutional review board

(IRB), to ensure research protocols are ethically appropriate. IRBs are responsible for protecting the rights and welfare of human research subjects. Under federal regulations and local institutional policies, an IRB can approve, require modifications to, or disapprove all research activities that are under its jurisdiction (Penslar & Porter, n.d.). All research endeavors must be approved by an IRB prior to conducting any type of research. Additional protocols are included in an IRB's review of research that investigates vulnerable populations such as prisoners, pregnant women, fetuses, and children. Although this watchdog group presents another barrier to research, it performs a valuable service to protect the integrity of research and the involved participants.

Suggested Health Promotion Strategies for Diverse Cultures

Promoting health in diverse populations is best accomplished when strategies that target three key areas are combined. Interventions should strive to strengthen the individual, strengthen the community, and reduce barriers to eliminate disparity in health care. Early work by the Task Force on Black and Minority Health (1985) provided the guiding principles for designing programs that better promote health in minority populations (CDC, 2007). The strategies offered here are reflections of the suggestions from the task force categorized by target area.

Strengthening the Individual

- Involve family, churches, employers, and community organizations as a support system for the individual to facilitate and sustain behavior change to a more healthful lifestyle. For example, although hypertension controls in African Americans depend on appropriate medical therapy, blood pressure control can be improved and maintained by family and community support of activities such as proper diet and exercise.
- Data suggest that health messages are more readily accepted if they do not conflict with existing cultural beliefs. Where appropriate, messages should acknowledge and incorporate existing cultural beliefs.

Strengthening the Community

- Channel efforts for minority communities through local leaders who could represent a powerful force for promoting acceptance and reinforcement of the central themes of health promotion messages.
- Encourage private organizations, such as religious and community organizations, clubs, and schools, to participate in developing minority support networks and other incentive techniques to facilitate the acceptance of health information and education.

Reducing Barriers

- Language barriers, cultural differences, and lack of adequate information on access to care can complicate health maintenance and treatment. Health educators must ensure that culturally sensitive information is available in many forms within a specific community. This information should not only be subject-specific, but also include basic explanations of *how* to determine services.

- Assess suitability of existing information and materials and/or develop new, culturally sensitive materials. Enlist the participation of professional and lay members of each minority group to determine the suitability of the materials.

Important points to consider before teaching and/or presenting to diverse populations follow:

- What is the precise ethnic mix of the class or audience? A description of *Hispanic* or *Asian* is probably not precise enough. Obtain as much specific information as possible.
- Find out more about the demographics of the group. Where do they live—in an urban, a suburban, or a rural setting? Do you have any information about educational levels or socioeconomic status?
- Consider the language proficiency of classes or groups. Is there a high proportion of recent immigrants who speak little English? Is a translator necessary, and, if so, can you find one?
- Are there any health problems unique to this group of which you should be aware? Research the health status of the group.
- Identify and consult individuals, perhaps school and community leaders, who are from, or at least familiar with, a specific race or culture.
- Adopt teaching or presentation strategies that will be culturally sensitive to specific groups. Your presentations will be much more effective and accepted better if the students/audience can closely relate to your style and content.
- Be aware of strong cultural influences within specific cultures, such as the family and the church. Gaining support and even cooperation from both these areas will add much credibility to the learning experience.

Objective: After reviewing the case study, the reader will provide justification for the necessity of researching the target population when selecting methods for interventions.

Case Study: Monica   Monica is a young and inexperienced community health educator presenting a workshop to a group of middle-aged Hispanic (Mexican American) women. The topic of the workshop is the importance of having a regular pelvic examination. Monica has been told that Hispanic women tend to report low rates of Pap smear screening, and Monica's main objective is to increase compliance with this important test. Monica believes that many women feel uncomfortable with their own bodies and has decided to begin the workshop with an exercise designed to reduce this discomfort. To the amazement of the group of Hispanic women, Monica lies down on the table at the front of the room, lifts up her dress, pulls off her underwear, and proceeds to identify her cervix with the aid of a mirror. Meanwhile, an assistant moves around the audience slowly, handing out similar mirrors to the stunned and silent group. Once the audience realizes the intention of the instructor, there is a mass exodus toward the nearest exit . . . . the workshop is over. (See Case Studies Revisited page 319.)

Questions to consider:

1. Was this appropriate strategy to use with any group? If not, why not?
2. How else could Monica have accomplished her objective?

Ethnicity and the Health Educator

One question that is often raised with regard to health education and race is whether the race of the health educator need always be the same as the race of the intended audience. This often becomes a moot point in that there are simply insufficient numbers of minority health educators to serve all populations. However, all things being equal, the consensus seems to be that a presenter/teacher of similar culture to the audience is preferable. Obviously, familiarity with a culture would avoid some major pitfalls in sensitivity, as, for example, were committed by the overzealous Monica in the case study. The issue of trust must also be considered. The Tuskegee study is an excellent illustration of why some cultures are suspicious of "external" interference. A more recent study seems to confirm the continuing suspicion of certain populations toward "outside influences." In a study of African American women attending a public health clinic, the researcher found that 21% of the women did not trust the federal government's reports on AIDS, and 54% were uncertain about them. In addition, when questioned as to whether they considered AIDS to be an act of genocide against the black race, only 52% disagreed with the notion (Sharon, 1992). Given this issue of mistrust, a same-race health educator would seem to be optimal. Ironically, among the women in the previously mentioned study, 70%, when asked if the race of the information "messenger" was of any consequence, responded that it was not.

For more information and tools related to this chapter visit
http://healtheducation.jbpub.com/strategies.

EXERCISES

1. Consider the case study where Monica's presentation to the Mexican American women went so poorly. You have been asked to perform the same 1-hour workshop for middle-aged Mexican American women on the importance of having a pelvic exam. Taking into account the features of this population, design a presentation plan (including behavioral objectives) that you think would be appropriate.

2. You have been asked to present a program on HIV/AIDS to an African American youth group (approximately 20 boys and girls ages 14–16 years). Write two objectives that you feel would be appropriate in this situation, then select two strategies/methods that you feel might be successful (keeping in mind what your objectives are). Justify your objective selection and choice of strategies.

3. In the light of what you know about the Tuskegee study and the more recent controversy concerning AIDS treatment studies in the third world, describe another contemporary minority health issue that might have the potential to cause some concern or suspicion within ethnic or racial minorities.

4. Selecting one of the areas of health targeted by the Initiative to Eliminate Racial and Ethnic Disparities in Health, briefly describe what you perceive to be the major barriers to effectively reducing discrepancies in the chosen area.

5. Using the guidelines provided in the chapter for promoting health literacy, design a pamphlet for promoting proper hand-washing techniques.

6. Define the term *cultural competency,* and briefly describe some practical measures that might increase the likelihood that cultural competency could be achieved.

CASE STUDIES REVISITED

Case Study Revisited: Susan

Susan had been presenting her important information to very homogenous groups and had not stopped to consider the culture of this latest group. Had she discovered the ethnic background of the participants beforehand, Susan could have identified levels of language, knowledge, and specific perceived needs of this population. Although advanced planning would not have removed the language issue, Susan could have taken steps to alleviate the problem. For example, she might have been able to identify a nurse or other health professional who was from that particular community and would have been willing to assist with the presentation, providing invaluable translation skills. (See page 288.)

Case Study Revisited: Denise

Although Denise's motives were laudable, she made some obvious mistakes based on erroneous assumptions. If a health educator has any doubts at all about a group or population with which he or she is unfamiliar, questions should be directed whenever possible to individuals within the group in question. Denise could have contacted some of the women leaders beforehand to familiarize herself with the group and assess what would be required to make the workshop successful. If this is not possible, perhaps there are fellow educators who have worked with these individuals or groups before who could provide information and advice. Working with diverse populations is not a simple matter, and we should all definitely avoid making assumptions based on what may not be true. (See page 310.)

Case Study Revisited: Monica   Monica's rather radical introduction to the workshop is a great example of poor method selection! This type of activity might have been problematic in many settings, and had Monica carried out the necessary research on this particular target population she would have realized that such a strategy was entirely inappropriate. Although Monica's intention was understandable, this type of overt and direct activity could not be successful with a population that is generally modest and self-conscious about sexuality. This rather disastrous workshop illustrates the necessity for thoroughly researching the characteristics of specific populations before designing intervention strategies. (See page 316.)

SUMMARY

1. Health educators need to have a good working knowledge of non-majority populations, including important information such as basic demographics and health disparities.

2. All individuals within minority populations are not the same. Appropriate methods of presentation must be considered to optimize the effectiveness of the program. Health educators can consult community members to help in developing potentially effective strategies.

3. The promotion of skills to develop health literacy will be critical in the elimination of health disparities.

4. Cultural competency is a concept designed to optimize the service and treatment received by racial and ethnic minorities within the healthcare system.

5. Health educators need to be aware of the influence of history on the receptiveness of racial and ethnic minorities to "outside" interventions.

REFERENCES AND RESOURCES

Agency for Healthcare Research and Quality. (2007). *Health Literacy, Program Brief.* AHRQ Publication No. 07-P010. Retrieved June 8, 2009, from http://www.ahrq.gov/research/healthlit.htm

Bowsworth, W. (2008). Discovering the Bronx: Using Census data to highlight social problems and achievements in a major urban area. Retrieved January 3, 2009, from http://www.lehman.edu/ deannss/ bronxdatactr/discover/bxtime.htm

Braunstine, J. B., Sherber, N. S., Schulman, S. P., Ding, E. L., & Powe, N. R. (2008). Race, medical researcher distrust, perceived harm, and willingness to participate in cardiovascular prevention trials. *Medicine (Baltimore)*, 87(1), 1–9.

Centers for Disease Control and Prevention. (1999). *HIV/AIDS Surveillance, U.S.* Atlanta, GA: Department of Health and Human Services, Public Health Service.

Centers for Disease Control and Prevention. (2002, August). Infant, neonatal, and postneonatal mortality rates by race and sex: United States, 1940, 1950, 1960, 1970, and 1975–2000. *National Vital Statistics Reports, 50*(15). Retrieved January 5, 2009, from http://www.cdc.gov/nchs/fastats/pdf/nvsr50_15 tb34.pdf

Centers for Disease Control and Prevention. (2005). Direct and indirect effects of routine immunization with 7-valent pneumococcal conjugate vaccine on invasive pneumococcal disease—United States, 1998–2003. *Morbidity and Mortality Weekly Report, 36*(9), 54.

Centers for Disease Control and Prevention. (2007a). Disease burden and risk factors. Office of Minority Health and Health Disparities (OMHD). Retrieved January 4, 2009, from http://www.cdc.gov/omhd/ AMH/dbrf.htm

Centers for Disease Control and Prevention. (2007b). *HIV/AIDS Surveillance Report, 2005.* (Vol. 17, rev ed.). Atlanta: U.S. Department of Health and Human Services, 1–46. Retrieved January 13, 2009, from http://www.cdc.gov/hiv/topics/surveillance/ resources/reports/2005report/default.htm

Centers for Disease Control and Prevention. (2008a). Disease infant mortality statistics from the 2005 period linked birth/infant death data set. *National Vital Statistics Reports, 57*(2). Table 2. Retrieved January 5, 2009, from http://www.cdc.gov/nchs/ data/nvsr/nvsr57/nvsr57_02.pdf

Centers for Disease Control and Prevention. (2008b). *HIV/AIDS Surveillance Report, 2006. Vol. 18.* Atlanta: U.S. Department of Health and Human Services. Retrieved January 13, 2009, from http://www .cdc.gov/hiv/topics/surveillance/resources/reports/ 2006report/default.htm

Centers for Disease Control and Prevention (2008c). HIV mortality (through 2005). U.S. Department of Health and Human Services, Division of HIV/ AIDS Prevention. Retrieved January 13, 2009, from http://www.cdc.gov/hiv/topics/surveillance/resources/ slides/mortality/slides/mortality13.ppt

Crave, C., & Delphin, M. (2006). Effective strategies for promoting systemic cultural competence. Cultural Competencies Presentation at the Washington Hilton Hotel, June 29, 2006. Retrieved

January 15, 2009, from http://www.nami.org/ Content/NavigationMenu/Inform_Yourself/Upcom ing_Events/Convention/2006_Highlights/Presenta tions4/Cultural_Competence-Cave_Thur.ppt

Doak, C., Doak, L., & Root, J. (1996). *Teaching Patients with Low Literacy Skills* (2nd ed.). New York: Lippincott.

Ellerbrock, J. V., Bush, T. J., Chamberland, M. E., & Oxtoby, M. J. (1991). The epidemiology of women with AIDS in the U.S. 1980–90. *Journal of the American Medical Association, 265*(22), 2971–2975.

Glynn, M., & Rhodes P. (2005). Estimated HIV prevalence in the United States at the end of 2003. National HIV Prevention Conference; June 12–15; Atlanta. Abstract T1-B1101. Retrieved January 13, 2009, from http://www.aegis.com/conferences/nhiv pc/2005/t1-b1101.html

Hamilton, B. E., Martin, J. A., & Sutton, P. D. (2003). Births: Preliminary data from 2002. *National Vital Statistics Reports, 51*(11), 1–20.

Harris, J., & Fletcher, M. (1997, September 17). Six decades later, an apology. *Washington Post,* A01.

Jones, J. (1981). *Bad Blood: The Tuskegee Syphilis Experiment—A Tragedy of Race and Medicine.* New York: Free Press.

Kaiser Family Foundation. (2008a). Distribution of U.S. population by race/ethnicity, 2000 and 2050. Retrieved January 3, 2009, from http://facts.kff.org/ chart.aspx?ch=364

Kaiser Family Foundation. (2008b). Uninsured adults vs. all adults, by education, 2007. Retrieved January 4, 2009, from http://facts.kff.org/chart.aspx?ch =776

Kelly, P. A. (2007). Physicians' overestimation of patient literacy: A potential source of health care disparities. *Patient Education and Counseling, 66*(1), 119–122.

Leonard, E. E. (2006). Race, ethnicity, culture and disparities in health care. *Journal of General Internal Medicine, 21*(6), 667–669.

Leslie, C. (1990). Scientific racism: Reflections on peer review, science and ideology. *Social Science Medicine, 31*(8), 891–912.

LeVeist, T. A. (ed.). (2002). *Race, Ethnicity and Health: A Public Health Reader.* San Francisco: Jossey-Bass, 701.

National Cancer Institute. (n.d.). *Pink Book—Making Health Communication Programs Work.* Washington, DC. Retrieved January 2, 2009, from http:// www.cancer.gov/pinkbook/page5

National Cancer Institute. (2008). Cancer disparities: Questions and answers. National Institutes of Health. Retrieved January 6, 2009, from http://www.cancer .gov/cancertopics/factsheet/cancer-health- disparities

National Commission on AIDS. (1990). Hearings on HIV disease in the African American Communities.

Nickens, H. W. (1995). The role of race/ethnicity and social class in minority health status. *Health Services Research, 30*(1), 151–162.

Osborne, N. G., & Feit, M. D. (1992). The use of race in medical research. *Journal of the American Medical Association, 267,* 275–279.

Parran, T. (1937). *Shadow on the Land: Syphilis.* New York: Reynal and Hitchcock.

Penslar, R. L., & Porter, J. D. (n.d.). IRB guidebook. Chapter 1. U.S. Department of Health and Human Services, Office for Human Research Protections (OHRP). Retrieved January 23, 2009, from http:// www.hhs.gov/ohrp/irb/irb_guidebook.htm

Raspberry, W. (1997, September 22). Shades of Tuskegee. *Washington Post,* A.19.

Savage, C. L., Anthony, J., Lee, R., Kappersser, M. L., & Rose, B. (2007). The culture of pregnancy and infant care in African American women: An ethnographic study. *Journal of Transcultural Nursing, 18*(3), 215–223.

Sharon, L. M. (1992). Assessing the AIDS education needs of black women in an urban epicenter for HIV infection: A descriptive analysis. Unpublished master's thesis, University of Maryland.

Smith, W. R., Betancourt, J. R., Wynia, M. K., Bussey-Jones, J., Stone, V. E., Phillips, C. O., et al. (2007). Recommendations for teaching about racial and ethnic disparities in health and health care. *Annals of Internal Medicine, 147*(9), 654–665.

Stolberg, S. (1997, September 18). U.S. AIDS research in poor nations raises outcry on ethics. *New York Times,* A.33.

Thomas, S. B., & Quinn, S. C. (1991). The Tuskegee syphilis study, 1932–1972: Implications for HIV education and AIDS risk education programs in the black community. *American Journal of Public Health, 81*(1503).

U.S. Census Bureau. (1999). Resident population of the United States: Middle series projections 2000–2050. Retrieved April 7, 1999, from http://www .census.gov

U.S. Census Bureau. (2007, October). Current population survey. Annual Social and Economic Supplement, Ethnicity and Ancestry Statistics Branch, Population Division. Retrieved January 3, 2009, from http://www.census.gov/population/socdemo/hispanic/ cps2006/2006_tab1.2a.xls

U.S. Census Bureau. (2008, August). An older and more diverse nation by midcentury. Retrieved December 26, 2008, from http://www.census.gov/population/ www/projections/files/nation/summary/np2008-t4.xls

U.S. Department of Health and Human Services. (n.d.). Quick guide to health literacy: Strategies. Improve the usability of health information. Retrieved January 2, 2009, from http://www.health .gov/communication/literacy/quickguide/healthinfo .htm

U.S. Department of Health and Human Services. (2000). *Healthy People 2010.* Washington, DC: U.S. Government Printing Office.

U.S. Department of Health and Human Services. (2005). Usability basics. Retrieved January 2, 2009, from http://www.usability.gov/basics/index.html

U.S. Department of Health and Human Services (2006). Clear communication: An NIH health literacy initiative. National Institutes of Health, Medical Research Agency. Retrieved January 2, 2009, from http://www.nih.gov/icd/od/ocpl/resources/clear communication/healthliteracy.htm

U.S. Department of Health and Human Services, Centers for Disease Control and Prevention, & National Institutes of Health. (2007). Midcourse review, Healthy People 2010. Retrieved January 6, 2009, from http://www.healthypeople.gov/data/mid course/html/focusareas/FA03TOC.htm

U.S. Department of Health and Human Services, Health Resources and Services Administration, Maternal and Child Health Bureau. (2007). Child Health USA 2007, Prenatal Care. Retrieved January 5, 2009, from http://mchb.hrsa.gov/chusa07/ hsfu/pages/309pc.html

U.S. Office of Minority Health. (1999). The initiative to eliminate racial and ethnic disparities in health. Department of Health and Human Services. Retrieved April 15, 1999, from http//www.omhrc.gov

U.S. Renal Data System. (2008). Annual Data Report: Atlas of Chronic Kidney Disease and End-Stage Renal Disease in the United States. National Institutes of Health, National Institute of Diabetes and Digestive and Kidney Diseases. Retrieved January 12, 2009, from http://www.usrds.org/2008/view/esrd_ 00b_hp2010.asp. Publications based upon USRDS data reported here or supplied upon request must include this citation and the following notice:

The data reported here have been supplied by the United States Renal Data System (USRDS). The interpretation and reporting of these data are the responsibility of the author(s) and in no way should be seen as an official policy or interpretation of the U.S. government.

U.S. Task Force on Black and Minority Health. (1985). *Secretary's Report.* Washington, DC: U.S. Department of Health and Human Services.

White House. (1997, May 16.) Remarks by President Clinton in apology for study done in Tuskegee. Press release, Office of the Press Secretary.

Williams, D. R. (1993). A framework for understanding the relationships between race and health. From *Race in the Health of America: Problems, Issues and Directions. Morbidity and Mortality Weekly Report,* 32(RR-10), 9.

Special Challenges

Entry-Level and Advance 1-Level Health Educator Competencies Addressed in This Chapter

Responsibility I: Assess Individual and Community Needs for Health Education
Competency A: Access existing health-related data.
Competency F: Infer needs for health education from obtained data.

Responsibility III: Implementing Health Education Strategies, Interventions, and Programs
Competency B: Demonstrate a variety of skills in delivering strategies, interventions, and programs.
Competency C: Use a variety of methods to implement strategies, interventions, and programs.

Responsibility VII: Communicate and Advocate for Health and Health Education
Competency B: Apply a variety of communication methods and techniques.
Competency D: Influence health policy to promote health.

Note: The competencies listed above, which are addressed in this chapter, are considered to be both entry-level and Advanced level 1 competencies by the National Commission for Health Education Credentialing, Inc. They are taken from *A Framework for the Development of Competency Based Curricula for Entry Level Health Educators* by the National Task Force for the Preparation and Practice of Health Education, 1985; *A Competency-Based Framework for Graduate Level Health Educators* by the National Task Force for the Preparation and Practice of Health Education, 1999; and *A Competency-Based Framework for Health Educators—The Competencies Update Project (CUP)*, 2006.

Method Selection in Health Education

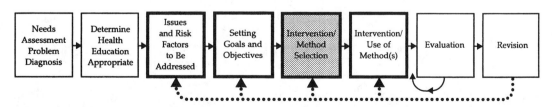

Heavy-bordered boxes indicate subjects addressed in this text; shaded boxes indicate subjects(s) of current chapter.

OBJECTIVES   After studying the chapter the reader should be able to:

- List populations that might require the health educator to prepare material differently for presentation.
- Describe health concerns unique to certain populations.
- Define terms related to disability and exceptionality.
- List some common mistakes when working with special populations.
- Describe strategies to enhance presentations for special populations.

KEY TOPICS

Culture	Exceptional populations
Literacy levels	Health knowledge levels
Language	Sources of health information
Political awareness	Presentation preparation

Just as health educators have to adapt their presentations to accommodate the needs of ethnically diverse populations, so must they do the same for groups or individuals who have particular special needs. Becoming an expert in all the subsets of populations that might utilize health education services is an unlikely and unrealistic proposition, yet health educators need to consider some of the challenges inherent when working in diverse settings. Simply considering and finding out about populations would be a solid first step in preparing more effective interventions. In some instances, unique factors that exist in certain populations may make little difference in how a presentation is made, yet the health educator needs to at least consider these factors in his or her preparation. It is beyond the scope of this text to focus in great depth on all different populations with special needs, so the intent of this chapter is simply to give health educators a glimpse into the worlds of individuals with whom they may at some point be working.

Objective: After reviewing the case study, the reader will suggest two potential methods available to reduce Kareem's narrow-minded thinking and increase his awareness of his target population and their needs.

Case Study: Kareem   Kareem, a community health educator, has been asked to make a presentation on contraception to students at a school for special students. He has made many such presentations to students in the local high schools on this topic but has never worked with an exceptional population. Kareem is surprised at the request, believing that such a population doesn't really need this type of education; after all, aren't they supervised most of the time? Maybe he could wait until next year, when many of the students will be placed in regular schools. Kareem really doesn't understand the point of covering such material with them. (See Case Studies Revisited page 353.)

Question to consider:

What do you think of Kareem's reaction?

Exceptional Populations

A much underserved and underconsidered population with regard to health education is one often labeled as **exceptional.** Exceptional learners are atypical in that their performance deviates from what is expected—either by a higher or lower performance. The needs of exceptional learners vary widely. They often require differing types, intensity, and frequency of services (Office of Program Policy Analysis and Government Accountability [OPPAGA], 2008). Mainstream health education students may be justifiably confused by descriptive labels related to this area, so some definition is necessary. The United Nations Educational, Scientific and Cultural Organization (n.d.) offers three fairly straightforward clarifications of often-used labels:

- **Impairment:** Refers to an abnormality in the function of organs or systems. Impairments are typically associated with a medical or organic condition, such as being near-sighted, heart conditions, cerebral palsy, or hearing disorders.
- **Disability:** Refers to the impact of impairment on functional ability. This might include total or partial behavioral, mental, physical, or sensorial loss of functioning. For example, as a consequence of a spinal cord injury, a patient may be unable to use her limbs and may use "mouthsticks" for most manipulations. A person with limited hearing, however, may be able to correct hearing loss with the use of hearing aids and thus has impairment but no disability. All disabled people are exceptional, but the reverse is not necessarily true.

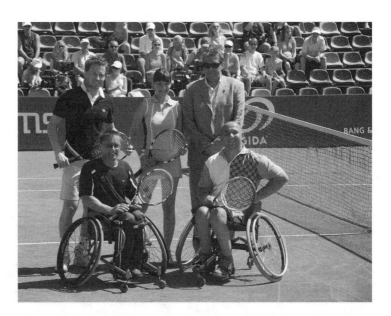

Health educators can expect to work with individuals from exceptional populations.

- **Handicap**: Refers to the social or environmental restrictions placed on a person's life as a result of a disability. Lack of environmental accommodation, such as wheelchair access ramps, handicap the ability of the disabled individual to perform. Although handicapped people are exceptional, not all disabled people are handicapped.

Beware, for the most sacred cow may become the tiger's breakfast.
—Mohan Singh

To illustrate the endless possibility of variations of exceptionality, consider the following case study. A 6-year-old boy named James was born with spina bifida, a condition where the spinal column fails to close and where the extent of disability can be extremely varied. James has limited use of his legs and has no bowel or bladder control. With regard to academic potential, he has been identified as gifted, and he attends a regular first-grade class. Table 9-1 shows how James would fit into the preceding definitions.

This profile clearly illustrates how labeling can be applied to specific conditions. However, although labeling serves a useful purpose in identifying the type of educational interventions that might prove optimal for individual development, the procedure is not without criticism. Labeling, or classifying an individual, has clearly been established as problematic for a variety of reasons (Hallahan & Kauffman, 2000; Markham, 2005; Meyen, 1978). The following summarizes a few of these:

1. All too often the label emphasizes the negative instead of stressing the positive. Specific learning disability labels can affect perceptions of the labeled individual (Hunt, 2006). This stresses the individual's limitations not strengths . . . what the person *cannot* do rather than *can*. This may become a self-fulfilling prophecy.
2. The accuracy of the label may be questionable. Often labels are simplistically given on the basis of single factors and, thus, may conceal a more complex causation. The individuality of the student may be lost as a student is viewed according to his or her disability, not as a student with a disability.

Table 9-1 Applications of Defined Terms

Exceptional: James is considered exceptional because he deviates from the norm (below average with regard to physical performance and exceeding the norm in intellectual performance).

Label	Corresponding Application
Impairment	The failure of the spinal column to close completely during gestation has resulted in a decreased ability of the spinal cord to function properly.
Disability	James is unable to walk or control bowel and bladder functions.
Handicap	James cannot move physically through his environment without assistance. In addition, he requires educational programs for the academically talented. (Although giftedness is not considered by most to be a handicap, it is the authors' opinion that gifted persons are socially handicapped in their superior abilities. For the most part, their abilities are not developed in most traditional educational programs.)

3. Labeling does not accurately account for differences within individual classifications. A broad range of disability can be found within any classification, a good example of this being hearing loss (discussed in this chapter).

4. Conditions of individuals rarely remain static, and classifications do a poor job of including this temporal concept. Individuals tend to change over time, as will their educational needs. Specific labeling, therefore, may no longer be accurate after a period of time.

As a result of these concerns about labeling, some propose abandoning the practice completely. In its place, educators should recognize individual differences and develop learning strategies that capitalize on learners' strengths, which empower them to be successful (Markham, 2005).

Categories of Exceptional Children

The passage of Public Law 94-142 in 1975 codified the rights of all exceptional children and youth to a free, appropriate education. In 2004, Public Law 108-446, known as the Individuals with Disabilities Education Act (IDEA), updated the guidelines outlined in PL 94-142. Exceptional children who are eligible by law for services through special educational placements are categorized as follows: autism, deaf-blindness, deafness, developmental delay, emotionally disabled, hearing impairment, mental retardation, multiple disabilities, orthopedic impairment, other health impairment, specific learning disabilities, speech/language impairment, traumatic brain injury, and visual impairment including blindness. These descriptors, or labels, are very broad, and to fully describe the population served by this law, a more precise definition is needed. The National Dissemination Center for Children with Disabilities (NICHCY, 2008) summarizes the rules and regulations of PL 108-446 and defines its labels as follows:

> **Autism** is considered a developmental disability, generally evident before age 3, that significantly affects verbal and nonverbal communication, social interaction, and educational performance. Other characteristics often associated with autism are engagement in repetitive activities and stereotyped movements, resistance to environmental change or change in daily routines, and unusual responses to sensory experiences.
>
> **Deaf-blindness** means concomitant hearing and visual impairments, the combination of which causes such severe communication and other developmental and educational needs that the person cannot be accommodated in special education programs solely for children with deafness or children with blindness.
>
> **Deafness** indicates a hearing impairment that is so severe that it diminishes a learner's processing of linguistic information through hearing—with or without amplification—and adversely affects a child's educational performance.
>
> **Developmental delay** occurs when children ages 3 through 9 experience a developmental disability as defined by the state and as measured by appropriate diagnostic instruments and procedures in one or more of the following areas—physical development, cognitive development, communication development, social or emotional development, or adaptive development—and who, by reason thereof, need special education and related services.

Emotionally disabled is considered a condition exhibiting one or more of the following characteristics over a long period of time and that adversely affects a child's educational performance to a marked degree:

- An inability to learn that cannot be explained by intellectual, sensory, or health factors
- An inability to build or maintain satisfactory interpersonal relationships with peers and teachers
- Inappropriate types of behavior or feelings under normal circumstances
- A general pervasive mood of unhappiness or depression
- A tendency to develop physical symptoms or fears associated with personal or school problems

Emotional disability includes schizophrenia. The term does not apply to children who are socially maladjusted, unless it is determined that they have an emotional disturbance.

Hearing impairment, whether permanent or fluctuating, adversely affects a child's educational performance, but is not included under the definition of deafness in this section.

Mental retardation includes significantly subaverage general intellectual functioning, existing concurrently with deficits in adaptive behavior and manifested during the developmental period, that adversely affects a child's educational performance.

Multiple disabilities means concomitant impairments (such as mental retardation–blindness, mental retardation–orthopedic impairment, etc.), the combination of which causes such severe educational needs that they cannot be accommodated in special education programs solely for one of the impairments. Multiple disabilities do not include deaf-blindness.

Orthopedic impairment includes a severe orthopedic impairment that adversely affects a child's educational performance. The term includes impairments caused by a congenital anomaly, disease (e.g., poliomyelitis, bone tuberculosis, etc.), and other causes (e.g., cerebral palsy, amputations, and fractures or burns that cause contractures).

Other health impairment means having limited strength, vitality, or alertness, including a heightened alertness to environmental stimuli, that results in limited alertness with respect to the educational environment and adversely affects a child's educational performance. This can be due to chronic or acute health problems such as asthma, attention deficit disorder or attention deficit hyperactivity disorder, diabetes, epilepsy, a heart condition, hemophilia, lead poisoning, leukemia, nephritis, rheumatic fever, and sickle cell anemia.

Specific learning disability is a disorder in one or more of the basic psychological processes involved in understanding or in using language, spoken or written, that may manifest itself in the imperfect ability to listen, think, speak, read, write, spell, or do mathematical calculations, including conditions such as perceptual disabilities, brain injury, minimal brain dysfunction, dyslexia, and developmental aphasia. Specific learning disability does not include learning problems that are primarily the result of visual, hearing, or motor disabilities; mental retardation; emotional disturbance; or environmental, cultural, or economic disadvantage.

Speech/language impairment is a communication disorder, such as stuttering, impaired articulation, or a language or voice impairment, that adversely affects a child's educational performance.

Traumatic brain injury means an acquired injury to the brain caused by an external physical force, resulting in total or partial functional disability or psychosocial impairment, or both, that adversely affects a child's educational performance. Traumatic brain injury applies to open or closed head injuries resulting in impairments in one or more areas, such as cognition; language; memory; attention; reasoning; abstract thinking; judgment; problem-solving; sensory, perceptual, and motor abilities; psychosocial behavior; physical functions; information processing; and speech. Traumatic brain injury does not apply to brain injuries that are congenital or degenerative, or to brain injuries induced by birth trauma.

Visual impairment including blindness means an impairment in vision that, even with correction, adversely affects a child's educational performance. The term includes both partial sight and blindness.

It is not practical, nor is it within the scope of this text, to describe in great detail all these categories of "exceptionality." The majority of mainstream health educators will have extremely limited contact with individuals included in some of these categories. Consequently, the remainder of this chapter will focus on the categories of exceptionality with which school and community health educators are likely to have the most frequent contact.

Visually Impaired

Definitions of visual impairment or blindness can be either legally or educationally based. Legal definitions are based on a technical evaluation, whereas educational definitions tend to be more pragmatic and simplified. Regardless, it is essential that an appropriate learning medium be carefully chosen no matter how much functional vision a student displays. This is an important population for the health educator to be familiar with, because many individuals with visual impairments are being mainstreamed in both school and community settings.

As with the deaf population, the effects of health education for visually impaired people depend to a great extent on the age of onset of visual impairment, the degree of any accompanying disability, and the availability of developmental opportunities. Identifying the extent of visual impairment is reasonably straightforward, but measuring secondary effects of impairment on such things as language development and cognition skills is more difficult, simply because most available instruments and standardized tests are written and are not available in braille. Even if they were available in braille, many participants could not use them, because not all visually impaired people know braille.

Individuals who are visually impaired are often restricted in their social and environmental experiences. The ability to move about the environment is particularly important, because it is this freedom that provides the sighted individual the opportunity for observation and experience. The absence of this opportunity will obviously affect the development of any individual. A concrete example of restricted experience is in the development of language. As most children develop, they take notice of what is happening around them. Children can then question a parent or other person about what they see . . . sometimes in an endless string of questions that only children can ask! A child who does not see a small animal or large gray raincloud has a compromised ability to ask questions and learn about the world. Vocabulary may then become limited, as will comprehension of the environment.

Objective: After reviewing the case study, the reader will suggest two or more ways Robert could enhance the effectiveness of his workshop for the exceptional participants.

Case Study: Robert   Robert is preparing to present a workshop on nutrition and fitness for college students. He has ascertained that approximately 35 students will attend. In anticipation of a workshop filled with a great deal of information, he has prepared a large number of overhead transparencies to facilitate teaching. As Robert is adjusting the focus on the overhead projector, he notices two students with canes carefully entering the classroom. They are obviously significantly visually impaired. Robert has a sinking feeling as he stares at his pile of overhead transparencies and wonders what to do next. (See Case Studies Revisited page 353.)

Question to consider:

What would you do next if you were in Robert's situation?

In its initial stages, motor development is dependent on vision. Seeing objects in the immediate environment stimulates an infant to raise a head or reach out a hand. If an infant is blind, the motivation to move may well be inhibited, and subsequently the visually impaired child cannot develop the experience of being able to move through his or her environment. The obvious lack of visual stimulation can lead some blind individuals to resort to **blindisms**, or primitive movements—perhaps a rocking back and forth motion, or excessive rubbing of the eyes (Blake, 2002). Providing visually impaired individuals with an environment that stimulates and encourages physical response will contribute to the development of motor and social skills.

Frazer and Maguvhe (2008) suggest some important principles that the teacher of any subject should consider when instructing visually impaired people:

1. Because all visually impaired people are not the same, instruction should be *individualized* as much as possible to capitalize on the strengths of the learner.

2. Teachers should stress, as much as possible, relationships between things in the environment that are not discernible to the blind. Strive to use concrete examples to show similarities and differences and avoid abstract things like light and darkness, black and white, beautiful and ugly.

3. Vary sources of stimulation—auditory, tactile, oral, olfactory, and visual—to attract and maintain attention.

4. Some visually impaired children must be taught to actively engage in the learning process. Children devoid of stimuli might tend to be somewhat passive and need to be taught how to become more involved. Professionals working with blind (and visually impaired) learners should incorporate multiple methods for delivery of educational experiences (e.g., collaborative learning, cooperative teaching, peer tutoring, and other innovative scheduling and planning activities) to yield better outcomes in teaching and learning.

Some valuable suggestions for individuals who might be teaching visually impaired people are offered by Mandell and Fiscus (1981) and Biggers (2002):

- Explain about and allow individuals to explore their physical environment—classroom, meeting room, and so on.
- Maximize the remaining vision of the visually impaired—consider adequate levels of light, classroom seating, using larger writing, and the like.
- In the school setting, give non-visually impaired children the opportunity to discuss blindness with the students who have vision problems.
- Provide learning opportunities that will actively include people who are blind. For example, slip items into the hands of the learner so she might "see" the heart model through the sense of touch.
- Ask other involved professionals, or in the case of children, ask parents, "What works?" Don't be afraid to ask for advice.
- In the classroom setting, be sure to orally repeat anything that is written on the blackboard.
- Verbally clarify any predominantly visual materials that you may be using (e.g., maps, charts, and graphs).
- Expand your explanations and descriptions to tell more about the item.
- If an individual is utilizing braille, allow additional time.
- Encourage individuals to utilize any alternative techniques and/or technology that might facilitate learning.

Learning Aids and Material for the Visually Impaired

Learning aids can basically be divided into two categories: optical and nonoptical. Examples of optical aids might be glasses and magnifiers; an example of a nonoptical aid would be the use of braille. Simply stated, braille consists of a series of raised dot patterns that represent elements of language. The dot patterns are placed within a six-dot cell to denote letters of the alphabet, numbers, and punctuation. (See Figure 9-1.) The braille characters are "read" by a person's fingertips.

An important point for educators to remember is that braille is more ambiguous than the printed word. Individuals who are blind and utilizing braille might take longer to read material than seeing people who are reading print.

a	b	c	d	e	f	g	h	i	j

k	l	m	n	o	p	q	r	s	t

u	v	w	x	y	z

Figure 9-1
Braille: A Nonoptical
Reading Aid

For example, in a study comparing the reading speeds of blind and seeing adults "the average print-reading rate ranged from 30% (oral reading) to 60% (silent reading) faster than the average braille-reading rate for the various reading tasks" (Wetzel & Knowlton, 2000, p. 152). Proficient readers of braille typically read with two hands, starting the line with the left hand and finishing it with the right (Whittle, 2005). Two-handed braille reading helps to increase reading speed; however, a time discrepancy may still exist. This time discrepancy must be acknowledged and considered when planning presentations or lessons.

Individuals who are blind may also write in braille. The two major options for doing this are a braillewriter, a machine somewhat similar to a typewriter in appearance that embosses paper with the braille code, and a slate and stylus. The latter device consists of a hinged frame within which paper is clamped. The writer presses down with the stylus, pushing the paper onto the

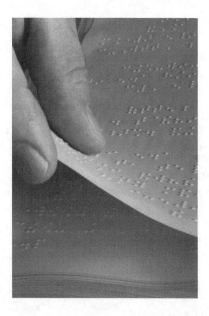

A person reading with braille might require additional time.

back of the frame, which contains six depressions arranged like dots in the braille cell. The writer thus creates the braille cells by hand as opposed to using a machine, the braillewriter, which performs this function more easily.

Additional and frequently utilized non-optical aids include audio forms of media such as CDs, MP3 players, or iPods. These media sources are relatively inexpensive and easy to use, providing the opportunity for the visually impaired to listen to a lecture, take a test from a tape, or even listen to a best-selling novel that has been downloaded to the individual's electronic device.

Assisting the Partially Sighted
Many individuals who are not blind, nevertheless have a vision impairment. Thus, they are able to only partially see. These individuals might be helped by taking the following simple steps, proposed by Rao (2005), to facilitate learning:

- Use specially adapted books with larger print (Figure 9-2).
- Use preferential seating to ensure the learner is placed where he or she sees well. Seating an individual at the front of the room might be helpful.
- Carefully consider background colors when preparing presentation materials. Ensure that print and graphics are clearly defined against the background. Clear contrast between the print and background is essential. Black print on white paper is usually best, and clarity is enhanced when there is contrast in print style and spacing of letters.

This is the type of font size that is often used in books and other written resources specifically developed for people with visual impairment.

Notice how different the above font size is to this example (Times 12), a font typically used for individuals without any form of visual impairment.

Figure 9-2
Enlarge Font Size to Help Those with Visual Impairments

- Ensure that adequate levels of lighting are available; reduce glare from windows by placing the learner's back to the windows as much as possible.
- Allow extra time for completion of work.
- Avoid using word games, puzzles, and graphs that may be inappropriate for low vision learners.
- For some individuals, listening might be a more effective learning device than reading. To that end, ensure that a quiet atmosphere exists that might be more conducive to learning.

One of the primary agencies providing resources for those with visual impairments is the American Printing House for the Blind in Louisville, Kentucky. For additional information, see the appendix.

Learning Disabled

Learning disabilities are more common than one might expect. Approximately one in five persons in the United States is considered learning disabled (NICHCY, 2008). Learning disabled individuals are generally of average or above average intelligence; however, a gap exists between the person's potential and actual achievement (Learning Disabled Association of Canada, 2004).

The label of **learning disabled** has become a somewhat amorphous term, often applied to any students who do not succeed in school. Some definitions include "slow learners" or "mentally retarded," and others incorporate "emotionally unstable" and even blindness. Other experts in this field believe that the label of "learning disabled" should be much more specific than failing to succeed in school. There are obviously many reasons why children might fail in school that would hardly be designated as a learning disability—lack of motivation, inappropriate or mediocre teaching methods, difficulties in the home life, poor nutrition, lack of sleep, and so on. Even the stigma of being labeled learning disabled could contribute to poor performance of a learner. According to Markham (2005), "The term *able* means the ability to do; if we add the prefix *dis-* meaning not, we identify these students as *not* being able to learn" (p. 6). Mandell and Fiscus (1981) suggest this yardstick: if learning difficulties can be overcome by a different type of instruction, then the child should *not* be considered learning disabled.

Perhaps following Markham's suggestion to think of learning disabled students as *students who learn differently* will enable the health educator to better design learning experiences for these learners.

A national definition of learning disabled was established in 1977 as a result of PL 94-142 (*Federal Register*, 1977):

> Specific learning disability means a disorder in one or more of the basic psychological processes involved in understanding or in using language spoken or written which may manifest itself in an imperfect ability to listen, think, speak, read, write, spell or to do mathematical calculations. The term includes

such conditions as perceptual handicaps, brain injury, minimum brain dysfunction, dyslexial and developmental aphasia. The term does not include children who have learning problems which are primarily the result of visual, hearing or motor handicaps, of mental retardation, of emotional disturbance, or of environmental, cultural or economic disadvantage.

Although this definition has remained fairly static since it was developed, regulations related to methodologies for evaluating students have been added. The Individuals with Disabilities Education Act (IDEA 2004) outlines the criteria to be used by states when determining whether a student qualifies as learning disabled. Both IDEA 2004 (effective July 1, 2005) and IDEA 2004 federal regulations (effective October 13, 2006) maintain the same definitions of SLD (specific learning disability) as PL 94-142; however, IDEA 2004 eliminates the requirement to show a "severe discrepancy" between intellectual ability and academic achievement.

Prior to IDEA (2004), the *Federal Register* considered seven areas where a severe discrepancy may exist between ability and achievement:

1. Oral expression
2. Listening comprehension
3. Written expression
4. Basic reading skill
5. Reading comprehension
6. Mathematics calculation
7. Mathematics reasoning

These categories are still used; however, altering the "severe discrepancy" requirement has helped to reduce late identification and misidentification of SLD students (Cotiella, 2006).

In order for a child to be eligible for special educational services, an evaluation team must agree that

- The child must exhibit learning difficulties in at least one of the seven areas just listed.
- The child has a severe learning achievement problem.
- The major reason for the discrepancy between achievement and ability is not other handicapping conditions or sociological factors.

IDEA 2004 federal regulations added the following criteria:

- Must *not* require a school to use a "severe discrepancy" between intellectual ability and achievement for learning disability determination
- Must allow the use of a process designed to determine if a student responds to scientific, research-based interventions or other alternative research-based procedures
- Must align with the criteria established by IDEA 2004 federal regulations, as stated above

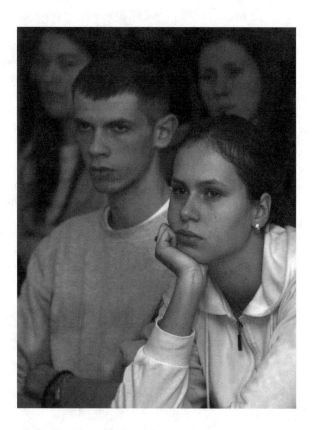

Learning disabilities can sometimes be difficult to detect.

Often the health educator, especially in the community setting, is not made aware of the presence of a learning disability in the individuals he or she is teaching. In school settings, information from the student's IEP (Individual Educational Program) should be provided to all teachers working with the student. School health education teachers also should consult with SPED teachers for appropriate strategies to work with various disabilities. The authors recommend becoming familiar with some of the more frequently cited characteristics of learning disabled children and adult learners. Being aware of some of the more prevalent characteristics might be useful to the health educator in considering health education methodology:

1. **Impairment of motor skills:** Experiencing difficulty reproducing information received through the senses. Difficulty with copying, problems with written information, identifying letters of the alphabet, reading from left to right, and reproducing basic shapes are characteristics of this impairment. Writing samples are often poor and laborious with bizarre spelling mistakes. One of the better known learning disabilities in this category is **dyslexia.**
2. **Limited attention and self-control:** A problem with focusing and holding attention for any length of time. Individuals might experience difficulty in completing tasks, are easily distracted, and often cannot remain seated for long periods of time.

3. **Speech and hearing impairments:** Some children who have a form of communication disorder might have a problem with using correct grammar, and articulating words and thoughts. Another indicator might be a repetition of the same phrases over and over, resulting from restricted language development.

4. **Memory:** Difficulty in memorizing information over long and short periods of time. Indicators might include an inability to remember basic information like the family's address and telephone number or being unable to remember things learned the day before.

5. **Emotional delay:** Some children might not have developed emotionally and socially to an age-appropriate level. This may result in a low threshold for frustration, difficulty with social interaction, and on occasion a temper tantrum. As a consequence, peer relationships may be limited or may be more common with younger groups.

6. **Literal interpretations:** Some children have a difficult time with abstract ideas, which makes them appear to be rigid, humorless, or gullible. For example, a learning disabled individual might misinterpret the meaning of the statement, "Wow . . . your hat is so cool" to mean that his hat is cold.

7. **Impulsivity:** These children rush into reactions or responses without any thought for the consequences. This characteristic could be manifested by writing down the first answer that comes to mind in a test or running out into the street after a ball without regard for traffic.

8. **Learning deficits in basic academic subjects:** These students may demonstrate a wide discrepancy in achievement between subjects. For example, a student might be a full grade level ahead in reading ability but two years below in math. Relevant terms in this section are
   Dyslexia: Problems in reading or a reading disability (commonly known as word blind)
   Dysgraphia: Problems in writing
   Dyscalcula: Problems with arithmetic (commonly known as number blind)

9. **Equivocal neurological signs:** *Equivocal* means questionable or uncertain. For children in this category, there is no direct evidence of neurological damage, yet the individuals demonstrate characteristics such as hyperactivity, poor attention, problems with concentration, distraction, impulsivity, or poor motor functioning.

Learning disabilities in adults often go undetected. As adults, these learners have developed coping mechanisms that often mask their disability. For example, they may choose to participate in oral discussions but make excuses to avoid producing written materials. Identifying an adult as learning disabled becomes a challenge. Some common indicators identified by the Learning Disabilities Association of Canada (2005) might include:

- Displays well-developed verbal ability but has difficulty expressing ideas on paper
- Likely to have poor skills related to reading, writing, or spelling
- Enjoys taking things apart and putting them back together
- Lacks social tact or displays socially inappropriate behavior
- Likely to have poorly developed peer relationships

- Appears to be irresponsible with personal belongings, time, or commitments
- Appears to be high-strung and lacking self-esteem

These indicators suggest that this type of learner will be more successful when methodologies are used that allow the learner to manipulate the content. A standard lecture is likely to be a less effective method than something like a discussion or simulation. Considering the disabled learner is important in the planning process, for it helps the health educator to plan the educational environment to meet the needs of all the participants.

Attention Deficit Disorder (ADD) and Attention Deficit Hyperactivity Disorder (ADHD)

On March 12, 1999, the federal government released the final regulations to the Individuals with Disabilities Education Act (IDEA). These regulations were an attempt to more tightly define and operationalize already established rules and regulations for ensuring educational access to all people and were intended to be incorporated into each state's existing standards. Prior to these new regulations, children with **attention deficit disorder** (ADD) or attention deficit hyperactivity disorder (ADHD) were eligible for special educational services only if their difficulties were accompanied by an additional qualifying disorder. Now ADHD (which includes ADD) alone can make a child eligible for special educational services. The Centers for Disease Control and Prevention (CDC, 2005) defines ADHD as a neurobehavior disorder characterized by pervasive inattention and/or hyperactivity-impulsivity resulting in significant functional impairment. The CDC estimates ". . . that 4.4 million youth ages 4–17 have been diagnosed with ADHD by a healthcare professional, and as of 2003, 2.5 million youth ages 4–17 are currently receiving medication treatment for the disorder. In 2003 7.8% of school-aged children were reported to have an ADHD diagnosis by their parent" (p. 1). Although a small percentage of ADHD students are taught in self-contained classrooms, the vast majority will spend at least part of a day in a regular setting. Thus, health educators are very likely to encounter children and adults with ADHD in both the school and community settings. When designing lessons to accommodate the ADHD learner, it is best to provide a structured and well-organized lesson that has clear expectations for learning. The U.S. Department of Education (2006) recommends a number of teaching-related practices that have been found especially useful in facilitating this process:

- **Provide an advance organizer.** Prepare participants for the lesson by quickly summarizing the order of various activities planned. Explain, for example, that you will use your handouts from the previous lesson to guide you in performing the Heimlich maneuver on the mannequin followed by a group evaluation of your performance.
- **Review previous lessons.** For example, remind learners that yesterday's lesson focused on how to clear a blocked airway in a choking victim. Review several problems before describing the current lesson.

- **Set learning expectations.** State what learners are expected to learn during the lesson. As mentioned in previous chapters of this book, stating the objective for learning is a fundamental practice. It becomes especially important, however, for organizing information for individuals with disabilities. For example, explain to students that the focus of today's session is to learn the sequence of steps for administering cardiopulmonary resuscitation (CPR).
- **Set behavioral expectations.** Describe how learners are expected to behave during the lesson. Tell the participants what they will be doing and how to accomplish their task. For example, "Today you will be working in groups of two. Take turns practicing your skills and helping each another practice the correct sequence of steps. If you need assistance, feel free to raise your hand and call me over."
- **State needed materials.** Identify all materials that the participants will need during the lesson, rather than leaving them to figure out on their own the materials required. For example, specify that participants will need alcohol wipes for cleaning and a barrier device—such as a pocket mask—for ventilating the mannequin.
- **Explain additional resources.** Tell participants how to obtain help in mastering the lesson. For example, refer learners to a particular page in the textbook for guidance on completing a worksheet.

Learning Disabilities With such a wide variety of potential problems, designing methods of instruction for this population can be extremely complicated, and there are no simple solutions for planning presentations. Hammel and Bartel (1978) believe that when constructing materials for teaching learning disabled students, instructors must consider three areas: design, methods, and practicality. The *design* component speaks to the basic organization of the material that the authors believe should be presented in logical, sequential building blocks. The *method* component considers whether the material should be used individually or in groups. Because of the variety of existing learning levels, a diversity of presentation methods is necessary, with a willingness to be flexible toward varying student responses. *Practicality* dictates that materials be "durable" (able to stand the test of time) and that they can be usable both independently and with supervision.

In an examination of instruction styles that seemed to produce better than expected results, the Learning Disabilities Association of America (2009) suggests that the most effective teachers/presenters:

- Broke learning into smaller, more manageable, and logical steps
- Made clear the objectives of the lesson/presentation
- Provided administrative probes and frequent quality feedback
- Used age-appropriate diagrams, graphics, and pictures to augment verbal information
- Modeled instructional practices and provided ample time to practice independently

- Developed a positive learning environment by engaging students in process questions like, "What are some ways you can use this information in another setting?"
- Provided prompts and modified instruction based on participant need

Westwood (1997) and Levin (2007) discuss the phenomenon of the *failure cycle*, experienced by all children but more acutely by the learning disabled child. The child attempts to master a specific skill but fails. Because other children seem able to perform this skill, even moderately, the child loses confidence, leading to a deliberate avoidance of the activity. This avoidance then ensures that no skill practice occurs, guaranteeing, in turn, that competency and proficiency are never attained. Constant failure leads to decreased self-esteem and a generalization of failure to nearly all activities. The basic message of this cycle is, "If at first you don't succeed, you don't succeed!" The implications of this concept are twofold. In order to avoid the possibility of early failure, presenters/teachers must plan and develop new activities with great clarity and provide enough assistance to the learners to make success extremely likely. Second, the only means of breaking the failure cycle is to develop ways in which participants can be successful and ultimately feel that they are improving. Rather than dwelling on the negatives of the child, on what he or she cannot do, educators are encouraged to focus on ways to allow the child to feel successful, using those gains as a springboard for future development and achievement.

Some health educators believe that it is particularly important for learning disabled students to receive sound information related to sex education. Like all human beings, individuals with learning disabilities have the same desires for love, companionship, and sexual activity. However, they may be lacking in the ability to process information and the social skills to practice safe and socially appropriate behaviors (Grieve, McLaren, & Lindsay, 2007). Providing sex education can help prevent sexual abuse and pregnancy while teaching handicapped learners how to express their sexual needs and how to engage in socially appropriate behaviors (McCammon & Knox, 2007). In the context of human sexuality, Rioux (2004) suggests the following guidelines for teaching learning disabled students:

- Use repetition; provide multiple exposures to the concept by using examples from different perspectives.
- Use materials that have a mature theme, after determining that a strong foundation exists in basic information. Many learning disabled students are of average or higher intelligence and may be bored or feel patronized by immature content and approach.
- Use interactive teaching methods to actively involve students in the learning process (role play, games, skits, etc.).
- Make material as relevant as possible to real-life situations. Using pictures or models is a good way to enhance the understanding.

- Practice skills including things like ways to appropriately express sexuality and competence in the ability to use refusal skills.
- With written materials, use simplified syntax, short sentences, and also short paragraphs with the main subject first.

Deafness

The deaf and hard of hearing are included in this chapter because they are truly minority populations in regard to language and culture. Many individuals might believe that people who are deaf or hard of hearing are exactly like hearing individuals, with the one obvious exception that they cannot hear. But this is a simplistic notion. The impairment in hearing has repercussions in various areas. Here are some important questions that health educators should consider in planning a presentation:

- Are the health needs of the deaf identical to the health needs of the hearing?
- Are the health knowledge levels of the deaf similar to the knowledge levels of the hearing?
- Is there any difference in health behavior between the deaf and hearing populations?
- How do knowledge levels, attitudes, and behaviors differ within the deaf and hard-of-hearing communities?
- Can health educators use the same methods of health education with deaf people as they do with hearing people?
- Can materials originally developed for hearing audiences be used effectively by deaf or hard-of-hearing audiences?

Objective: After reviewing the case study, the reader will recommend two strategies Jill might have implemented to better meet the needs of her deaf or hard-of-hearing participants.

Case Study: Jill   Jill was a community health educator who had been asked to present a 1-hour workshop on safer sex to a group of 30 new students at a local community college. The organizer had mentioned the possibility that one or two students who were either deaf or hard of hearing might attend the workshop. Jill gave the matter little further consideration, feeling that if the students did attend they could be seated at the front of the room and that she would attempt to speak louder and enunciate more clearly. Two deaf students did indeed attend, and after seating them in the front row Jill proceeded with the workshop, taking great care to speak loudly and clearly, facing the deaf students as much as possible. Part of the workshop included a short videotape on safer sex practices, and when the two deaf students left the room 5 minutes into the film, Jill supposed that the students had been offended by the explicit nature of what they had seen. Jill completed the workshop oblivious to her mistaken assumptions and beliefs. (See Case Studies Revisited page 353.)

Question to consider:

What do you think the real problem was, and what steps could Jill take should this issue arise again?

Before attempting to address some of these questions, it is essential for the health educator to understand some basic information related to deafness.

Deaf Culture   Like any true subculture or minority group, people who are deaf adhere to certain cultural norms that are passed on from one generation to the next. Most cultures pass on their beliefs within the family unit. However, the deaf community is unique in the way that its culture is perpetuated. Because 90% of deaf children have two hearing parents, only a minority of deaf individuals acquire their cultural identity and social skills in the home. For many, learning the culture of the deaf occurs when they become part of the deaf community—commonly referred to as capital "D." Not all deaf people are members of a D community; however, it is the common conditions of deafness and the use of visual language that unite its members.

Social etiquette within the deaf community can be slightly different from that of the hearing community. For example, although the hearing culture generally considers staring to be rude, deaf culture has no prohibition against this, because staring is necessary for effective sign communication.

As with all cultures, it is equally important that health educators demonstrate cultural sensitivity with the deaf or hard of hearing. For example, time and punctuality are important concerns, because arriving early to large scale events enables those with limited hearing to secure seating with the best visual clarity. Ensuring that auditory cues are received by those with limited hearing while controlling for distracting movements will better foster an effective learning environment (Mindess, 2006). As a non-deaf practitioner, one should be aware of the recommended guidelines for working with and in the presence of a deaf or hard-of-hearing person. Deaf Ministeries Worldwide has codified these guidelines as the Ten Commandments of Deaf Culture. (See Figure 9-3.)

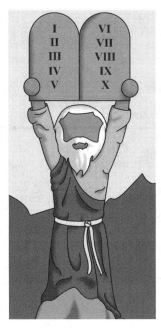

I.   You shall not put "hearing culture" above deaf culture.

II. You shall not lose eye contact when communicating.

III. You shall communicate in sign language at all times.

IV. You shall not be the deaf person's sign language teacher.

V.   You shall not be the deaf person's English or grammar teacher.

VI. You shall not be the deaf person's speech therapist.

VII. You shall not be the deaf person's comedian, telling non-deaf jokes and puns.

VIII. You shall not be the deaf person's mother.

IX. You shall view deaf as an ethnic group not as handicapped people.

X.   You shall believe deaf can do all things.

Figure 9-3
The Ten
Commandments
of Deaf Culture
Source: Deaf Ministries
Worldwide. Adapted with
permission.

Professionals who have studied the deaf culture have isolated and defined some common characteristics and values; a few of these summarized by The National Academy, Gallaudet University, 1990, are presented here:

1. There is a heavy emphasis on vision. **American Sign Language (ASL)**, a visual mode of communication, is the language used within the deaf community. Members gain the vast majority of their information through their eyes and make a point of observing closely what is happening around them. Lip-reading is considered to be an ineffective means of communication for most in the D community. According to Jeff Pollock, teacher of ASL and "Deafolympic" snowboarder, only about 30% of speech originates in the spoken word, making the interpretation of what is being said mostly guesswork (Jarvik, 2007).

2. There is a specific set of social norms. Members follow certain social habits that are somewhat different from those of general society. Among these are the following:

   a. Members do not generally use their voices with deaf friends even if they do so with hearing friends. Some members of the deaf community purposely refrain from using their voices in order to dissociate themselves from speech.

   b. Attention-getting behaviors are considered socially appropriate. Members will wave, create a vibration by tapping objects, throw a small piece of paper, or point at another person to attract the person's attention. Even lightly tapping a deaf person on the shoulder is a suitable practice.

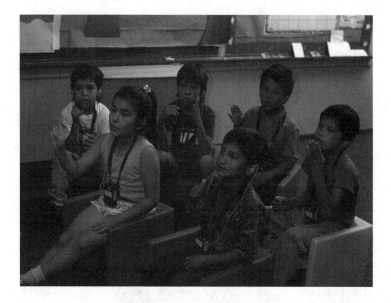

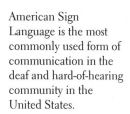

American Sign
Language is the most
commonly used form of
communication in the
deaf and hard-of-hearing
community in the
United States.

When working with groups in the D community, it is acceptable to flick
the lights on and off to gain the attention of the entire group.

c. Maintaining direct eye contact is considered an essential part of communication.

d. Members use a variety of devices to replace ordinary alarm clocks,
door bells, telephones, fire alarms, etc.

3. Members place a strong emphasis on fostering and maintaining social
ties within the community.

The two most common descriptors related to individuals who have a hearing loss are *deaf* (cannot make use of residual hearing for the purposes of
communication) and *hard of hearing* (can use residual hearing to assist in
communication). The term *hearing impaired* is often avoided for two reasons.
First, as with many other contemporary issues, deafness is influenced by its
own political agendas, and for some deaf individuals the word "impaired"
suggests that something is "broken." This descriptor, therefore, is viewed as
inaccurate and undesirable by many in the deaf community. Second, this terminology does not usefully distinguish between "deaf" and "hard of hearing"
and so has limited practical use. Keeping up with terms that are constantly
changing is not easy, particularly when individual health educators live
outside many of the cultures in which they are asked to work. However, the
educators should make every possible attempt to remain current in order to
prevent offending individuals and to maintain crucial credibility.

Deafness can be divided into two types: *congenital* (deaf from birth) and
acquired (becoming deaf after birth because of illness or accident). Acquired
deafness can then be divided into *prelingual* (becoming deaf before spoken
language skills had been developed) and *postlingual* (becoming deaf after
spoken language had been developed) categories. (See Figure 9-4.)

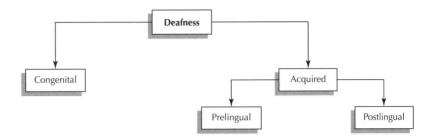

Figure 9-4
Forms of Deafness

Although at first glance these distinctions might seem subtle, they carry important implications for health educators as they approach program and material development. Those individuals who are congenitally or prelingually deaf will not have been exposed to the more typical methods of language development—repetition of the spoken word, constantly hearing words and sounds, and learning to read by hearing written words spoken aloud. As a result, congenitally or prelingually deaf individuals may struggle with written and spoken English. Studies have shown that many deaf and hard-of-hearing students read at lower than the norm grade levels for their age. Findings from a 30-year study conducted at Gallaudet Research Institute (n.d.) revealed that of the children with hearing loss, half of them graduated with a fourth-grade reading level.

Unfortunately, many individuals mistakenly equate reading levels with intelligence, and health educators must be careful not to make this assumption. Although deaf and hard-of-hearing individuals might indeed read at lower grade levels, their I.Q. scores do not differ greatly from the hearing population. However, because of this lack of comprehension of both written and spoken language, communication can become a major barrier between deaf and hearing people . . . a barrier of which the health educator must be aware. Consideration must be given as to how to overcome the barrier in effectively educating the deaf and hard-of-hearing communities about important health issues.

Here are some examples of questions addressed to the health educator of a college for the deaf via the computer/mail system (Morrone-Joseph, 1992). Take note of the wide range of linguistic ability among students.

Example 1   *Hi . . I want to know and curious. Suppose I did period on the end of the month at Feb . . later in the two weeks and the sperm did in the vagina. But the period will come on the end of march . . is it possible to be pregnant or not . . . please let me know this week so I can aware that . . .*

Example 2   *There are two questions I need to know . . . I am 20 years old female. Am I suppose to take pap-smear and breast check up? Or is it too early for me to test? Can you tell me the difference between the pap-smear and breast check up?*

Example 3   *Which days are safe to have sex without getting pregnant, without using any method of birth control? I was told that the time before ovulation is safe.*

These three examples above clearly represent a cross-section of written-English levels. Although the writing levels are very different, it is interesting to note that all of these excerpts do effectively communicate their questions. It is often necessary to read for content and not be put off by "strange" English. The health educator must be aware that all deaf individuals are *not* the same, nor do they operate at identical levels of communication. This factor must be taken into account when developing and planning programs.

If I Speak in a Clear Manner, Can't They Read Lips?

The foregoing is a common misconception about communicating with the deaf. Remember, in the case study, Jill assumed that speaking in a loud voice with clear enunciation was sufficient accommodation for her deaf and hard-of-hearing students. But the notion that a good way to communicate with the deaf is for them to read lips is a myth. There are many reasons why reading lips is fraught with problems, not the least of which is that the English language has many words that look the same on the lips. Here are some examples of words with very different meanings but identical appearances on the lips:

MAIL	MALE
BAIL	BALE
PAIL	PALE
SAIL	SALE

In addition, factors such as distance from the speaker, people in between, poor lighting, head movements, and poor speech patterns all contribute to making lip-reading an ineffective mode of communication. It is perhaps ironic to note that because they have developed speech and language through hearing, the best lip-readers are in fact hearing individuals (Lowell, 1958).

Couldn't I Take a Quick Course in Sign Language?

The idea that a hearing person could take a brief course in sign language and then effectively communicate with a deaf person is, unfortunately, as common as it is absurd! Imagine that in one month you will be expected to present a 1-hour workshop on stress management to a group of 30 Russian immigrants who speak no English. In preparation for this, you will polish your presentation material and then take a short course in Russian! As absurd as this example might appear, the comparison is not inaccurate. Many people believe that deaf individuals communicate in a language that is essentially English transformed into signs. This is not the case. American Sign Language (ASL), which is the native language of most culturally deaf Americans, is not English. This visually based language bears little relationship to English, particularly in grammar and syntax. An interpreter who is signing for a deaf person is not always signing what is being said word for word. Rather, concepts and ideas are signed.

Most cultures have a colloquial element to their language that all of us outside that specific culture find difficult to follow. People from the northern regions of the United States often find expressions unique to the south impossible to understand, and vice versa. Also, many of us who have taken French in school or college have experienced the horrors of visiting Paris or other French cities and been left wondering just what language *are* these people speaking?! This problem with understanding colloquialisms is no less important in communicating with the deaf. Here are just a few examples of idioms that hearing health educators would probably not hesitate to use under normal circumstances but that might prove to be dysfunctional in the communication process with the deaf:

pulling my leg	check it out
really hits home	sink or swim
cut the light	hooking up
hit on her	a no-brainer

Health educators must be aware that many deaf individuals are in an almost identical situation to foreigners . . . English is a *second* language to them. This does not mean that they are less intelligent or able. It simply means that efforts to communicate will be compromised unless this factor is taken into account and measures are implemented to compensate for it.

Sources of Information   Very little data exist to assist the health educator in comprehending the world of deaf people. Do deaf individuals gain most of their health information in the same manner as their hearing peers, or do they follow an alternative route? Practitioners who work with the deaf postulate that, at least in the area of sexuality, deaf individuals, because of their lack of hearing, are denied access to all the usual agents contributing to sexual knowledge and awareness (Berke, 2008; Denny, Getch, & Young, 1998; Fitzgerald & Fitzgerald, 1980). For example, young people in the hearing world gain information in a multitude of ways: talking with others, watching television, going to the movies, listening to the radio, attending classes in school, reading, and personal experience. Deaf individuals typically are denied these *incidental learning* opportunities that hearing individuals take for granted. Very few films are captioned, radio is not an option, limited language skills often make reading difficult, and even observations can lead to mistaken impressions.

Fitzgerald and Fitzgerald (1980) relate the story of the 11-year-old deaf boy who on entering the classroom began to share his packet of Certs with the girls in the class. It quickly became obvious that the young man was expecting to be kissed by the girls in return for the Certs! The boy had seen the televised Certs commercial without the benefit of sound, had missed the verbal communication related to breath freshness, and had come to the very reasonable conclusion that anyone who was given a Cert was expected to respond with a kiss.

It is the contention of Reaves-Fitzgerald and Fitzgerald (1998) that without the benefit of incidental learning, deaf individuals might rely on personal experience more than their hearing counterparts. The pitfalls and dangers of learning through experience are obvious for most areas of health but are particularly acute in the arena of contemporary sexuality, given the threat of AIDS and other sexually transmitted diseases as well as unintended pregnancy. Findings from a study of deaf college students indicated that they had significantly less knowledge about HIV/AIDS than their hearing peers (Heuttel & Rothstein, 2001). Their findings are particularly alarming in light of the fact that deaf college students are better educated than the general deaf population. An earlier study comparing deaf and hearing college students found that although hearing students scored higher than deaf students on sexual knowledge items, both populations had low levels of sexual knowledge, and gender was a more accurate predictor than hearing status of age at first intercourse, number of sexual partners, and preventive health practices. This study also reported that a significantly higher rate of forced sexual intercourse existed in the deaf community (Sawyer, Desmond, & Joseph, 1996).

In addition to missing the benefits of incidental learning, deaf individuals are less likely to have the opportunity to attend formal sexuality education courses. Sexual knowledge for many deaf individuals, therefore, might often be derived from personal experience. There is insufficient research to demonstrate whether this one finding could be generalized to other populations or even other areas of health. However, it does suggest that a health education approach of assuming that deaf individuals have identical health interests, concerns, and behaviors to hearing individuals might be unwise.

Teaching Methods and Strategies

Research into the effectiveness of health education teaching methodology for the deaf is scant. Tomasetti, Beck, and Clearwater (1983) compared the effectiveness of three different types of teaching methods used in cardiopulmonary resuscitation (CPR) education for both the hearing and deaf populations. Three deaf groups each received a different teaching method: standard course through signed instruction; standard instruction with a captioned videotape; and standard instruction with uncaptioned videotape, signed by an interpreter. The hearing group, which received a standard course, performed the best of all groups on psychomotor skills in an immediate posttest. However, in a 4-month retest, the deaf group that had received a signed videotape performed better on psychomotor skills than any of the other groups, including the hearing group. It is not clear why the signed film was more effective than the captioned. One possibility might be that poor reading levels compromised the participants' ability to comprehend the captions, or perhaps the presence of an interpreter caused the students to identify with the instructor, thus influencing retention levels.

An interesting addition to this study would have been a group instructed by a deaf health educator who was able to sign. Whether or not levels of learning are enhanced by having an educator from the same community as the group receiving the education is a subject worthy of further research. This concept would seem no less important to the deaf community as it would in the African American or Latino populations. However, the limited number of minority health educators underlines the necessity for nonminority health educators to be educated about other cultures.

Beck and Tomasetti (1984) make an important contribution to health education teaching methodology for the deaf in their description of a safety training program. The authors describe the preparation for teaching a special population and the adaptations they made to successfully complete the workshop. Many of their recommendations are included here in suggestions for working with the deaf.

The almost complete absence of research related to the health education needs, knowledge, attitudes, and behavior of the deaf means that health educators working with this population must really give a great deal of thought to method selection. As emphasized in this text, not all deaf or hard-of-hearing individuals are alike, and some effort by the educator should be made to discover specific information about individuals and their needs. Here are some suggestions that might facilitate working with the deaf:

- Make no assumptions! Obtain as much information you can about the hearing levels, reading levels, and so forth of the individuals involved.
- Come to terms with the idea that most presentations will require an interpreter. Forget about depending on your audience's ability to read lips . . . get an interpreter.* Some organizations will provide them, some deaf individuals will bring their own . . . make some inquiries! Often the expense or shortage of interpreters continues to limit deaf people's access to health education.
- When using an interpreter, speak directly to the learner, not to the interpreter. This will enable the learner to interpret nonverbal cues.
- Do not expect a deaf person to look at printed information and the interpreter at the same time. Allow time for the participants to look over any printed information before resuming the discussion.
- If you're using any method where the lights are dimmed, give some thought to the interpreter. Provide a side light for him or her, or turn the lights back on between slides or transparencies to discuss information.
- Take a "hands on" approach to learning. This move away from the lecture format necessitates less translation, and in addition may be a more effective means to facilitate comprehension.

---

*Title I of the Americans with Disabilities Act of 1990 prohibits private employers, state and local governments, employment agencies, and labor unions from discriminating against qualified individuals with disabilities in job application procedures, hiring, firing, advancement, compensation, job training, and other terms, conditions, and privileges of employment. The ADA covers employers with 15 or more employees, including state and local governments. It also applies to employment agencies and to labor organizations. The ADA's nondiscrimination standards also apply to federal sector employees under section 501 of the Rehabilitation Act, as amended, and its implementing rules. An employer is required to make a reasonable accommodation to the known disability of a qualified applicant or employee if it would not impose an "undue hardship" on the operation of the employer's business. To that end, presentations performed by public agencies (e.g., state, local, and community) must provide and pay for interpreters if requested. In addition, private agencies (e.g., a health maintenance organization) must also provide and fund any reasonable accommodation, including an interpreter, if requested.

NOTEWORTHY   **Myths About Deafness**

Like all minority groups, deaf people are the target of stereotyping. Some myths about deaf people follow:

MYTH: *All hearing losses are the same.*
FACT: The single term *deafness* covers a wide range of hearing losses that have very different effects on a person's ability to process sound and thus to understand speech.

MYTH: *All deaf people are mute.*
FACT: Some deaf people speak very well and clearly; others do not because their hearing loss prevented them from learning spoken language. Deafness usually has little effect on the vocal cords, and very few deaf people are truly mute.

MYTH: *People with impaired hearing are "deaf and dumb."*
FACT: The inability to hear affects neither native intelligence nor the physical ability to produce sounds. Deafness does not make people dumb in the sense of being either stupid or mute. Deaf people, understandably, find this stereotype particularly offensive.

MYTH: *All deaf people use hearing aids.*
FACT: Many deaf people benefit considerably from hearing aids. Many others do not; indeed, some find hearing aids to be annoying and choose not to use them.

MYTH: *Hearing aids restore hearing.*
FACT: Hearing aids amplify sound. They have no effect on a person's ability to process that sound. In cases where a hearing loss distorts incoming sounds, a hearing aid can do nothing to correct this and may even make the distortion worse.

MYTH: *All deaf people can read lips.*
FACT: Some deaf people are very skilled lip-readers, but many are not. This is because many speech sounds have identical mouth movements. For example, *p* and *b* look exactly alike on the lips.

MYTH: *Deaf people are not sensitive to noise.*
FACT: Some types of hearing loss actually accentuate sensitivity to noise. Loud sounds become garbled and uncomfortable. Hearing aid users often find loud sounds, which are greatly magnified by their aids, very unpleasant.

MYTH: *Deaf people are less intelligent.*
FACT: Hearing ability is unrelated to intelligence. Lack of knowledge about deafness has often limited educational and occupational opportunities for deaf people.

MYTH: *Deaf people are alike in abilities, tastes, ideas, and outlooks.*
FACT: Deaf people are as diverse in their abilities, tastes, ideas, habits, and outlooks as any other large group of people.

- Practical demonstrations rather than descriptions and handouts can facilitate learning when poor reading comprehension levels exist. Use models and pictures.
- Films should be captioned or an interpreter used. Here again, the absence of good, captioned materials continues to be a major problem in program delivery.
- The use of games as a teaching method can be an effective way to involve participants in an interactive manner.
- Be aware that programs might take more time with a deaf audience, and allow for this difference. The extra time allows individuals to feel less pressure and permits the educator to reiterate and consolidate important points. Issues requiring more complex levels of comprehension can be covered more than once.
- Never ask, "Do you understand?" The likely response will be an affirmative nod of the head. Always use the "check back" technique, asking for a review of information understood.

Communication Tips   Following are some tips for communicating with deaf and hard of hearing people that were developed for use by health professionals at Gallaudet University for the deaf and hard of hearing (2003).

Helpful Tips for Speaking

- Face the deaf person.
- Maintain eye contact with the deaf person.
- Be sure that there is a light source in front of you. Avoid having your back to any light source because it causes a glare.
- Speak slowly and clearly.
- Avoid distracting background noise (conversations, printers, etc.); move to another location if necessary.
- Do not exaggerate your mouth movements.
- Keep objects/hands away from your mouth.
- Isolate or emphasize key words when appropriate.
- Give the deaf person as many visual cues as possible.
- Consider your choice of words carefully.

Helpful Tips for Getting the Person's Attention

- Call the person by name or title (such as "sir").
- Tap the person on the shoulder or arm.
- Wave your hand (but not frantically).
- Make sure the person is looking at you before you speak.
- Tap on the table or counter.

Helpful Tips for Communicating Through Writing/Drawing

- Keep your writing brief and to the point.
- Look for meaning in the deaf person's message; ignore any grammatical errors.
- When appropriate, use a drawing in addition to your written message.
- Use open-ended questions.
- Face the deaf person after you have written your messages, and ask for a communication check.

- Often, requesting that the deaf person rephrase what he or she has understood is the best way to identify and prevent potential misunderstandings.

Helpful Tips for Working with an Interpreter

- Stand or sit close to the interpreter.
- Place graphics or models near you and the interpreter.
- Speak at a reasonable pace.
- Look at the deaf person(s).
- Address the deaf person(s) directly. Do not say to the interpreter, "Tell her . . ."
- Leave time for the interpreter to finish because the interpreter will likely be a few words behind.
- Adjust lighting appropriately.
- Allow time for the deaf person(s) to ask and respond to questions.
- Say only what you want interpreted; remember that it is the interpreter's job to interpret *everything* you say and *everything* the deaf person signs.

Helpful Tips When Working in Groups

- Make sure the deaf or hard of hearing person is in the best location possible to satisfy communication needs. (The best location may vary depending on the setting. Ask!)
- Avoid pacing and other distracting movements.
- Make sure you face the deaf or hard-of-hearing person when you speak.
- Use visual aids.
- Allow the audience time to look at visual aids before speaking.
- Prepare written instructions and handouts.
- Repeat questions/comments from audience members.
- Use hands-on activities.

Helpful Tips for Hosting a Program or Meeting

- Be aware there are different types of interpreting and ask users what they need.
- Schedule interpreters well in advance (at least 2 weeks).
- Provide the interpreter with copies of handouts and with the names of program/meeting participants and spelling of any technical terms or jargon before the program begins.
- Make sure all arrangements (lighting, seating, interpreter preferences, client preferences, etc.) are worked out before the program/meeting begins.
- If the interpreter is working alone, give adequate breaks.

Although this chapter focuses narrowly on only four exceptional populations—the visually impaired, the learning disabled, those with ADHD, and those who are deaf or hard of hearing—the health educator needs to have an awareness of these challenges when preparing health interventions or delivering presentations. It is obvious that this surface approach only creates an awareness of the scope and complexity of the adaptations necessary for effective teaching and implementation of intervention strategies.

For more information and tools related to this chapter visit
http://healtheducation.jbpub.com/strategies.

EXERCISES

1. A group of deaf college students (approximately 15 male and female students, ages 19–23 years) has requested a speaker on birth control. You have been given the assignment. With your newfound knowledge of people who are hearing impaired or deaf, describe the steps you would take to plan for this presentation. Then list some presentation methods related to contraception education that might be appropriate with this group.

2. You are teaching a combination ninth/tenth-grade high school health education course. You have been informed that 3 of the 25 students are special education students. Describe the steps you would take to accommodate these students in your course, both in preparation for teaching and during individual classes. (You can either respond in general terms or select specific learning disabilities.)

3. Jennifer, one of the students in your seventh-grade health education class, is visually impaired. Describe the steps you would take to discover the extent of the impairment, and make some suggestions as to how you would accommodate Jennifer in your class.

CASE STUDIES REVISITED

Case Study Revisited: Kareem

Kareem is in need of some education and perhaps sensitivity training. Unfortunately, many educators when faced with special population groups make equally unfounded assumptions. No health educator can be an expert concerning every exceptional population, but even a small amount of research and investigation on the health educator's part would go a long way to reduce the likelihood of Kareem's type of aberrant thinking. (See page 324.)

Case Study Revisited: Robert

Robert could take the easy way out and just continue with his prepared lecture. But if he has some initiative, he will take steps to alleviate a possible problem. The most obvious initial step would simply be to welcome the visually impaired participants and before beginning the lecture ask them if there is anything that he can do to make the workshop more effective. Would seating arrangements make a difference—perhaps closer to the front of the room? Ask yourself whether Robert should make a greater effort to verbalize the written material to facilitate understanding. Would written materials like pamphlets be useful for participants to take home after the workshop so that someone could read them to the visually impaired participants or perhaps even translate them into braille? Obviously, there is a limit to what Robert can do at such short notice, but these simple steps would be reasonable in an attempt to accommodate all his workshop participants. (See page 330.)

Case Study Revisited: Jill

Jill was fortunate enough to have gained the information that deaf students might be attending her workshop *before* the event took place. Had she done some basic research into the deaf population, Jill could have avoided some very basic mistakes. Her first thought should have been to find out if an interpreter was needed, and if so, seek help in making such an arrangement. The presence of an interpreter could have prevented the whole problem. Jill also believed the myth that if you speak loudly and clearly enough, a deaf person will understand you. As this chapter explains, lip reading is not an easy or efficient means of comprehension for the vast majority of deaf or hearing impaired people. Jill made the assumption that the deaf students left during the videotape because of its sexually explicit nature. Although this could have been the case, a more obvious explanation would be that the students could simply not hear the narration and therefore had little understanding of what was occurring. This case study illustrates the need for a greater knowledge of special populations when planning health education interventions. (See page 341.)

SUMMARY

1. Health educators need to have a good working knowledge of special populations, including important information such as basic demographics and health problems unique to specific populations.

2. Health educators must familiarize themselves with the laws relating to the provision of services for special populations.

3. As the trend to mainstream exceptional individuals continues, the health educator is more likely to have to be prepared to devise presentation methods that will optimally include these individuals in the learning process.

4. Health educators need to familiarize themselves with available resources specifically designed to meet the needs of exceptional populations.

REFERENCES AND RESOURCES

Aukerman, R. (1972). *Reading in the Secondary Classroom.* New York: McGraw-Hill.

Beck, K. H., & Tomasetti, J. A. (1984, May). Safety training for the deaf. *Professional Safety,* 20–23.

Berke, J. (2007). Teaching deaf kids the birds and the bees. About.com. Retrieved February 7, 2009, from http://deafness.about.com/cs/parentingarticles/a/sex education.htm

Biggers, E. (2002). Tips for classroom teachers with a visually impaired student. *See/Hear Newsletter,* 7(3). Retrieved February 1, 2009, from http://www.tsbvi .edu/Outreach/seehear/summer02/tips.htm

Blake, S. J. (2002). Beating blindisms. *See/Hear Newsletter,* 7(2). Retrieved February 1, 2009, from http:// www.tsbvi.edu/Outreach/seehear/spring02/blindisms .htm

Centers for Disease Control and Prevention. (2005). Attention-deficit/hyperactivity disorder (ADHD). Retrieved February 3, 2009, from http://www.cdc.gov/ ncbddd/adhd

Clements, S. D. (1966). *Minimal Brain Dysfunction in Children: Terminology and Identification, Phase 1 of a Three-Phase Project.* Washington, DC: U.S. Department of Health, Education & Welfare, Public Health Service Bulletin No. 1415.

Cotriella, C. (2006). IDEA 2004 close up: Evaluation and eligibility for specific learning disabilities. Retrieved February 2, 2009, from http://www.great schools.net/cgi-bin/showarticle/3063

Cratty, B. J. (1971). *Movement and Spatial Awareness in Blind Children and Youth.* Springfield, IL: Charles Thomas.

Deaf Culture. (1990). Handout prepared by College for Continuing Education, National Academy, Gallaudet University.

Denny, G., Getch, Y., & Young, M. (1998). Sexuality education for students who are deaf: Current practices and concerns. *Sexuality and Disability, 16*(4), 269–281.

Federal Register (Part IV). (1977). Washington, DC: Department of Health, Education, and Welfare, 163, 42.

Fitzgerald, D., & Fitzgerald, M. (1980, September). Sexuality and deafness—An American overview. *British Journal of Sexual Medicine,* 30–34.

Fraser, W. J., & Maguvhe, M. O. (2008, September). Teaching life sciences to blind and visually impaired learners. *Journal of Biological Education, 42*(2), 84–89.

Gallaudet Research Institute. (n.d.). Stanford Achievement Test. (9th ed). Form S. Norms Booklet for Deaf and Hard of Hearing Students. Washington, DC: Gallaudet University. Retrieved February 7, 2009, from http://gri.gallaudet.edu/Literacy

Gallaudet University. (2003). Communicating in the library with people who are deaf or hard of hearing. Retrieved February 13, 2009, from http://library.gallaudet.edu/Library/Deaf_Research_Help/Communication_Tips_for_Librarians.html

Goldstein, H., Arkell, C., Ashcroft, S. C., Hurley, O. L., & Lilly, M. S. (1975). Differentiating learning disability. In N. Hobbs (Ed.), *Issues in the Classification of Children.* San Francisco: Jossey-Bass.

Gordon, S. (1973). *The Sexual Adolescent.* North Scituate, MA: Duxbury Press.

Grive, A., McLaren, S., & Lindsay, W. R. (2007). An evaluation of research and training resources for the sex education of people with moderate to severe learning disabilities. *British Journal of Learning Disabilities, 35*(1), 30–37.

Grossman, S. (1972). *Sexual Knowledge, Attitudes and Experiences of Deaf College Students.* Unpublished master's thesis, George Washington University.

Haight, S. L., & Fachting, D. D. (1986). Materials for teaching sexuality, love and maturity to high school students with learning disabilities. *Journal of Learning Disabilities, 19*(6), 344–350.

Hallahan, D. P., & Kauffman, J. M. (2000). *Exceptional Learners: Introduction to Special Education* (8th ed.). Needham Heights, MA: Pearson Education.

Hammel, D. D., & Bartel, N. R. (1978). *Teaching Children with Learning Disabilities and Behavior Problems.* Boston, MA: Allyn & Bacon.

Harlan, L. C., Bernstein, A. B., & Kessler, L. G. (1991). Cervical cancer screening: Who is not screened and why? *American Journal of Public Health, 81*(7), 885–890.

Heuttel, K. L., & Rothstein, W. (2001). HIV/AIDS knowledge and information resources among deaf and hard of hearing college students. *American Annals of the Deaf, 146*(13), 280–286.

Hogan, D. (1997). ADHD: A travel guide to success. *Childhood Education, 73,* 3.

Hunt, F. (2006). The effects of labeling and social desirability on perceived success of a learning disabled student. *Journal of Undergraduate Psychology Research, 1,* 9–12.

IDEA. (2004). Building the legacy: A training curriculum on IDEA 2004. Retrieved February 2, 2009, from http://www.nichcy.org/Laws/IDEA/Pages/BuildingTheLegacy.aspx

Jarvik, E. (2007). What is it like to be Deaf with a capital D? *Deseret Morning News.* Retrieved February 7, 2009, from http://www.deseretnews.com

Learning Disabilities Association of America. (2009). Successful strategies for teaching students with learning disabilities. Retrieved June 19, 2009, from http://www.ldanatl.org/aboutld/teachers/understanding/strategies.asp

Learning Disabilities Association of Canada. (2005). LD in depth. Retrieved February 4, 2009, from http://www.ldac-taac.ca/InDepth/child_indicators-e.asp

Levin, B. (2007). The failure of failure. *Phi Delta Kappan,* 8–9(3), 234–235.

Lowell, E. L. (1958). *John Tracey Clinic Research Papers III–VII.* Los Angeles, CA: John Tracey Clinic.

Lowenfeld, B. (1962). Psychological foundations of special methods of teaching blind children. In P. A. Zahl (Ed.), *Blindness.* New York: Hafner.

Mandell, C. J., & Fiscus, E. (1981). *Understanding Exceptional People.* St. Paul, MN: West.

Markham, D. (2005). The language of labels. *Teaching Exceptional Children Plus, 2*(2). Retrieved February 1, 2009, from http://escholarship.bc.edu/education/tecplus/vol2/iss2/art1/

McCammon, S. L., & Knox, D. (2007). Choices in sexuality. (3rd ed.). Manson, OH: Thompson Learning.

McFarland, D. L., Kolstad, R., & Briggs, L. D. (1995). Educating attention deficit hyperactivity disorder children. *Education, 115*(4), 597–603.

Meyen, E. L. (1978). *Exceptional Children and Youth.* Denver: Love.

Mindess, A. (2006). *Reading Between the Signs: Intercultural Communication for Sign Language Interpreters*. Boston, MA: Intercultural Press.

Morrone-Joseph, J. (1992). Personal files. Gallaudet University, Washington, DC.

Myers, E., Ethington, D., & Ashcroft, S. (1958). Readability of braille as a function of three spacing variables. *Journal of Applied Psychology, 42*, 163–165.

National Dissemination Center for Children with Disabilities. (2008). Part B of IDEA: Services for school-aged children, subpart A: General provisions. Title 34, Section 300.8, July. Retrieved January 30, 2009, from http://www.nichcy.org/Laws/IDEA/Pages/subpartA-PartBregs.aspx#34:2.1.1.1.1.1.36.7

Office of Program Policy Analysis and Government Accountability. (2008). Steps taken to implement the exceptional student education funding matrix, but more monitoring needed. Report number 08-24. Retrieved January 29, 2009, from http://www.oppaga.state.fl.us/reports/pdf/0824rpt.pdf

Rao, E. (2005). Considerations for low vision students in a classroom. *See/Hear Newsletter*. Retrieved February 1, 2009, from http://www.tsbvi.edu/Education/low-vision-student.htm

Reaves-Fitzgerald, D., & Fitzgerald, M. (1998). A historical review of sexuality education and deafness: Where have we been this century? *Sexuality and Disability, 16*(4), 249–268.

Rioux, J. (2004). Sex education for youth with intellectual disabilities. Retrieved February 6, 2009, from http://www.sexualityandu.ca/teachers/tools-10-1.aspx

Sawyer R. G., Desmond, S. M., & Joseph, J. M. (1996). A comparison of sexual knowledge, behavior and sources of information between deaf and hard of hearing university students. *Journal of Health Education, 27*(3), 144–152.

Tomasetti, J. A., Bech, K. H., & Clearwater, H. E. (1983, August). An analysis of selected instructional methods on CPR retention competency of deaf and non-deaf college students. *American Annals of the Deaf*, 474–478.

Trybus, R. J., & Karchmer, M. A. (1977). School achievement scores of hearing impaired children: National data on achievement status and growth patterns. *American Annals of the Deaf Directory of Programmes and Services, 122*, 62–69.

United Nations Educational, Scientific and Cultural Organization. (n.d.). Inclusive education: Labels and terminology. Retrieved January 29, 2009, from http://cms.unescobkk.org/index.php?id=2953

U.S. Department of Education, Office of Innovation and Improvement, Office of Non-public Education. (2008). The Individuals with Disabilities Education Act (IDEA) Provisions Related to Children with Disabilities Enrolled by Their Parents in Private Schools. Retrieved on June 19, 2009, from http://www.ed.gov/admins/lead/speced/privateschools/index.html

U.S. Department of Education, Office of Special Education and Rehabilitative Services, Office of Special Education Programs. (2006). 2006 Annual Report to Congress on the Individuals with Disabilities Education Act, Part D. Retrieved June 19, 2009, from http://www.ed.gov/about/reports/annual/osep/2006/part-d/idea-part-d-2006.doc

West, J. (1991). *The Americans with Disabilities Act: From Policy to Practice*. New York: Milbank Memorial Fund.

Westwood, P. (1997). *Commonsense Methods for Children with Special Needs*. London: Routledge.

Wetzel, R., & Knowlton, M. (2000, March). A comparison of print and Braille reading rates on three reading tasks. *Journal of Visual Impairment and Blindness, 94*(3), 146–154.

Whittle, J. (2005). Building braille reading speed: Some helpful suggestions. National Federation for the Blind Nebraska. Retrieved February 1, 2009, from http://www.nfb.org/images/nfb/Publications/bm/bm08/bm0808/bm0808.htm

Controversial Topics: Sexuality Education

Entry-Level and Advanced 1 Health Educator Competencies Addressed in This Chapter

Responsibility I:	Assess Individual and Community Needs for Health Education
Competency A:	Assess existing health-related data.
Competency C:	Distinguish between behaviors that foster or hinder well-being.
Responsibility II:	Plan Health Education Strategies, Interventions, and Programs
Competency A:	Involve people and organizations in program planning.
Responsibility III:	Implement Health Education Strategies, Interventions, and Programs
Competency B:	Demonstrate a variety of skills in delivering strategies, interventions, and programs.
Competency C:	Use a variety of methods to implement strategies, interventions, and programs.
Responsibility IV:	Conduct Evaluation and Research Related to Health Education
Competency E:	Interpret results of evaluation and research.
Competency F:	Infer implications from findings for future health education activities.
Responsibility VII:	Communicate and Advocate for Health and Health Education
Competency A:	Analyze and respond to current and future needs in health education.
Competency B:	Apply a variety of communication methods and techniques.
Competency D:	Influence policy to promote health.

Method Selection in Health Education

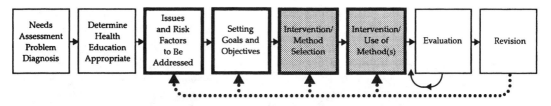

Heavy-bordered boxes indicate subjects addressed in this text; shaded boxes indicate subjects(s) of current chapter.

Note: The competencies listed, which are addressed in this chapter, are considered to be both entry-level and Advanced 1 competencies by the National Commission for Health Education Credentialing, Inc. They are taken from *A Framework for the Development of Competency Based Curricula for Entry Level Health Educators* by the National Task Force for the Preparation and Practice of Health Education, 1985; *A Competency-Based Framework for Graduate Level Health Educators* by the National Task Force for the Preparation and Practice of Health Education, 1999; and *A Competency-Based Framework for Health Educators—The Competencies Project (CUP)*, 2006.

OBJECTIVES

After studying the chapter the reader should be able to:

- Describe the potential problems inherent in planning, implementing, and evaluating programs concerning controversial topics.
- Provide a justification, or rationale, for implementing human sexuality and drug abuse prevention programs.
- Develop meaningful, realistic goals and objectives in human sexuality and drug abuse prevention programs.
- Describe the major concerns of sexuality education opponents.
- List the most common mistakes that occur when presenting programs on sexuality education.
- Describe a diversity of approaches to sex and drug education.

KEY ISSUES

Goals and objectives	Defending a program
Educational philosophy	Effects of programming
Educational approaches	Political correctness
Opposition concerns	

The **health education field** today deals with many topics and issues that are sometimes considered controversial. One obvious difficulty with this area is trying to define what exactly is meant by the term *controversial*. What might be considered sensitive, difficult, or even dangerous material by some people may be considered by others as mundane, basic, and unthreatening. Although most health educators certainly tend to subscribe to the less threatened mindset, they should not be oblivious to the fact that many **health education programs** can attract certain constituencies who will inevitably have a problem with either material or approach. Working with various types of issues on a daily basis can sometimes lead to the health educator becoming desensitized to the material, and he or she should always remember that the general public might well feel less comfortable about many areas.

Obviously, sex education/human sexuality comes immediately to mind when controversy is mentioned. The fact that many **school health education** programs and **school health services** feel the necessity to camouflage even the name "sexuality" by using the more comfortable euphemism **family life** speaks volumes for the potential difficulties surrounding this topic. A second major topic that has drawn almost as much criticism is that of alcohol and other drug education. In fact, almost any health topic can become controversial!

Objective: After reviewing the case study, the reader will be able to justify the need for analyzing multiple sources of information when preparing for presentations in health education.

Case Study: Todd   Todd is a recently appointed health educator who has been asked to attend an upcoming PTA meeting to discuss the proposed implementation of a new sex education component in the school system's curriculum. Todd is a fervent believer in the necessity of sex education and puts together an impressive set of overhead transparencies that explains the curriculum. He intends to strengthen his presentation by citing national data on the prevalence rates of adolescent STIs, HIV infection, and unintended pregnancy. Todd's initial enthusiasm as he sees large numbers of parents at the meeting quickly turns to dismay as his presentation is largely ignored and some very vocal parents barrage him with questions and comments that he is not adequately prepared to answer: "Why do we need sex education in our town . . . our community doesn't have these problems," "These programs only increase sexual activity, don't they?" "Can you say that your program will reduce pregnancy rates?" "Why don't you teach some type of moral values?" "Why don't you stay out of this . . . this type of education should happen in the home, not the school." The meeting deteriorates into a shouting match, Todd is unable to make any progress, and the evening ends without any type of resolution. (See Case Studies Revisited page 396.)

Questions to consider:

1. Should Todd have been surprised at the meeting's outcome?
2. How could Todd have been better prepared to face such a volatile situation?
3. Who should Todd seek assistance from to gain support for his program?

Because of the focus of this text, this chapter will concentrate mainly on sex education as an example of how to anticipate and minimize potential controversy. Covering other controversial topics in any great depth is beyond the scope of this text because it is not intended to be a content book. However, the health educator should be aware that even the areas within health education that appear at first glance to be benign are sometimes fraught with problems. For example, nutrition, particularly when concerned with dieting, has become an area that can stir emotions, and achieving a consensus about weight management is often very difficult. The topic of death and dying is considered by many to be sufficiently sensitive that the home is the only place to deal with the issue. Also one of the most contentious recent topics to receive a great deal of attention and discussion has been violence prevention, particularly in light of the tragic shootings at Columbine High School in Littleton, Colorado, in 1999, Virginia Tech in 2007, and Northern Illinois University in 2008.

It is interesting to note that drug education and sex education seem to have followed a very similar evolutionary direction in regard to the development of strategies and methods of education. In the 1960s, when many of the first sexuality and drug education programs were being implemented, the focus was clearly on disseminating factual information. The rational but simplistic triad of knowledge, attitude, and behavior was being routinely utilized, the hypothesis being that if we give individuals the "facts" (knowledge), then their attitudes will change for the better, and ultimately the individuals will cease their risky and dangerous health behaviors. This type of approach then dictated that the methods of educating about these subjects would take a biological/physiological direction. It is interesting to note that as long ago as 1919 the U.S. Government Printing Office published a text titled, *A High School Course in Physiology in Which the Facts of Life Are Taught* (Means, 1992). No need to guess the method utilized in this approach to sexuality! In the drug area, nearly 20 years later, the element of fear was added to the educator's arsenal in the form of a new film intended to depict the evils of marijuana use. The now classic 1936 film *Reefer Madness* showed how paragons of normalcy could be transformed into crazed perpetrators of rape and murder after a single exposure to marijuana (Anderson, 1973). Although this type of hysterical approach can be viewed as ridiculous by today's more sophisticated youth, elements of this method still survive today as health educators struggle to stimulate just the right amount of anxiety (Taqi, 1972).

In more contemporary times, health educators began to realize that facts alone would not change human behavior. Sex education in the form of "plumbing" that stressed biology and drug education that focused on pharmacology seemed to have little relevance to the lives of young people. The trend that seems to characterize contemporary methods in both drug and sex education is that of decision making. Most of the newer curricula, although still including factual information, tend to focus on the more abstract practice of decision making. For example, in drug education a plethora of school-based programs has been developed that stresses skills of saying "No" to drugs and actively resisting the pressures to use drugs (Battjes, 1985; Botvin, 1983).

One example of a much utilized school-based drug education program is the DARE program. This program, at one time, adopted in as many as 49 states, relies on the cooperation of specially trained uniformed police officers and combines factual information with a major emphasis on the resistance of societal and peer pressures to use drugs (Ringwalt, Ennett, & Holt, 1991). Students are actively encouraged to participate in the development and practice of measures of resistance. Methods and strategies with this type of program necessitate more innovative learning opportunities than the simple exchange of facts. However, despite the ubiquity of the DARE program, research has seriously questioned DARE's ability to have any significant effect on the drug-related behaviors of its participants (Lynam, 1999), reinforcing the notion that curriculum programs alone are likely to be less effective than a **comprehensive school health program**.

Sexuality education has traveled a similar road to drug education in its diversion from straight facts to individual and group process, incorporating decision making. The whole field of sexuality education has taken on a broader perspective, with more organizations involved in the process, more children being exposed to education at an earlier age, and the development of programs that address the emotional as well as the physical components of the issue (Greenberg & Bruess, 1981). Statistically, there does appear to have been an increase in the prevalence of sex education. In 1980 only 3 states mandated sex education, compared with 47 states in 1993 that required or *recommended* sex education (*Time*, 1993). Unfortunately, the onus is on "recommended," as a 1998 analysis of a state-by-state review of mandated sexuality education demonstrated (SIECUS, 1998). The data, originally collected by NARAL (National Abortion and Reproductive Rights Action League), indicated that in fact in 1998, only 20 states mandated sexuality education, with even fewer states (13) including contraception education in the mandate. Thirty-six states mandated HIV/STD education, suggesting perhaps that HIV/AIDS was viewed as a more acceptable and maybe a more pressing topic, the omission of which would be difficult to justify. As of 2007, 20 states plus the District of Columbia (DC) mandated sex education (only 9 states required coverage of contraception), and 35 states plus DC mandated STD/HIV education (Guttmacher Institute, 2008).

However, states do not mandate any minimum number of **contact hours**, nor does any state monitor carefully to ensure that existing requirements are fully implemented. Specifically, these data cannot report how much of the recommended sexuality education actually occurs, or describe the quality or amount of teaching in this area. In an era of educational accountability through testing, a major problem for health and sexuality education is the absence of standardized tests. Health and sexuality education are not part of the testing process, so little or no incentive exists for principals and administrators to fully **implement** such programs. Table 10-1 shows the states that are required to provide sexuality or HIV/AIDS education.

This increase in exposure to sexuality education remains well below the levels that most sexuality experts believe is needed to achieve minimally effective educational levels. For example, Popham (1993) suggests that for an AIDS education unit to have the slightest possible chance of influencing behavior, it must consist of a number of 3–5-hour instructional activities in early grades, 10–15 hours of education in grades 9 or 10, followed by one or more 3–5-hour booster sessions after the main AIDS unit has been concluded . . . all, by the way, taught by the most talented, first-rate teachers. How do these minimal standards compare with common AIDS education practices in our public schools?

The AIDS epidemic is undoubtedly responsible for allowing sexuality educators to gain access to hitherto unreachable audiences, and most states

Table 10-1 State Policy Requirements for Sexuality, STD, and HIV/AIDS Education, 2007

Schools Required to Provide Both Sexuality Education and STD or HIV/AIDS Education

Delaware	Montana
District of Columbia	Nevada
Florida	New Jersey
Georgia	North Carolina
Hawaii	Oregon
Iowa	Rhode Island
Kansas	South Carolina
Kentucky	Tennessee
Maine	Utah
Maryland	Vermont
Minnesota	

Schools Not Required to Provide Either Sexuality Education *or* STD or HIV/AIDS Education

Alaska	Mississippi
Arizona	Nebraska
Arkansas	North Dakota
Colorado	South Dakota
Idaho	Texas
Illinois	Virginia
Louisiana	Wyoming
Massachusetts	

Source: Guttmacher Institute. (2008). State policies in brief: Sex and STI/HIV education. Retrieved February 13, 2008, from http://www.guttmacher.org/statecenter/spibs/spib_SE.pdf

and regions have mandated some compulsory AIDS education programming. Despite this temporary acceptance of the need for increased awareness, sexuality education continues to meet much opposition from individuals and groups who are opposed either to the approach taken by educators or to the idea that such education should even exist. Health educators involved with human sexuality, **sex educators**, should at least acknowledge the strong possibility of individual and community opposition to such programming.

Justification of Program Development

Developing a rationale for program development is a crucial factor in gaining support and acceptance for new or continuing programs. Even a cursory glance at the scope of problems related to sexuality and drug abuse reveals little argument against the necessity for program development. During the past decade, although there is evidence of a reduction in the use of illicit drugs, the following data concerning drug and alcohol use among *high school students,* summarized from the 2005 *Youth Risk Behavior Survey* (Centers for Disease Control and Prevention, 2005), should still be of major concern:

- 74.3% of students had at least one alcoholic drink during their life.
- 43.3% of students had at least one drink in the 30 days preceding the survey.
- 25.5% of students had five or more drinks on a single occasion in the 30 days preceding the survey.
- 38.4% of students had used marijuana at least once in their lifetime.
- 20.2% of students had used marijuana in the 30 days preceding the survey.
- 7.6% of students had used any form of cocaine at least once in their lifetime.
- 6.3% of students had used Ecstasy at least once in their lifetime.
- 54.0% of students had tried cigarette smoking at least once in their lifetime.
- 9.4% of students had smoked cigarettes on ≥ 20 of the 30 days preceding the survey.

Data taken from the American College Health Association/*National College Health Assessment* (ACHA/NCHA, 2006), examining the alcohol and other drug-related behaviors of college students reflect continued usage into early adulthood (see Table 10-2).

Table 10-2 Drinking Practices Among College Students

Reported number of drinks consumed the last time students "partied"

	Male (%)	Female (%)	Total (%)
≤ 4	51.3	68.7	62.7
≤ 5	59.1	78.8	72.0
≤ 6	66.3	85.8	79.1

Reported number of times college students consumed five or more drinks in a sitting within the last two weeks

	Male (%)	Female (%)	Total (%)
None	52.9	68.2	62.9
1–2 times	23.9	20.7	21.8
3–5 times	16.8	9.2	11.9
6 or more times	6.3	1.8	3.4

Source: American College Health Association/*National College Health Assessment*. (2006). National College Health Assessment. Retrieved February 15, 2008, from http://www.acha-ncha.org/pubs_rpts.html

Sexual Behavior   Data chronicling the sexual behavior of young people are also difficult to ignore. The *Youth Risk Behavior Survey* (Centers for Disease Control and Prevention, 2005) paints a clear picture of the sexual behavior of *high school students:*

- 33.9% of students had sexual intercourse during the 3 months preceding the survey.
- 37.2% of students had not used a condom at last intercourse.
- 14.3% of students had four or more different sexual partners in their lifetime.

Data examining the sexual behavior of *college students* reinforces the concept that young people are both sexually active and placing themselves at risk for various sexually related problems (ACHA/NCHA, 2006). (See Table 10-3.)

Table 10-3 Sexual Practices Among College Students

College students reported the following within the last 12 months

	Male (%)	Female (%)	Total (%)
Having had no sexual partner	32.5	33.0	32.8
Having had 1 sexual partner	41.3	43.8	42.9
Having had 2 sexual partners	10.2	11.4	11.0
Having had 3 sexual partners	6.2	5.4	5.7
Having had 4 or more sexual partners	9.8	6.3	7.6

Oral sex in past 30 days	Male (%)	Female (%)	Total (%)
Never did this	30.1	32.2	31.5
Have not done this in past 30 days	25.6	24.6	25.0
Did this 1 or more times	44.3	43.2	43.5

Vaginal sex in past 30 days	Male (%)	Female (%)	Total (%)
Never did this	35.4	36.0	35.8
Have not done this in past 30 days	20.6	16.5	17.9
Did this 1 or more times	44.0	47.5	46.3

Anal sex in past 30 days	Male (%)	Female (%)	Total (%)
Never did this	72.8	80.1	77.7
Have not done this in past 30 days	21.4	16.2	18.0
Did this 1 or more times	5.8	3.6	4.4

Sexually active students reported

Type of behavior	Oral (%)	Vaginal (%)	Anal (%)
Using a condom last time they had sex	3.9	54.0	26.6

Source: American College Health Association/*National College Health Assessment.* (2006). National College Health Assessment. Retrieved February 15, 2008, from http://www.acha-ncha.org/pubs_rets.html

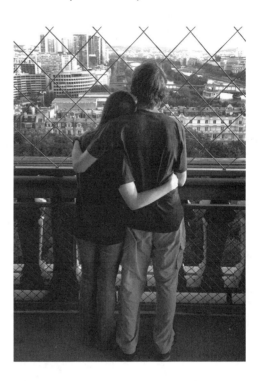

Despite recent improvement, U.S. teen pregnancy rates are the highest in any Western industrialized nation.

Obviously, substantial numbers of young people who are sexually active translate to a significant potential for increased health problems. Again, an abundance of available data reflect the problems inherent in widespread, often unsafe sexual activity.

The Bad News   **Unintended Pregnancy**

Since the early 1980s the United States has led the Western world in unintended-pregnancy rates. Compare the following teen pregnancy rates for women ages 15–19 years of age (Ventura et al., 2001):

United States	79.8 per 1,000
France	20.2 per 1,000
Germany	16.1 per 1,000
Sweden	35 per 1,000
Holland	8.7 per 1,000

Although there is evidence that teen pregnancy rates are decreasing, in general, the problem continues, costing the United States an estimated $9.1 billion a year (National Campaign to Prevent Teen Pregnancy, 2006). Consider the following statistics:

- There are over 750,000 teen pregnancies annually (Guttmacher Institute, 2006b).

- Eight in 10 teen pregnancies are unintended (Guttmacher Institute, 2006b).
- Eighty-one percent of the pregnancies are to unmarried teens (Guttmacher Institute, 2006b).

Sexually Transmitted Infections (STIs)

Sexually active American youth are at high risk for many sexually transmitted infections; direct medical costs are estimated to exceed $8 billion annually. Although young adults represent only 25% of the sexually active population, 15- to 19-year-olds account for nearly half of all STI diagnoses each year (Weinstock, Berman, & Cates, 2004). Approximately 9.1 million new cases of STIs occurred in 2000 among 15- to 24-year-olds. (See Table 10-4.)

The Good News   A trend analysis of sexual behavior among high school students demonstrates that some small but positive changes are occurring (Centers for Disease Control and Prevention, 2007).

- "Ever had sex before"

1991	1993	1995	1997	2005
54%	53%	53%	48%	47%

- "Had intercourse with 4 or more partners"

1991	1993	1995	1997	2005
18.7%	18.7%	17.8%	16%	14.3%

- "Currently sexually active . . . within last 3 months"

1991	1993	1995	1997	2005
37.4%	37.5%	37.9%	34.8%	33.9%

- "Condom used at last intercourse"

1991	1993	1995	1997	2005
46.2%	52.8%	54.4%	56.8%	62.8%

Table 10-4 STIs Among Young Adults

STI	New Cases
HPV	4.6 million
Trichomoniasis	1.9 million
Chlamydia	1.5 million
Genital herpes	640, 000
Gonorrhea	431,000
HIV	15,000
Syphilis	8,200
Hepatitis B	7,500

Source: Guttmacher Institute. (2007). Facts on Sexually Transmitted Infections in the U.S. Retrieved February 15, 2008, from http://www.guttmacher.org/pubs/2009/06/09/FIB_STI_US.pdf

- Teenage women's contraceptive use at first intercourse increased from 48% to 65% during the 1980s, almost entirely because of a doubling in condom use. By 1995 contraceptive use at first intercourse reached 78%, with two-thirds of it being condom use (Guttmacher Institute, 1998).
- The pregnancy rate among U.S. teens ages 15–19 has declined steadily, from 117 pregnancies per 1,000 women in 1990 to 75 per 1,000 women in 2002 (Guttmacher Institute, 2006b). Approximately 14% of this decline is ascribed to teens delaying initial intercourse or having intercourse less often, whereas 86% is credited to more frequent and consistent contraceptive use (Santelli et al., 2007).

Current Issue: Abstinence Versus Responsibility

Like all topics in health education, particularly controversial issues such as human sexuality or drug education, nothing remains static, and different approaches to education come and go. One of the current dilemmas in approaching sexuality education in both the school and community can be categorized as *abstinence versus responsibility* (see Figure 10-1). Should we teach young people from the perspective that if only they would remain or become sexually abstinent, then they would not have to be concerned with sexual problems? Or should we take a more pragmatic approach, acknowledge that whether adults like it or not, many young people are sexually active, and therefore we need to talk about sexual responsibility.

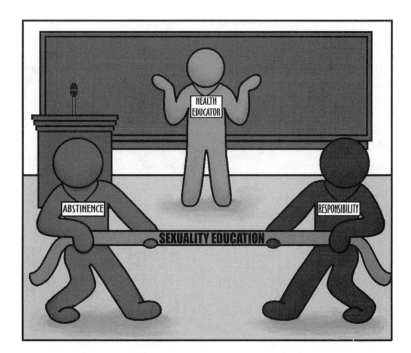

Figure 10-1
Opposing Views on
Sexuality Education

There is no question that much sexuality education is politically and religiously motivated and that during the 1980s and early 1990s the message was clearly one of abstinence, beautifully depicted in the slogan, "Just Say No!" Nearly 20 years ago Congress appropriated money for the development of abstinence education programs, and since then abstinence-based programs like *Sex Respect* were adopted in several states (*Wall Street Journal*, 1992). Many school districts adopted such programs in the belief that traditional types of programming had not been effective. Students were schooled in the virtues of chastity and taught that premarital sex could lead to emotional turmoil, disease, pregnancy, and guilt. The *Sex Respect* curriculum included a chart that marked a prolonged kiss as "the beginning of danger" and the course uses the slogan, "No petting if you want to be free" (*Wall Street Journal*, 1992). Students were encouraged to create bumper stickers that read "Control Your Urgin'/ Be A Virgin" and to consider alternative activities to sex, such as bicycling, dinner parties, and playing Monopoly (*Time*, 1993).

Opponents of abstinence curricula argue that such an approach does little but cause extremely negative ideas about sex. In addition, because such curricula do not include information about preventing pregnancy, HIV infection, and STIs, they may have disastrous effects on sexual behavior. In 1993 Planned Parenthood of Northeast Florida and local citizens in Duval County, Florida, sued the local school board for rejecting a broad-based sex education curriculum in favor of an abstinence-only program from Teen-Aid of Spokane. Also, in Shreveport, Louisiana, a district judge ruled that the abstinence-only text of *Sex Respect* was biased and inaccurate, ordering its removal from the Caddo Parish junior high schools (*Time*, 1993). Concern

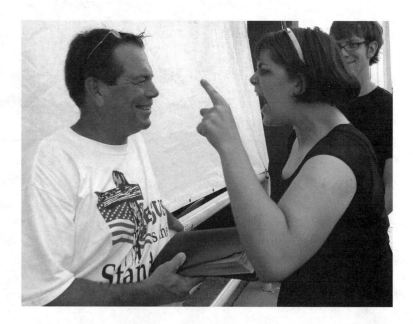

Sexually related issues can create passionate and heated disagreements.

about the accuracy of abstinence-only programs continued into the 21st century, culminating in a 2004 congressional staff analysis, chaired by Representative Henry Waxman. The analysis reported that 11 of the 13 most commonly used abstinence programs in the United States contained "unproven claims, subjective conclusions or outright falsehoods" (Connolly, 2004).

It is ironic that in the 21st century, when sexuality education may be playing a part in helping to increase contraceptive usage in general (also, specifically at first intercourse) and decrease the rate of teenage abortions, a major, politically driven economic initiative has developed aimed at ensuring the survival and promotion of abstinence-only sex education. Congress fueled the continuation of this movement with a $50 million yearly allocation in federal funds for abstinence-only-until-marriage programs each year for federal fiscal years 1998 to 2002. Since 1996, the federal government has spent over half a billion dollars on Title V abstinence-only-until-marriage programs, despite the fact that numerous evaluations demonstrate their ineffectiveness (SIECUS, 2007a). This is a classic example that serves to illustrate for new health educators how many policy decisions are made based on political and religious agendas rather than existing scientific data. Although educational curriculum decisions are ordinarily made at the local level, such large federal funds are difficult for states to turn down. A political groundswell occurred based on the unfounded premise that if talking about sex has caused all the previously mentioned teenage sexual pathologies, then talking *only* about abstinence must surely decrease the problems. Debra Haffner, then president of SIECUS, fittingly commented:

> If the Congress and the states are serious about helping young people delay sexual behaviors and grow into healthy, responsible adults, they will support a comprehensive approach to sexuality education that has a proven track record in accomplishing these goals. There are no published studies in the professional literature indicating that abstinence-only-until-marriage programs will result in young people delaying intercourse. (SIECUS, 1998)

In 1998 all but two states accepted the federal funding for abstinence-only education, and five states passed state laws requiring that sexuality education programs teach abstinence-only-until-marriage as the standard for school-age children (SIECUS, 1998). Just as objective indicators appeared to demonstrate a positive shift toward more responsible teenage sexual behavior, a multimillion-dollar federally funded abstinence initiative, based solely on political and religious beliefs, challenged the more comprehensive, inclusive, and evaluated approaches to sexuality education. As more empirical evidence of the failure of abstinence-only programs has grown, additional states are rejecting federal dollars, with 14 states refusing or planning to refuse such monies in 2008 (SIECUS, 2007b). Unfortunately, the result of denying teenagers comprehensive sexuality education has already had a deleterious effect on knowledge of contraception. By 2002, one-third of teens had not received any formal instruction about contraception; more than one in five adolescents (21% of females and 24% of males) had received abstinence education without any instruction about birth control in 2002, compared with 8–9% in 1995; and in 2002 only 62% of sexually experienced female teens had received contraceptive education before they first had sex, compared with 72% in 1995 (Lindberg, 2006).

Europe . . . a Different Approach
European sexuality educators should be forgiven if they look across the Atlantic Ocean and shake their heads in disbelief. Western industrialized nations, having lifestyles not substantially dissimilar to that of the United States, seem to take a very different approach to sexuality, and if objective data such as unintended pregnancy and teenage birth rates are anything to go by, their approaches are much more successful. A U.S. fact-finding mission that examined the European approach to teenage sex, characterized by more open attitudes and greater availability of contraception, reported some very interesting findings (Advocates for Youth, 1997). Despite the exposure to more open and often explicit sexual information, European teens tended to *delay* sexual initiation later than their American counterparts. For example, the average age at first intercourse in Holland was 17.0 years, 16.2 in Germany, and 16.8 in France, compared to 15.8 in the United States. In addition, the teen birth rate in the United States of 52 per 1,000 teenage women was found to be much higher than in Germany (13 per 1,000), France (9 per 1,000), or Holland (6 per 1,000) (UNICEF, 2002). Some of the major differences reported between the European countries and the United States with regard to teenage sexuality follow:

- Teen reproductive health is treated as a public health issue, not a political or religious one.
- Research drives public policy to reduce unintended pregnancies, abortion, and STIs.
- Adolescents have convenient, confidential access to contraception and sexual health information and services, which are usually free.
- Teens receive open, honest, consistent messages about sexuality from parents, grandparents, media, schools, and healthcare providers.
- The governments fund massive, consistent, and long-term public education campaigns that utilize television, radio, billboards, dance clubs, pharmacies, and clinics to deliver clear, explicit portrayals of responsible sexual behavior.
- Mass media is a partner, not a problem (Advocates for Youth, 1997).

One of the greatest distinctions that seems to come through when comparing cultures is the *consistency* of messages in European cultures and the *inconsistency* between media messages and political/educational messages in

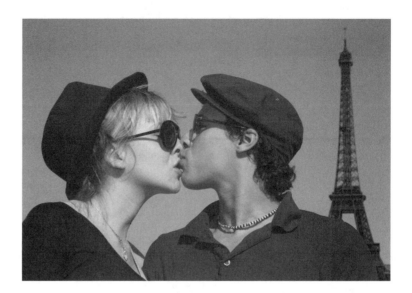

European teen sexuality is characterized by lower rates of pregnancy, births, and abortion.

the United States. In referring to the federally funded abstinence-only education, James Wagoner, president of Advocates for Youth, stated, "It is ironic that the United States is the only industrialized nation to have an official government policy of no sex until marriage, yet our teenagers initiate sexual activity at an earlier age than their European counterparts. Instead of encouraging sexual activity, the European openness results in safer and more responsible sexual behavior" (Advocates for Youth, 1997). Clearly, comparing different cultures is a difficult issue, and detractors could suggest that European educational approaches would not be equally effective in the United States. Nevertheless, these examples from European countries provide empirical, scientific proof that exposure to openness, access to contraception, and explicit, frank sexuality information do *not* result in greater levels of sexual pathology . . . just the opposite.

Despite any amount of persuasive information that clearly points to the fact that American youth has a problem with both alcohol or other drug abuse and sexuality issues, the health educator should not be surprised when individuals and groups do not share his or her vision of the situation. Opponents of education on these issues may acknowledge that a national problem exists, but they tend to see the problem in a vacuum—that is, one that does not involve their particular family. To that end, when beginning a program, the cooperation of local experts and respected community leaders who can speak forcefully in favor of programming is absolutely essential. Also, in addition to national statistics, the health educator should make a concerted effort to obtain local data that can be used more effectively to personalize an issue to specific communities.

NOTEWORTHY **Why Do Sexuality Education Programs Create Such Controversy?**

Vincent et al. (1999) cite five important factors that seem to add fuel to the fire of sexual controversy:

- *Sexuality education is not a priority in public school education.* This subject is seen as peripheral to the major educational goal of the school, somewhat like art, music, and physical education. In a contemporary atmosphere of time constraints, accountability, and external testing, sexuality education becomes a low priority.
- *Most people have a limited perception about what constitutes sexuality education.* Very few individuals understand the full scope of sexuality education; many fear that their children are being taught *how* to have intercourse.
- *Sexuality education is perceived as direct admonitions by adults.* Adults are often comfortable with the "direct" approach to adolescent/parent interaction ("do as you're told") and expect sexuality education to take the same simplistic and directed approach—an admonition to "just say no." Anything outside this realm is viewed with deep suspicion.
- *Fear of inquiry, objectivity, and development of critical thinking skills.* Teaching students to think critically about sexuality is viewed by many as a sure way to confuse adolescents, undo their values, and usurp parental control. The interesting idea that children "don't need to learn what they shouldn't be doing anyway" falls into this category.
- *Adults have a high degree of discomfort regarding the language of sex, sexual growth and development changes, and their views of appropriate sex role socialization and gender roles.* Most parents have little or no formal training in sexuality and feel distinctly uncomfortable with the whole issue. This discomfort is exacerbated by having to consider their children as sexual beings, making open and honest communication understandably problematic. In addition, much of this informally acquired sexuality education has left some adults with a very negative outlook toward sex in general and a particularly skeptical attitude toward sexuality programming.

Developing Goals and Objectives for Sexuality Education

One of the most difficult and sometimes dangerous components of sexuality education is developing meaningful, useful, and attainable objectives. Just what will the program accomplish? What will happen to the students after they experience such a program? Developing unattainable objectives in this area can give the opponents of sexuality programming ammunition with which to challenge the legitimacy of sex education. Reasonable, achievable objectives must be formulated, or the health educator will be literally ensuring failure.

For example, at first glance, the following behavioral objective for a high school sexuality class does not seem unreasonable: *As a result of a recently developed sex education class, there will be fewer pregnancies at All American High School.* In the community setting, developing an objective for HIV education might look like this: *Following a 2-hour presentation on "safer sex" the participants will report higher levels of condom usage.* In both cases, the objectives developed are almost certainly doomed to failure.

School   In isolation, very few human sexuality courses have ever been effective enough to significantly reduce rates of unintended pregnancy. So if an objective is written to reduce such rates and no decrease occurs, then the objective has not been reached, and many will judge the class to be a failure. Reducing overall pregnancy rates might be a sound *goal* of any sexuality class, and as such it should be included; however, decreased pregnancy rate is not a reasonable, attainable objective under these conditions.

Community The possibility that condom usage will increase significantly after a 2-hour presentation is almost nonexistent! As with most behaviors related to sexuality, condom usage is a complex psychosexual dynamic unlikely to be influenced in such a short period of time. If increased condom usage is written as an objective, then the likelihood of failure, or not achieving the objective, is almost certain. Again, increased condom usage might be a realistic *goal* to set, but under the present conditions it is a very unrealistic behavioral objective.

So what are some reasonable objectives that can be developed in sexuality education? Some educators have made a definite attempt to avoid the pitfalls just outlined by purposely designing objectives that are *not* easily measurable. For example, Kirby et al. (1979a) suggest the following objectives:

> *To provide accurate information about sexuality.*
> *To facilitate insights into personal sexual behavior.*
> *To reduce fears and anxieties about personal sexual developments and feelings.*
> *To encourage more informed, responsible, and successful decision making.*
> *To encourage students to question, explore, and assess their sexual attitudes.*
> *To develop more tolerant attitudes toward the sexual behavior of others.*
> *To facilitate communication about sexuality with parents and others.*
> *To develop skills for the management of sexual problems.*
> *To facilitate rewarding sexual expression.*
> *To integrate sex into a balanced and purposeful pattern of living.*
> *To create satisfying interpersonal relationships.*
> *To reduce sex-related problems such as venereal disease and unwanted pregnancies.*

The authors of these objectives have cast their net very wide in order to include most of the major facets they consider germane to sexuality education. Under the terminology used in this text these "objectives" would be better characterized as "goals." These goals are obviously a far cry from

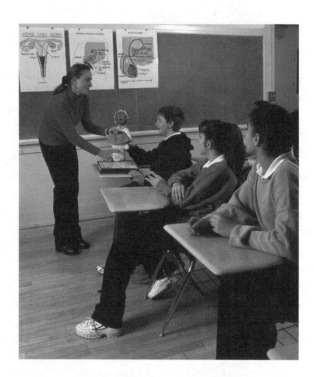

Human sexuality
objectives should be
both meaningful and
attainable.

objectives/goals that might have been generated for the "plumbing" sexuality course. The major advantage to this type of objective/goal is that the educator can promote very generalized aims instead of being restricted to more narrow, specific, and quantifiable projections. This certainly facilitates the avoidance of developing objectives that are unreasonable and likely to remain unattainable. However, this same strength is often viewed by opponents as a definite weakness. If objectives/goals are developed without an eye to some type of evaluation, how is program effectiveness then determined? In times of economic difficulty, particularly in education, accountability has become a crucial factor in funding. As thorough and appropriate as the objectives/goals developed by Kirby et al. might be, most program developers would make an attempt to include objectives that relate to specific sexuality issues and that are quantifiable.

To that end, as in most disciplines, quantifiable behavioral objectives can be confidently written in the cognitive domain. A significant increase in knowledge is often the criteria for evaluating any classroom performance, and human sexuality is no exception.

Examples

1. *The students will be able to list in order of effectiveness four methods of contraception, as described in class.*
2. *The students will be able to describe orally three factors that might precipitate date rape, according to the video viewed in class.*

These types of objectives are valid, easily measurable, and attainable. A sound, well-taught class/workshop should be able to achieve objectives like these without much difficulty.

Objectives in the affective domain are more difficult to achieve than their cognitive counterparts. Nevertheless, affective domain objectives should be a reasonable inclusion when planning programs in sexuality. Given that the field of human sexuality has now expanded to be considered more than mere "plumbing," an attempt to consider affective concerns is crucial. One of the simplest ways to evaluate attitudinal changes is by using a pretest/posttest. Give the participants a short questionnaire before the workshop or unit and then have them complete a similar questionnaire at the conclusion of the unit.

Be aware that this procedure raises two important concerns: How valid is the instrument you are using? Won't any changes in attitude that might arise be only short-term in nature? The first concern is of prime importance, but one remedy would be to use an already developed instrument with proven levels of reliability and validity. This is not always possible, but an increasing number of instruments are available as more evaluation is performed in this field (Davis, Davis, & Yarber, 1988). In regard to the second concern about short-lived effects on attitude change, it would be unrealistic to assume that as a result of a single unit or workshop any changes would be long-term. Only consistent follow-up programming would be likely to maintain attitude change, and that is not always possible. Health educators have to be prepared to take small gains where they can, and there is nothing wrong with the idea of "planting a seed." Accordingly, writing behavioral objectives that would address only immediate attitude change is not so unreasonable.

Examples 1. As a result of the unit on AIDS, the students will demonstrate higher levels of perceived susceptibility to HIV infection as measured in a pre/posttest.
2. As a result of the workshop on safer sex, participants will report on a post-workshop survey a higher level of acceptance of using a condom.

Both of these examples reflect affective objectives that are reasonable and attainable. AIDS education should include components intended to personalize the issue to students who fail to see themselves at risk, and one of the most important factors in increasing condom usage is having individuals feel comfortable in accepting condom use. Both these objectives are also measurable, and by using a pretest/posttest questionnaire educators can gain a sense of what might have been accomplished.

As discussed earlier, addressing specific behavioral objectives related to behavior change is a difficult undertaking that might be better written as a less specific program/unit goal. Given the extremely limited time students spend in a sexuality education classroom, or that individuals spend in community workshops, it would not be fair or reasonable to expect changes in sexual behavior such that pregnancy rates or STI rates would dramatically decline. Should a student who has studied French once a week for 50 minutes during one semester be able to pass fluency tests? Suppose the French class was taught by the physical education teacher who had, after all, taken a 2-day course in preparation for this teaching assignment! Sexuality educators should try to ensure that their programs are not evaluated by criteria used to measure other courses. One way to avoid such unfair scrutiny, though, is to avoid writing unreasonable behavior objectives that could guarantee failure. One study found that the goals of various school districts were as follows:

- Promoting rational and informed decision making about sexuality: 94%
- Increasing students' knowledge of reproduction: 77%
- Reducing the sexual activity of teenagers: 25%
- Reducing teenage childbearing: 21% (Hofferth, 1981)

It is interesting to note that in this particular study, "plumbing" was superseded by a decision-making focus and much smaller percentages of school districts than before made mention of behavior change, even as goals.

Opposition to Sexuality Education

Even the rivers of ignorance contain clever crocodiles.
—Mohan Singh

Since the inception of widespread sexuality education, opposition groups have attempted to discredit and, in many cases, remove existing programs. A long history of such opposition is beyond the scope of this chapter, but a knowledge of some of the major complaints might prove useful to those planning or maintaining programs. The same principles apply to any area of study.

Majority or Minority?

Many opponents of sexuality education would have us believe that they are in the majority . . . that most Americans oppose sexuality education. However, objective barometers of this issue, various national polls, clearly demonstrate that the majority of Americans have consistently favored some form of organized sexuality education. One poll carried out in 1986 (Louis Harris & Associates, 1988) found that 85% of U.S. adults favored sexuality instruction in schools, up from 76% in 1975 (National Opinion Research Center, 1982) and 69% in 1965 (Gallup Poll, 1976). Surveys conducted in the 1990s continued to reinforce the large majority of support for comprehensive sexuality education (Clark, Houser, & Powell, 1995; *Gallup Poll Monthly*, 1991), and, in 2006, 82% of individuals polled supported comprehensive sex education over abstinence-only approaches (MSNBC, 2006). In addition, studies have demonstrated that a large majority of teachers are also in favor of sexuality education in schools (Forrest & Silverman, 1989). More recently, a 2005 Harris poll reported 87% of the public supported sex education. Evidently, opponents of some form of sexuality education have never been in the majority! Unfortunately, as with many other issues, the "squeaky wheel" gathers all the attention, disproportionate to the size of the group. The lesson is clear. Those people in favor of sexuality education should be proactive in order to maintain the gains made over the past 20 years, and should not take for granted what has been achieved.

Common Opposition Arguments

Following is a discussion of some common arguments against sexuality education.

1. **Sex education increases sexual activity.** Perhaps the most common claim made by opponents of sexuality education is that such education will result in and encourage increased sexual behavior. Professional educators, or even those of us with a memory that stretches back to those halcyon days of adolescence, might marvel at the notion that without sex education, teenagers would not think about sex at all! As facile as that idea might seem, many opponents view sex educators as the source of their child's first thought about sex. Opponents view high rates of teen pregnancy, pandemic levels of STIs, and, of course, the AIDS epidemic as clear evidence that sex educators have corrupted today's youth.

Contrary to these subjective and sometimes hysterical beliefs, objective evaluation of sexuality programs does not reveal increased sexual activity. Studies on the effects of sex education demonstrate that it increases knowledge levels of young people, increases the likelihood of contraceptive usage, and in some cases delays the onset of initial sexual intercourse. There is absolutely no empirical evidence that sexuality education encourages young people to initiate or increase sexual activity (Baldo et al., 1993; Dawson, 1986; Louis Harris & Associates, 1986; Marsiglio & Mott, 1986; Sawyer and Gray-Smith, 1996; Zelnik & Kim, 1982). In addition, how many American teens actually receive regular, consistent dosages of sex education, sufficient to ruin their souls? A large national study performed in the late 1970s placed that figure at no more than 10% (Kirby et al., 1979b), and a more recent study showed a modest increase to a maximum of 15% (Sonenstein & Pittman, 1984). Pregnancies and pandemic levels of STIs can hardly be blamed on comprehensive sexuality education when only tiny percentages of American youth are receiving such education! To make matters worse, for the past decade abstinence-only education had dominated sexuality programming, greatly compromising the flow of useful, accurate information.

Figure 10-2 illustrates the many influences related to sexuality experienced by young people today. Note that formalized sex education plays only one small part. Given that all schooling takes up only 8% of an individual's life, and that sex education is just a tiny fraction of that amount, the idea that sex education is responsible for a mountain of social ills is not grounded in reality (Finn, 1986).

2. **Sex education doesn't work.** A major criticism leveled at sex education is that it simply doesn't work. Since sex education has become more common in schools in the United States, there has been little reduction in teenage pregnancy and rates of STI transmission. As discussed earlier, blaming sex education for exacerbating sexual problems is simply not logical

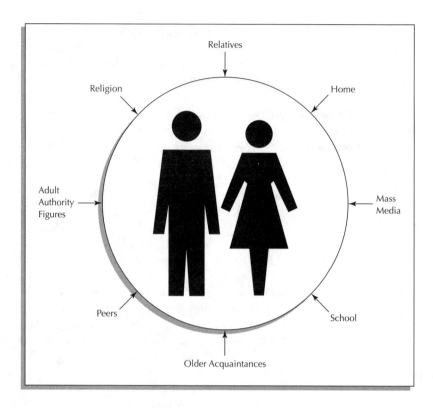

Figure 10-2
Influences on a
Teenager's Life

when so few children receive any meaningful sex education. However, sex educators need to be able to defend against this type of criticism as programs come under closer scrutiny. Sex educators can help prevent some of this criticism by not promising more than can be realistically delivered. Be extremely cautious about writing behavioral objectives promising to reduce rates of pregnancy and STIs. Sex education on its own will not achieve these objectives.

Individuals who claim that sex education does not work need to be "educated" to the reality that little or no meaningful sex education exists in our schools today, so it is unfair to expect a minimalistic approach to have any meaningful effects. Also, other subjects in school are not held to the same levels of outcome accountability as sex education. Should schools abandon teaching civics because fewer than 50% of the population votes in presidential elections and vast numbers of adolescents cannot name the vice president? One study found that nearly one-half of the nation's 17-year-olds did not know that each state has two senators (National Assessments of Educational Progress, 1976)! Foreign language education provides another fitting example of the double standard to which sexuality education is held. Despite the fact that most students take at least 2 to 3 years of a foreign language, usually taught several times a week by a language specialist, how many students can hold a reasonable conversation in that foreign tongue, let alone reach levels of fluency? How, therefore, can we expect sexuality education taught a few times a week for a total of about 3 weeks (often taught by an unqualified individual) to result in some type of complex behavior change? Obviously, very few people would suggest that American schools discontinue teaching civics or foreign languages because of these dismal findings, but the unfairness and disparity in how programs are evaluated should be noted.

A more tangential but valid response to this criticism would be that objectives of sexuality education are about more than just pregnancy, STI, and AIDS prevention. For example, the Sex Information and Education Council of the U.S. (SIECUS) defines sexuality this way:

> Human sexuality encompasses the sexual knowledge, beliefs, attitudes, values, and behaviors of individuals. Its various dimensions involve the anatomy, physiology, and biochemistry of the sexual response system; identity, orientation, roles, and personality; and thoughts, feelings, and relationships. Sexuality is influenced by ethical, spiritual, cultural, and moral concerns. All persons are sexual, in the broadest sense of the word. [*Source:* SIECUS Position Statement. (2009). Available at: www.siecus.org/index.cfm?fuseaction=Page.viewPage &page Id=494&parentID=472]

Obviously, such a broad definition suggests an educational experience in which sexual health plays only one particular role. Even a cursory glance at the position statement formulated by SIECUS to address sex education (see the box) affords a good example of how education in this area is not concerned with sexual health alone.

3. **Abstinence education curricula work.** In 1981 the American Family Life Act was passed, creating Title XX funds that were intended to develop abstinence-based sexuality programs that were expected to result in delaying the onset of sexual activity. Despite rhetoric to the contrary, in five studies of the major abstinence-until-marriage programs (Sex Respect, Success Express, and An Alternative National Curriculum on Responsibility), students who had participated in the programs 1 to 2 years earlier showed no significant increases in maintaining abstinence over a control group (Christopher & Roosa, 1990; Weed & Olsen, 1990). A 1997 study of the abstinence curricula confirmed earlier findings that such programs have not been found to have consistent or significant effects on the onset of intercourse (Kirby, 1997). The most comprehensive and rigorous evaluation performed by Mathematica in 2007 confirmed the failure of abstinence-only programs.

4. **Mixing abstinence education with curricula that include contraceptive information and skills building ("abstinence plus") gives students a "mixed message" and encourages sexual behavior.** In studies of "abstinence plus" programs (Postponing Sexual Involvement, Reducing the Risk, and Skills for Life), students surveyed 1 to 2 years after the programs maintained levels of abstinence longer than students in a control group (Howard & McCabe, 1990; Kirby et al., 1991; Vincent et al., 1987).

> **NOTEWORTHY**   **Sexuality Education**
>
> Sexuality education is a lifelong process that begins at birth. Parents/caregivers, family, peers, partners, schools, religious organizations, and the media influence the messages people receive about sexuality at all stages of life.
>
>   All people have the right to accurate information and age- and developmentally appropriate education about sexuality. Sexuality education should address the biological, sociocultural, psychological, and spiritual dimensions of sexuality within the cognitive learning domain (information), the affective learning domain (feelings, values, and attitudes), and the behavioral learning domain (communication, decision-making, and other skills).
>
> Source: Copyright © Sex Information and Education Council of the United States, Inc. (SIECUS). 90 John Street, Suite 704, New York, NY 10038. Reprinted with permission.

There is something I don't know that I am supposed to know I don't know what it is I don't know. And yet I am supposed to know. And I feel I look stupid if I seem both not to know it and not know what it is I don't know. Therefore I pretend I know it. This is nerve-racking since I don't know what I must pretend to know. Therefore I pretend to know everything. I feel you know what I am supposed to know but you can't tell me what it is because you don't know that I don't know what it is. You may know what I don't know, but not that I don't know it, and I can't tell you. So you will have to tell me everything.
—R.D. Laing (1972)
(Reprinted by permission)

5. **Teaching about contraception encourages students to become sexually active.** There is empirical evidence to suggest that historically many teenagers have sexual intercourse for the first time *before* using contraception and in fact only begin contraceptive use because of a pregnancy or pregnancy scare. The length of time of unprotected sex before contraceptive use can range from 6 to 18 months (Pollack, 1992). Additionally, no evidence supports the idea that making contraceptives available hastens or increases sexual activity (Kirby, 1997).

6. **Teaching students about contraception increases the likelihood that they will become pregnant.** There is clear evidence to the contrary, particularly in European countries, where educators routinely include contraceptive information in school sexuality programming. U.S. teens initiate sexual activity at earlier ages than their European counterparts and also experience higher rates of pregnancy and births (Advocates for Youth, 1997; Guttmacher Institute, 1994).

7. **Because contraceptives fail so frequently, we should simply teach abstinence.** Although rates of teenage sexual activity and teen pregnancy have dropped over the past decade, contraceptives, correctly used, are still preventing pregnancy for those adolescents who do not choose abstinence.

8. **Condoms have a high failure rate and so are minimally effective.** Most of the failure associated with condoms is related to *user* failure and not any flaw in the condom itself. For example, many individuals reporting condom failure only use them sporadically, only put them on after they have had intercourse but immediately prior to ejaculation, leave no room at the tip to collect semen, or don't hold them during withdrawal. Condom failure rates hover around the 2% mark, with the vast majority of failure owing more to lack of education or motivation than to manufacturing defects (Trussell, 2007).

9. **Sex education should be done in the home.** Many opponents of sex education vehemently state that sex is a private matter and children should be educated in the home by the parents. A sex educator would be foolish to deny such a claim, and indeed the statement prepared by SIECUS (see the box) clearly endorses parental responsibility in this area. However, the fact remains that although many parents do a wonderful job of educating their children about sexuality, some parents pass on harmful myths and partial truths, and some parents do nothing. The ideal sex education is one that begins at home and is then augmented by many individuals and agencies, one of which is the school. The reality of the situation is that for some children, the *only* sexuality education they receive is performed by the school (Sawyer & Gray-Smith, 1996).

10. **People who teach sex education are not qualified.** Unfortunately, this is one area where sexuality education does seem vulnerable to criticism. Although there are numerous well-trained, qualified individuals currently teaching human sexuality, there are also too many others who have unwillingly accepted responsibility for this area, lacking both enthusiasm and expertise. There is little or no consistency nationally in the type of preparation individuals receive to teach human sexuality.

One of the few examples of an attempt to standardize sexuality education training is the American Association of Sex Educators, Counselors, and Therapists (AASECT), which developed standards for granting certification to sex educators. The Guttmacher Institute performed a large survey to identify who is teaching sex education in our schools (Guttmacher Institute, 1989). It is interesting to note that this study identified the greatest proportion of sex education teachers as primarily physical education specialists. Figure 10-3 indicates the breakdown by responsibility area. This study revealed

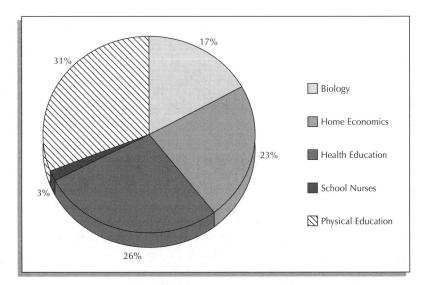

Figure 10-3
Sex Education Teachers
by Specialty

that about 60% of sex education teachers are women, half are over 40 years old, and nearly half have been teaching sex education for at least 8 years. The majority of these individuals have received some type of preparation to teach sex education, although any type of state or local certification in human sexuality education is rare. Thus, a good proportion of sex education teachers are mature and experienced individuals who have received professional preparation. However, given that there is little quality control in the types of preparation available, school districts and individual schools would be very wise to ensure that any individuals who are asked to teach sex education have adequate training in this field and that they teach within the accepted curricular framework. To do any less than this would make a school and/or school district extremely vulnerable to complaint and criticism, and ultimately jeopardize an entire program.

Obstacles to Teaching Sex Education

Although sexuality education has now existed for quite some time, and despite the fact that the AIDS epidemic has legitimized the need for sex education for at least some people, many obstacles still exist that impede the development and implementation of comprehensive programming. More than one in five sex education teachers report that they face curriculum limitations. A similar proportion report that they experience negative pressure from parents and community groups. One in three feels that their school administration is nervous about negative community reactions, and one in five believes that their school administrators do not support them (Guttmacher Institute, 1989).

On the surface, with more states mandating AIDS education it would seem that sexuality is now an accepted part of educational programming and that obstacles are diminishing. However, the concerns of the teachers just mentioned clearly paint a different picture—a picture of an uneasy and potentially volatile truce between (1) school administrators, who have to do *something* because of the new mandates; and (2) the opponents of sexuality education, who are ever vigilant for mistakes that could provide ammunition for their cause. Often the result of such a situation is that the administrator, in an attempt to avoid offending anyone, restricts and dilutes the sexuality curriculum to the degree that it becomes ineffectual.

Another way to effectively "lose" sex education is to have small segments taught in various classes by regular classroom teachers. This way state requirements are met and yet no one actually realizes that sex education took place . . . and given the level of expertise by many teachers unprepared in this area, sex education did not take place!

In 1989, Peter Scales identified five major barriers that sex educators must overcome in order to make sexuality education flourish (Scales, 1989). Given what has happened in the United States since 1989, Scales's words are almost prophetic.

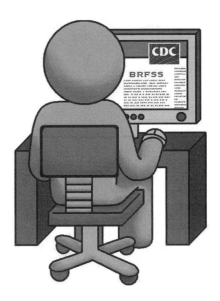

Figure 10-4
Creating Educational
Strategies

Barrier 1. Taking a narrow view of sexuality education.
Within this context Scales describes how sex educators must avoid the temptation to "oversell" the impact of sexuality education. As described earlier, sex education in isolation cannot achieve major behavioral changes, and these changes should not be expected.

Sexuality education should not be evaluated solely on the basis of its short-term *measurable* impact. Instead, included in an assessment of the value of sexuality education should be a component of sex education's intrinsic value to the development of the total human being. This would necessitate an acceptance that sex education plays a fundamental role in defining a holistic viewpoint of "being educated."

Instead of a "back to basics" approach, Scales believes educators need to move forward in order to prepare children for a different and complex world. Children will need to develop critical thinking skills to cope with a new and challenging world environment. The current high-tech Internet-dominated society must be considered when creating educational strategies.

Barrier 2. Failure to understand the importance of self-efficacy.
Although sex educators have historically held the opinion that self-esteem is pivotal in sexual decision making, Scales argues that perhaps a more relevant component for behavioral change is self-efficacy. However, Scales would argue that neither self-esteem nor self-efficacy can really be taught, so educators and policy makers should attempt through social action to create conditions in which self-efficacy can flourish.

Barrier 3. Failure to resolve the role of public schools as "surrogate parents."
Schools today are asked to do much more than the "three Rs" of education. As we adapt to new demands and pressures, sexuality education must also change to contribute more to students' broader education. Scales describes

how sexuality education must go beyond mere pregnancy prevention to tackle issues of sexism, racism, homophobia, and social action.

Barrier 4. AIDS and the decline of pluralism.

AIDS prevention of late has included a rather anti-sex message, which Scales argues is causing a decrease in a national acceptance of pluralism and diversity. Acceptance of different ideas and values is seen as a central premise to modern sexuality education, and Scales suggests that all sex educators, whether conservative or liberal, should strive to maintain a flexible and pluralistic approach to the field. Certainly, the past decade of using a narrow and confining abstinence-only approach would hardly qualify as either flexible or pluralistic.

Barrier 5. Inadequate political skills.

Although the political savvy of sex educators has improved over the years, Scales sees much room for improvement in the following three areas: translating beliefs into budgets, setting the right agenda, and speaking for ourselves. These areas speak to the importance of realizing that political battles are about resource allocation and that educators must translate ideas and beliefs into funding; that the "right agenda" is much more than just having greater numbers of better trained sex educators; and, finally, that sexuality education advocates must be proactive and not just allow others to say what they think advocates believe.

The observations of Scales are a far cry from the early concerns of sexuality educators and certainly reflect a wider and more visionary perspective of sexuality education. There is no doubt, though, that the politicization of issues like abortion, contraception, AIDS, and sexual orientation will necessitate that teachers of human sexuality be continuously aware that their educational efforts will receive a unique form of public scrutiny. To that end, political awareness should now be considered a prerequisite for teachers involved in sexuality education.

There is no doubt that the implications of making mistakes while implementing a sexuality curriculum can be far more severe than making errors in other subject areas. Even minor examples of poor judgment could compromise an entire program, particularly when administrators might exhibit little or no support for sexuality education.

Avoiding Trouble in Sexuality Education

Sources of problems in implementing sexuality education follow:

1. **Inadequate knowledge and background:** Just as with any subject, an ill-prepared teacher or presenter will inevitably experience great difficulty in providing solid, correct information in a meaningful way. However, the implications of poor preparation in human sexuality are potentially disastrous for the recipients of the program, the teacher/facilitator, and the program itself. In the school setting, where the participants are often immature and impressionable, incorrect information could lead to disastrous consequences.

Then the entire program will very quickly lose credibility, and the next step will be the abandonment of the program.

Ideally, individuals teaching in this area should have the utmost preparation and strive to keep "current" in a field that is always changing. Pragmatically, particularly in the school situation, it is unlikely that this ideal situation will occur. Teachers are often coerced into teaching sex education or have an interest in the area but have very little professional background. If programs are to survive, administrators must ensure that they select individuals who at least have an interest in the subject, and that these individuals receive sufficient training to enable them to be effective. This means they need to be able to attend continuing education workshops and courses that will keep them up to date on new information and teaching methods.

Community health sexuality educators need to be no less qualified and prepared. The organizations they represent, whether they are private or public agencies, will be judged by the response to their presentations, and community groups can be every bit as critical and volatile as parent groups in the school setting. Whenever possible, school and community sex educators should not accept assignments for which they know they are unprepared. The damage could be irreparable.

2. **Unrealistic curriculum goals and objectives:** As mentioned earlier, a major criticism by sex education opponents is that sex education simply does not work. To minimize such attacks, sexuality educators must be very prudent when designing course goals and objectives. Do not write behavioral objectives that are unrealistic. Most sex educators would laugh if a fellow educator wrote as an objective for a 10-week course that their students would discover a cure for AIDS! And yet some of these same sex educators will happily promise to miraculously reduce unintended pregnancy as the result of a once-a-week, for 10 weeks, sex education course. By all means write broad, generalized, **long-range goals** that might include pregnancy reduction or higher rates of condom usage. However, specific behavioral objectives, which must all be *measurable*, should be far more realistic and attainable. Objectives promising knowledge gains, for example, are entirely appropriate. Sexuality educators should not promise what they have no hope of producing.

3. **Not being prepared to defend the program:** Unlike other areas of school curriculum or community health topics, sexuality education is consistently placed under the microscope of scrutiny. Despite the publicity and awareness surrounding the AIDS epidemic, sexuality education remains in many communities a commodity to be either grudgingly tolerated or viewed with intense suspicion. Although studies mentioned earlier in this chapter clearly demonstrate that opponents of sexuality education are in the minority, these groups continue to be a voluble and persistent nuisance. Therefore, both sex educators and administrators of such programs should be prepared to defend programming in the face of intense criticism. Preparation should include a knowledge of the major opposition arguments (these have not changed greatly over the years), a rebuttal to these arguments, a developed support system within the community to help bolster acceptance of the program, and a

major effort to ensure that the sex educators are well trained and teaching within the accepted curriculum guidelines. Of course, not all criticism of programming will be irrational and unreasonable. Administrators should be honest enough to accept valid criticism and be prepared to alter program guidelines in an attempt to improve programming standards and overall quality.

Objective: After reviewing the case study, the reader will be able to describe the major reason for Jennifer's failure to connect with the audience, according to information in this chapter.

Case Study: Jennifer

Jennifer works for a county health department. At the request of the local middle school's PTA group, she is making a presentation to parents on the benefits of the Gardasil immunization. Jennifer introduces herself and begins her presentation by providing a great deal of factual information about the prevalence of human papillomavirus (HPV), the dangers of cervical cancer, and the protective benefits of Gardasil. Although most parents are listening attentively, a small group of individuals starts to aggressively question Jennifer on why their children would need to have the immunization, and how the immunization will only encourage young girls to be promiscuous. Jennifer struggles to maintain control and continues to restate the effectiveness of the immunization. A very uncomfortable atmosphere has been created, and at the end of the evening Jennifer is left with the feeling that perhaps the presentation could have gone a lot better. (See Case Studies Revisited page 396.)

Questions to consider:

1. What should Jennifer's objectives look like?
2. What types of problems should Jennifer have anticipated?
3. What alternate approach could Jennifer have taken?

4. **Inappropriate materials or assignments:** More ammunition for opponents of sexuality education and a very quick way to lose program credibility is for the sex educator to use inappropriate materials. The difficulty here is with the definition of "inappropriate." There may be nothing intrinsically wrong with the materials themselves, but it is the setting in which they are to be used that will determine appropriateness. The school setting allows for less discussion than the community environment, because most school districts have fairly strict policies about "sensitive" materials. A committee will preview a video and determine its acceptibility. Of course, frustration occurs when the teacher feels that the material is acceptable and useful, but the committee in its infinite wisdom thinks otherwise! The teacher has little choice but to accept the committee's decision, other than perhaps approaching the committee members individually to lobby for their support and a possible re-review. Most school districts have a catalogue or list of accepted materials that is well publicized and to which the area teachers must conform.

The community health situation is much less regulated, and if the sex educator is at all uncertain about the acceptability of materials, then people living in or familiar with the targeted community should preview them and provide feedback before any presentations are made. If the community health educator is actually working as a guest speaker in a classroom, it is most important to ensure that materials and content are acceptable in that particular school.

The question of appropriateness is obviously more relevant to school health but could also occur in a community health environment. Asking students to visit a drugstore to purchase condoms is one example of an assignment that would likely cause an uproar with many parents and school administrators. Setting the same assignment for a youth or church group in a community setting would inspire a similar negative reaction. The point is that the assignment itself is perhaps not a bad one, but it is simply inappropriate in many settings. Problems like this can be minimized if the sexuality educator consults administrators or community leaders *before* the damage is done. Also, many of these problems would not arise if all or even most sexuality educators were professionally trained and adequately prepared (see #1).

5. **Using materials without preview:** Using materials without previewing them is never a good idea in school or community health. At least in the school situation, if the educator is using materials from the approved catalogue, the worst that might happen is the students would not understand the material or, more likely, would become incredibly bored. Of course, using nonapproved sexuality materials in the school with or without preview is grounds for dismissal, so such an action could have severe implications. In the community setting—again, where few regulations exist—the sexuality educator certainly needs to preview the materials to evaluate their appropriateness and usefulness. Beware of using something recommended by a friend or colleague without evaluating it yourself. Once the sex educator has previewed the materials, having students or any intended audience also preview the materials can provide useful feedback. Educators can easily fall into the trap of assuming that because they think materials are great, their audiences will feel the same way . . . not always the case!

6. **Inappropriate guest speakers:** Just as certain materials will be deemed by communities and organizations to be "inappropriate," using guest speakers can potentially raise the same concerns. For example, if a school sex educator is fortunate enough to be able to explore sexual orientation as a topic, how will the school and community react if the teacher invites a homosexual or lesbian to speak to the class? How will the community church group react when the sex educator schedules a panel on AIDS that includes a bisexual, a prostitute, and a drug abuser who are all HIV-positive? As valuable and educational as both these examples might be, are they worth potentially placing the programs in jeopardy?

As stated before, experience in this field usually prevents this type of problem from occurring, but there are some simple safeguards the sex educator can take. In the school setting, the teacher can check to see if there is a list of approved guest speakers already in existence. If not, or if the desired speaker is not on the list, the teacher should consult a school administrator to seek official approval. In this way, if there is any fallout following the guest speaker's presentation, the teacher has protected him- or herself and the administrator will handle the conflict. In the community setting there will be few, if any, formal regulations. As with the materials discussed earlier, the community sex educator should consult a few community leaders in an attempt to solicit their opinions regarding the guest speaker. Individuals within the community setting will have a much more accurate reading on how their peers will react to certain types of speakers than will the health educator.

Regardless of the setting, the educator should always discuss with the speaker beforehand just what the speaker is going to present. Similarly to previewing audiovisual materials, ideally the educator should have heard the guest speaker present before an invitation was extended. An important concern should not only be *what* the individual is going to say but *how well* he or she is going to say it! There are many health experts or individuals who have important messages to send who are such poor speakers that the value of their presence is minimized. In the school setting, where attention spans are often very short, a stunningly boring speaker will quickly be "tuned out" regardless of the quality of the information.

7. **Personal bias in teaching:** All teachers and communicators have some types of biases, no matter how subtle. This is a crucial issue for sexuality educators to consider, because biases related to so many sensitive issues could potentially cause major problems for the educator and overall program. For example, the sex educator who is "pro-choice" in the volatile abortion issue, and provides a one-sided and very subjective view of the issue, can cause many problems. Obviously, those participants who would describe themselves as "pro-life" will be greatly offended by a pro-choice speaker, as perhaps would those individuals who are undecided. Many school sexuality education programs do not allow any discussion about abortion, but for those that do, if the sex educator merely promotes his or her own subjective views, the school will quickly hear about it! Once again, sexuality educators must take great care not to do anything that might place the entire program at risk. There is nothing wrong with having personal biases, and there are very few human beings who have none. The important point is that the well-prepared sexuality educator should be aware of and sensitive to his or her own biases and ensure that they do not influence how material is presented. The well-prepared and experienced sexuality educator should have achieved this higher level of self-awareness.

8. **Using slang:** For many students and participants, in both the school and community setting, using correct clinical terms to describe reproductive anatomy and sexual behavior will be a new experience. The sexuality educator will play an important role in modeling and normalizing the use of correct terminology, particularly in the school setting. Because there are so many different cultures in the United States, slang terminology will be extremely varied; therefore, if slang is used, communication becomes very complicated. There is nothing wrong with addressing the slang issue

early in the class or presentation, where "translations" can be made and the correct terminology established. But for the sake of accuracy and consistency, correct terminology should be used whenever possible. Community health educators, when dealing with specific subcultures, might argue that correct terminology is only an unnecessary diversion, and to some extent that might be true. For example, in regard to a single inner-city, ethnic minority student who is an intravenous drug abuser, to insist that the educator use the correct terminology in attempting to encourage condom usage would seem overzealous, and quite possibly dysfunctional. Community sexuality educators must therefore use their best judgment, using correct terminology whenever possible, but being sensitive to the need for exceptions.

9. **Sharing personal sexual experience:** A more generalized term for this issue might be *self-disclosure*. How much of his or her own experiences does the sexuality educator share? At first glance this would appear to be a simple issue—the sexuality educator should *never* disclose any personal information. But perhaps we are defining *sexual experience* in too narrow a fashion. Look at the following examples, and consider whether or not the disclosures are appropriate:

> A *female sex educator, while teaching about menstruation to a class of sixth-grade girls, relates how she had felt about her own period beginning.*

> A *male sex educator, while discussing relationships in a coed senior high school class, describes how he felt when his "first love" ended their relationship in high school.*

> A *female sex educator, presenting a workshop for community youth on becoming sexually active, describes her own fears of having sex for the first time when she was a teenager.*

> A *female sex educator describes her own experience with* inorgasmia *(inability to orgasm) to an adult community group interested in sexual dysfunction.*

> A *male peer sexuality educator, during a workshop on date rape, explains how he had previously had sex with a women after she had said "No."*

Clearly, the gratuitous use of graphic depictions of personal sexual experiences has no place in sexuality education. However, as you consider the preceding examples, you might gain a sense that not all personal revelation in the area of sexuality needs to be viewed as negative and forbidden. There is no doubt that in many instances, self-revelation by the educator places the participants at greater ease, thus encouraging more meaningful contributions. Self-disclosure allows the participants to perceive the "expert" or educator as not being so different from them, and the environment for participant disclosure as being safe.

Again, experience and training will help the educator avoid trouble, and a good rule of thumb, particularly in the school setting, is that if there is any doubt as to the appropriateness of the disclosure, decide against it. Do not feel duty bound to answer every question that you are asked.

For example, suppose that while discussing decision-making skills related to becoming sexually active, a student asks, "How old were you when you had sex for the first time?" How should you respond? This is probably not an appropriate question, nor an appropriate issue about which to self-disclose. A possible reply might be, "That is a personal issue which I would prefer to remain private. I will respect your privacy about such issues and I won't ask you personal questions, and I'd be grateful if you would respect me in the same way." In the school setting students will always ask inappropriate questions . . . that's their job! The sexuality educator, therefore, must always be alert to possible problems that might arise from impulsive self-disclosure, and be prepared to politely but firmly decline to answer certain questions.

10. **Behind closed doors:** All individuals who work with youth are placed in a position of trust—a trust that they will not abuse by using their positions of power to take advantage, in any way, of young persons placed in their care. To many individuals, sexuality educators are a little "suspect" anyway, as a result of the sensitive nature of the material that they teach. Ironically, students often view the sexuality educator as a warm, caring individual and one of few adult figures with whom they can discuss personal concerns and problems. There is no question that in the school setting, good, effective sexuality educators will frequently be consulted by students on many diverse issues. Some of the issues may be simple clarification of fact; others may range from disclosure of the students about unintended pregnancy, STIs, and even sexual abuse. There is no simple formula or recipe for dealing with these issues, but the sexuality educator must balance genuine concern for the student with an awareness of the dangers that advising students on personal matters may pose to the educator's professional reputation and the integrity of the entire program.

To minimize the potential for problems, do not meet students in "private places" outside class. There is nothing wrong with having a private conversation, but have it in an office or classroom, where the wrong assumptions are less likely to be made. If a student wants to relate something in confidence, explain that there are certain issues that the law requires an educator to report, child sexual abuse, for example. Many sexuality educators, because of the types of individuals they are, can provide an incredibly important outlet for student concerns, and this invaluable service should not be compromised. However, the educator needs to be aware of potential misinterpretations and take preventive measures against them.

Assumptions to Avoid   Mary Krueger (1993) provides an interesting and thought-provoking list of *assumptions to avoid* when discussing sex education, particularly in the classroom. Some of the following ideas may seem obvious, but they are definitely worthy of our attention:

1. **All students come from traditional families:** With divorce rates of over 50%, the "traditional" family is no longer the norm. Make no assumptions about home situations.

2. **All students are heterosexual:** Whatever the rate of homosexuality/bisexuality in our society, alternate sexual orientations certainly exist. Include all segments of society in the educative process.

3. **All students are sexually involved:** Not all young people are sexually active, so do not present information as if being a virgin is somehow abnormal and undesirable.

4. **No students are sexually involved:** Alternatively, avoid the assumption that *no one* is sexually active, which often leads to an emphasis on abstinence, a concept to which some sexually active individuals might have difficulty relating.

5. **All students' sexual involvements are consensual:** Given the prevalence of sex abuse in our society, particularly with school-aged individuals, an educator should assume that some students/participants are experiencing or have experienced sexual exploitation. Sexuality educators can expect to be approached about this type of issue and should be prepared to give aid and advice.

6. **Students who are "sexually active" are having intercourse:** There are many different forms of sexual behaviors that do not include penis/vagina intercourse. In fact, adolescents are more likely to be participating in oral sex than vaginal intercourse (CDC, 2002). Therefore, discussion should not be confined to preventing pregnancy and STI/HIV transmission but should incorporate other behaviors such as masturbation, mutual masturbation, oral sex, petting, and kissing and hugging.

Establishing a Curriculum or Program in a Controversial Area

Whether you are establishing a potentially controversial program in sexuality, drug education, nutrition, or any other subject matter, it is important to follow procedures that will minimize complaints and address the standards of the environment in which you are working. Following the procedures previously discussed in conducting a needs assessment will be very important. Establishing a process to ensure that representatives of the community are involved and that community standards are represented is vital to the success of any program. A common method that has proved successful for developing a curriculum or program involves the establishment of two committees. In this **two-committee system**, one committee is made up of professionals who are charged with writing the curriculum, and the other is advisory in nature to give some guidance and reaction to the first committee's work before it is presented to a school board or community agency.

Writing Committee   The *writing committee* should be composed of professionals in the area of study. If this is a school curriculum, this committee should be made up of employees of the school district only. The size is very important, because the charge of the committee is to write or adapt materials for use. Therefore, it is recommended that the committee never exceed eight members, with the optimal size being six members. The writing committee has final say on what is submitted to the supervising board for approval. School districts generally have a school board, and health agencies have some type of board of directors.

Advisory Committee   The *advisory committee* is to be composed of citizens from the community who have an interest in the subject matter to be addressed. The charge is to react to materials developed by the writing committee and to make suggestions. This can be a large committee, because it is advisory in nature and reacts to the work of the professional committee. Care should be taken in membership to ensure proportionate representation of the community. It is generally a good idea to place a representative of the opposition on the committee. This will demonstrate there is nothing secret and there is a willingness to listen to all sides. However, it is important not to let this person or group dominate the discussions; the selection of a strong chair can help with this issue. This is a lay advisory group but might include ministers or other religious leaders, physicians, and other appropriate members of the medical community, parents, community leaders, police, and community organization leaders.

Characteristics of Effective Sexuality and HIV Education Programs

After a great deal of research examining attributes common to sexuality programs that seemed to be the most effective, Kirby (2001) listed the following characteristics that should be included whenever possible:

- Focus on reducing one or more sexual behaviors that lead to unintentional pregnancy or STIs, including HIV.
- Deliver and consistently reinforce a clear message about abstaining from sexual activity and/or using condoms or other forms of contraception.
- Provide basic, accurate information about the risks of teen sexual activity and about ways to avoid intercourse or to use methods of protection against pregnancy and STI.
- Include activities that address social pressures that influence sexual behavior.
- Provide examples of and practice with communication, negotiation, and refusal skills.
- Incorporate behavioral goals and teaching methods and materials that are appropriate to the age, sexual experience, and culture of the students.
- Employ teaching methods designed to involve participants and have participants personalize the information.
- Deliver programs based on theoretical approaches that have been demonstrated to influence other health-related behaviors and identify specific important sexual antecedents to be targeted.

- Select teachers or peer leaders who believe in the program and then provide them with adequate training.
- Programs should last an adequate length of time, not be one-off or multiple interventions that last for only a few hours.

This list is certainly not exhaustive, but knowledge about the attributes of programs that have demonstrated effectiveness through quality evaluation would be a great place to start when considering beginning or enhancing program delivery.

Political Correctness and the Health Educator

Political correctness (PC) . . . myth or reality, fact or fiction? Does any such phenomenon exist, or is PC just an epithet used to describe an imaginary influence? Although the term "PC" is heard less frequently today than in the last decade, many of the negative attributes of this phenomenon still exist. But what does PC mean? Is it good or bad? Should we embrace the positive, worthwhile tenets of the PC movement (if, of course, it exists), or should we struggle to free ourselves from the ties of such a stifling, censorial monster? A chapter on controversial topics would not be complete without a mention of this phenomenon, which has actually become a controversial topic in its own right.

A 1991 study by the American Council on Education surveyed university administrators on campus trends and suggested that "reports of widespread efforts to impose politically correct thinking on college students and faculty appear to be overblown" (Dodge, 1991). Reinforcing these data is the sentiment of UCLA professor Alexander Astin that "the PC thing is a kind of Christmas tree the Right has chosen to hang on all the things it doesn't like about higher education today . . . there's no thought control occurring" (Daniels, 1991). An opposite position was taken by Yale president Benno Schmidt, who stated when discussing the effects of PC, "The most serious problems of freedom of expression in our society exist on our campuses" (Cheney, 1992). Even presidents have voiced an opinion related to this issue. When ex-President George H. W. Bush addressed the graduates of Michigan University in 1991, he warned that "the notion of political correctness replaces old prejudices with new ones. It declares certain topics off-limits, certain expressions off-limits, even certain gestures off-limits. What began as a crusade for civility has soured into a cause of conflict and even censorship" (Daniels, 1991).

Unlike education in general, very little attention has been paid to PC in the field of health education, which, given the sensitivity of many health-related topics, is somewhat surprising. One area of PC that is particularly relevant to health education is the use of language. Zola (1993) reflected on the power and importance of language in an article that discussed the linguistics of disability. Zola compares the linguistic terms used in regard to the disability issue and describes the negative connotations and inferences that some of the terms carry. Zola also decries the overt criticism suffered by individuals who use the "wrong" or un-PC terminology and suggests that such reactions are unproductive. In addition to disability, use of appropriate language is often scrutinized in the areas of ethnicity, gender, and sexual orientation.

Undergraduate students, for example, often full of youthful zeal and desperate for others to embrace their cause, often seem oblivious to the fact that their ideas, values, concepts, and approach will not be uniformly accepted. When the nonacceptance accelerates to a personal challenge against the type of health education message or the messenger's style of delivery, the neophyte health educator risks intimidation and bewilderment. Conceding that most of us have found that experience (albeit painful) is the best teacher, protecting students from unnecessary criticism and harm through professional preparation would seem the ethical thing to do. After polling both graduate and undergraduate health education majors, it became clear to this author (RGS) that there was absolutely no consensus as to the definition of PC or whether or not the whole concept of PC was positive or negative. Perhaps arriving at an agreed-upon definition, or even establishing whether or not such a phenomenon exists, is less important than ensuring that students at least consider the possible implications that PC might hold in the practice of health education.

For example, as someone who has taught human sexuality for a number of years, this author has observed a definite decline in willingness to share ideas and attitudes that do not conform to what has been recognized as the PC position. Specifically, very few males in sexuality and communication presentations are willing to publicly voice any sentiments that might be labeled "traditionally male." Some of the men sheepishly shuffle up to the teacher after the presentation to say that they would have liked to have contributed during the discussion, but they were tired of being ridiculed and berated for their opinions. When program participants all adhere to the "party line" and keep their real opinions to themselves, we achieve nothing save a sanitized and hollow version of what could have been a meaningful, honest, and open discussion. However, one could argue against that position by stating that maybe men's attitudes have really changed. Another argument might be that men are not feeling comfortable enough to deliver what could be construed as sexist, misogynistic comments is actually a positive thing because their silence demonstrates society's successful lack of tolerance for "antisocial" speech. The important point here is not who is right or wrong, PC or un-PC, but rather that the health educator be aware of the potential presence of "outside influences" when planning and conducting programs.

Objective: After reviewing the case study, the reader will describe orally several issues related to political correctness that Paul should consider when developing his workshop according to this chapter.

Case Study: Paul   Paul, a newly qualified health educator, has been tasked with designing a date rape workshop for college students. Being fresh out of college, Paul remembers his "methods" course and vaguely recalls that such a topic might include some sensitive issues that he should consider. Before sitting down to write objectives and consider appropriate strategies, Paul decides to develop a list of any potential PC issues that might be relevant to this particular situation.

Before seeing what Paul came up with, why don't you jot down some issues that you consider might have some relevance here, then compare your list with Paul's thoughts. When you are ready, see Case Studies Revisited page 397.

Questions to consider:

1. Think about your objectives.
2. Consider your audience/population.
3. Anticipate what type of problems could occur.

For more information and tools related to this chapter visit http://healtheducation.jbpub.com/strategies.

EXERCISES

1. You have been asked by your rather reluctant high school principal to design a one-semester human sexuality course that may become mandatory for all 10th-grade students. Consider what you think is feasible, then construct relevant goals and objectives that you will present to the principal.

2. You have been given the onerous task of speaking for the development of a human sexuality program in the local school system. The public evening meeting is expected to be volatile and opposition to the proposed program very vocal. Describe the steps you will take in preparing your presentation and on which points you will focus your discussion.

3. Anystate University, where you are employed as a health educator, has an obvious alcohol problem. You have been asked by your supervisor to design a workshop for incoming freshmen about alcohol use and abuse. Consider your own philosophy, likely university administration philosophy, and the current political climate before briefly describing your approach to such a workshop. Which goals and objectives would you choose? What types of strategies/methods would you utilize?

4. You are a community health educator responsible for designing and implementing a sexuality program for a local youth group (ages 14–16 years). While you are describing the program to the parents of the prospective participants, one parent becomes extremely antagonistic and demands to know why "responsible sex" is even mentioned, because abstinence is the only message that should be given. Briefly describe how you would respond to such an attack, and justify your reasoning.

5. You are a community health educator working in an inner-city clinic that deals mostly with unintended pregnancy, STI treatment, and HIV testing. A 13-year-old girl tells you that she has been having sexual intercourse regularly during her period and cannot understand why she has not become pregnant. She explains that she "needs" to get pregnant in order to keep her boyfriend, who has threatened to leave her unless she has his baby. You try the predictable counseling route of the difficulties of a 13-year-old raising a baby, not finishing school, the boyfriend leaving anyway . . . all the rational reasons why she should not get pregnant. None of these arguments makes a difference, and the girl demands to know what she is doing wrong. How will you respond? Will you help her to become pregnant, or is it ethically all right to suggest that she keep having sex during her period? Does the end truly justify the means? Respond briefly to this situation, and justify your answers.

6. You are a community health educator working for a local office of Planned Parenthood. The principal of a nearby high school has asked you to meet her to discuss the possibility of your teaching a short unit (three 1-hour classes) on "Responsible Sexuality" to ninth-grade students. The principal has asked you to prepare a basic course outline, including goals and objectives. Consider how you would approach this request and complete a brief outline that includes goals and objectives.

Responding to these last two exercise questions will not be easy. Health education students must realize that because they deal with sensitive issues, they will invariably become involved in real-life, personal problems, not just the abstract design of objectives or workshop protocols. Thinking through your own ideas and listening to the philosophies of others will prepare you, at least in some small way, to handle extremely difficult situations.

CASE STUDIES REVISITED

Case Study Revisited: Todd   Todd had allowed his own belief and enthusiasm in sex education to blind him to the realization that many individuals are extremely opposed to the inclusion of sex education in the school curriculum. Setting up new programs is one of the most difficult facets of sex education, and health educators who are involved in any controversial programming should be as prepared as possible to defend against a sometimes vociferous opposition. As health educators we sometimes forget that although responses to health concerns appear obvious to us, many individuals will greet our propositions with great skepticism. To that end, an ever increasing role played by the health educator is that of politician, who must carefully prepare the ground for innovative ideas that might be met by strong public opposition. Support for programming must be carefully but consistently developed with influential community individuals, and opposition arguments must be anticipated and appropriate responses prepared. (See page 359.)

Case Study Revisited: Jennifer   From a purely health education perspective, Jennifer's approach was perfectly logical. She concentrated on extolling the factual virtues of an immunization product that could reduce rates of cervical cancer by as much as 75%—why should that be a problem? However, considering her presentation was connected to sexuality, Jennifer was a little naïve, and in planning her presentation she should have considered possible opposition to her message and what issues those opposing views might reflect. Instead of beginning her presentation with the facts about HPV and Gardasil, had Jennifer first acknowledged the existence of concern about encouraging sexual activity, and the denial by certain parents that their child would ever need the immunization, she could have immediately countered the concerns with relevant information and data. Of course, we all understand that some individuals will never let facts get in the way of their own beliefs, but Jennifer may have at least partially headed off some of the problems that troubled the remainder of her presentation. Always try to anticipate opposing arguments and be prepared to present an alternate opinion based on current available research. (See page 386.)

Case Study
Revisited: Paul

- Use of language—"women" rather than "girls."
- Inclusion—if designing scenarios of sexual situations, include a same-gender situation.
- Stereotypes—consider including scenarios that are not so stereotypical, such as a woman pressuring a man to have sex.
- Gender—does the gender of the presenter(s) influence the presentation, and if so, how? Is there a preferred format with regard to gender?
- Many men tend not to actively participate in such discussions for fear of criticism. What can you do to draw them out?
- This topic might stimulate some students to be very "political" in their interaction. How would you handle that?

This list is by no means exhaustive, but generating the list might be useful in helping health educators realize that even the most straightforward assignments can be fraught with potential problems. Once the potential difficulties have been established, possible responses or solutions can be developed. (See page 395.)

SUMMARY

1. There are many controversial issues within the discipline of health education.

2. Sexuality education and drug education have traced parallel paths with regard to the evolution of teaching strategies.

3. An ever increasing number of "canned," or commercially prepared, programs are being utilized in both the drug and sexuality areas.

4. Health educators must be prepared to defend the existence of programming in controversial areas.

5. The accurate development of feasible, attainable objectives is of crucial importance when developing programs in controversial areas.

6. Health educators must be knowledgeable about the existence and tactics of opposition groups.

7. Health educators must be aware of the major obstacles to developing a sexuality education program.

8. Health educators must be aware of and avoid some of the more common pitfalls in teaching/presenting sex education.

9. The current struggle in sex education, particularly in the schools, is the adoption of abstinence-versus-responsibility curricula.

10. Developers of potentially controversial programs should consider the two-committee strategy of development.

11. Political correctness is an issue that health educators should consider, regardless of individual definitions or even disagreements over actual existence.

REFERENCES AND RESOURCES

Advocates for Youth. (1997). Differing European/US approaches to teen sex show surprising results. Press release. Retrieved April 16, 1999, from http://www .advocatesforyouth.org/NEWS/index.php?option= com_contentandtask=viewandid=419andItemid=336

American College Health Association/National College Health Assessment. (2006). National College Health Assessment. Retrieved February 15, 2008, from http://www.acha-ncha.org/pubs_repts.html

Anderson, P. (1973, January 21). The pot lobby. *New York Times Magazine*, 8–9.

Baldo, M., Aggleton, P., & Slutin, G. (1993). *Does Sex Education Lead to Earlier or Increased Sexual Activity in Youth?* Geneva: World Health Organization Global Programme on AIDS.

Battjes, R. J. (1985). Prevention of adolescent drug abuse. *International Journal of Addiction, 20,* 1113–1134.

Botvin, G. J. (1983). Prevention of adolescent substance abuse through the development of personal and social competence. In: Glynn, T., Leukefeld, C., & Ludford, J. P. (Eds.), *Preventing Adolescent Drug Abuse: Intervention Strategies.* Rockville, MD: NIDA.

Centers for Disease Control and Prevention. (1993). Update: Barrier protection against HIV infection and other sexually transmitted diseases: Editorial note. *Morbidity and Mortality Weekly Report, 42,* 590.

Centers for Disease Control and Prevention. (2002). National Survey of Family Growth. Retrieved January 23, 2008, from http://www.cdc.gov/nchs/nsfg .htm

Centers for Disease Control and Prevention. (2005). Youth Risk Behavior Surveillance. Retrieved February 13, 2008, from http://www.cdc.gov

Centers for Disease Control and Prevention. (2007). Trends in HIV-related risk behavior among high school students, U.S. 1991–2005. Retrieved September 15, 2009, from www.cdc.gov/mmwr/preview/ mmwrhtml/mm5531a4.htm

Cheney, L. V. (1992). Beware the PC police. *Executive Educator, 14,* 31–34.

Christopher, F. S., & Roosa, M. W. (1990). An evaluation of an adolescent pregnancy prevention program: Is "just say no" enough? *Family Relations, 39,* 68–72.

Clark, J. E., Houser, C. M., & Powell, K. D. (1995). *We the People* Charlotte, NC: Pregnancy Prevention Coalition of North Carolina, p. 5.

Connolly, C. (2004, December 2). Some abstinence programs mislead teens, report says. *Washington Post,* p. A01.

Daniels, L. A. (1991, September/October). Diversity, correctness, and campus life. *Change,* 16–20.

Davis, C. M., Davis, S. L., & Yarber, W. L. (Eds.). (1988). *Sexuality Related Measures: A Compendium.* Lake Mills, IA: Graphic Publications.

Dawson, D. A. (1986). The effects of sex education on adolescent behavior. *Family Planning Perspectives, 18,* 162–170.

Dodge, S. (1991). Few colleges have had "political correctness" controversies, study finds. *Chronicle of Higher Education, 37*(47), A23–A24.

Finn, C. (1986). Educational excellence: Eight elements. *Foundations News, 27*(2), 40–45.

Forrest, J. D., & Silverman, J. (1989). What public school teachers teach about pregnancy prevention and AIDS. *Family Planning Perspectives, 21,* 65–72.

Gallup Poll. (1976, January 23). *Growing Number of Americans Favor Discussion of Sex in the Classroom.* News release, Princeton, NJ.

Gilbert, G. G. (1979, September/October). Easy ways of getting into trouble when teaching sex education. *Health Education,* 31–32.

Greenberg, J. S., & Bruess, C. E. (1981). *Sex Education; Theory & Practice.* Belmont, CA: Wadsworth.

Guttmacher Institute. (1989). *Risk and Responsibility.* New York: Alan Guttmacher Institute, p. 7.

Guttmacher Institute. (1994). *Sex and America's Teen-agers*. New York: Alan Guttmacher Institute, p. 76.

Guttmacher Institute. (2006a). Facts on sexually transmitted infections in the United States. Retrieved February 13, 2008, from http://www.guttmacher .org/pubs/fb_sti.html

Guttmacher Institute. (2006b). U.S. teenage pregnancy statistics: National and state trends and trends by race and ethnicity. Retrieved February 19, 2008, from http://www.guttmacher.org/pubs/2006/ 09/11/USTPstats.pd

Guttmacher Institute. (2007). Facts on sexually transmitted infections in the U.S. Retrieved September 15, 2009, from http://www.guttmacher.org/pubs/ 2009/ 06/09/FIB_STI_US.pdf

Guttmacher Institute. (2008). State policies in brief: Sex and STI/HIV education. Retrieved February 13, 2008, from http://www.guttmacher.org/statecenter/ spibs/spib_SE.pdf

Harris Poll. (2005). Support for sex education. Retrieved January 22, 2008, from http://www.harrisin teractive.com/harris_poll/index.asp?PID=608

Hofferth, S. L. (1981). Effects of number and timing of births on family well-being over the life cycle. Final report to National Institute of Child Health and Human Development (Contract # 1-HD-82850).

Howard, M., & McCabe, B. (1990). Helping teens postpone sexual involvement. *Family Planning Perspectives*, 22, 21–26.

Kirby, D. (1997). *No Easy Answers: Research Findings on Programs to Reduce Teen Pregnancy*. Washington, DC: National Campaign to Prevent Teen Pregnancy.

Kirby, D. (2001). *Emerging Answers: Research Findings on Programs to Reduce Teen Pregnancy*. Washington, DC: National Campaign to Prevent Teen Pregnancy.

Kirby, D., Alter, J., & Scales, P. (1979a). *An Analysis of U.S. Sex Education Programs and Evaluation Methods*. Springfield, VA: National Technical Information Service.

Kirby, D., Alter, J., & Scales, P. (1979b). Executive Summary. In *An Analysis of U.S. Education Programs and Evaluation Methods*. Atlanta, GA: U.S. Department of Health, Education and Welfare.

Kirby, D., et al. (1991). Reducing the risk: Impact of a new curriculum on sexual risk taking. *Planning Perspectives*, 23, 253–262.

Krueger, M. M. (1993). Everyone is an exception: Assumptions to avoid in the sex education classroom. *Phi Delta Kappan*, 74, 596

Laing, R. D. (1972). *Knots*. New York: Random House, p. 56.

Lindberg, L. D. (2006). Changes in formal sex education: 1995–2002. *Perspectives on Sexual and Reproductive Health*, 38(4), 182–189.

Louis Harris and Associates. (1986). *American Teens Speak: Sex, Myth, T.V. and Birth Control*. New York: Planned Parenthood.

Louis Harris & Associates. (1988, November 18). Public attitudes toward teenage pregnancy, sex education & birth control. H. Quinley of Yankelovich Clancy Shulman, memorandum to all data users regarding Time/Yankelovich Clancy Shulman Poll Findings on Sex Education, p. 24.

Lynam, D. R., Milich, R., Zimmerman, R., Novak, S., Logan, T., Martin, C. (1999). Project DARE: No effects at 10-year follow-up. *Journal of Consulting and Clinical Psychology*, 67(4), 590–593.

Marsiglio, W., & Mott, F. L. (1986). The impact of sex education on sexual activity, contraceptive use and premarital pregnancy among American teenagers, *Family Planning Perspectives*, 18, 151–162.

Mathematica Policy Research. (2007, April). *Impacts of Four Title V, Section 510 Abstinence Education Progams: Final Report*. Trenton, NJ: Author.

Means, R. K. (1962). *A History of Health Education in the U.S.* Philadelphia: Lea & Febiger.

MSNBC. (2006). Few Americans favor abstinence-only sex ed. Retrieved June 19, 2008, from http://www .msnbc.msn.com/id/156037641

NARAL. (1998). *A State by State Review of Abortion and Reproductive Rights*. Washington, DC: Author.

National Assessment of Educational Progress. (1976). *Bicentennial Citizenship Survey*. Denver.

National Campaign to Prevent Teen Pregnancy. (2006). By the numbers: The public costs of teen childbearing. Retrieved January 22, 2008, from http:// www.thenationalcampaign.org/costs/pdf/report/BTN _National_Report.pdf

National Institute on Drug Abuse. (1986). *National Survey on Drug Abuse*. DHHS Pub. No. (ADM) 84-1356. Washington, DC.

National Institute on Drug Abuse. (1991). *High School Senior Survey*. Washington, DC.

National Opinion Research Center. (1982). *General Social Surveys, 1972–1978: Cumulative Code Book*, Chicago: Author.

Pollack, A. E. (1992). Teen contraception in the 90s. *Journal of School Health*, 62, 288–293.

Popham, W. J. (1993, March). Wanted: AIDS education that works. *Phi Delta Kappan, 559–562.*

Ringwalt, C., Ennett, S. T., & Holt, K. D. (1991). An outcome evaluation of project DARE. *Health Education Research, 6*(3), 327–337.

Santelli, J. S., Lindberg, L. D., Finer, L., Singh, S. (2007). Explaining recent declines in adolescent pregnancy in the United States: The contribution of abstinence and improved contraceptive use. *American Journal of Public Health, 97*(1), 1–7.

Sawyer, R. G., & Anastasi, M. C. (1998). Political correctness and the professional preparation of health educators. *Journal of Health Education, 29*(4), 240–243.

Sawyer, R. G., & Gray-Smith, N. (1996). A survey of situational factors at first intercourse among college students. *American Journal of Health Behavior, 20*(4), 208–217.

Scales, P. (1989). Overcoming future barriers to sexuality education, theory into practice. *Health Education, 28*(3), 172–176.

Sex in America. (1991). *Gallup Poll Monthly, 56,* 1–9, 71.

Sexuality Information and Education Center of the United States. (1998). *Between the Lines: States' Implementation of the Federal Government's Section 510(b) Abstinence Education Program in Fiscal Year 1998.* New York: SIECUS.

Sexuality Information and Education Center of the United States. (1999). Position statement on human sexuality. Retrieved May 5, 1999, from http://www.siecus.org

Sexuality Information and Education Council of the United States. (2006). Sex education and abstinence-only-until-marriage programs in states: An overview. Retrieved January 23, 2008, from http://www.siecus.org/policy/states/2006/analysis.html

Sexuality Information and Education Center of the United States. (2007a). Federal abstinence-only-until-marriage programs not proven effective in delaying sexual activity among young people. Retrieved February 13, 2008, from http://www.siecus.org/index.cfm?fuseaction=feature. Show Feature. Feature ID = 955

Sexuality Information and Education Center of the United States. (2007b). SIECUS applauds New Mexico's refusal of Title V funding. Retrieved February 13, 2008, from http://www.siecus.org/

Sonenstein, F. L., & Pittman, K. J. (1984). The availability of sex education in large school districts. *Family Planning Perspectives, 16,* 19–25.

Taqi, S. (1972). The drug cinema. *Bulletin on Narcotics, 24,* 19–24.

Time. (1993, May). How should we teach our children about sex? 60–66.

Trussell, J. (2007). Contraceptive efficacy. In Hatcher, R. A., Stewart, F., Nelson, A., Cates, W., Guest, F., Kowal, D. (Eds.). *Contraceptive Technology* (19th rev. ed.). New York: Ardent Media, p. 221–252

UNICEF. (2002). Innocenti Research Centre. Retrieved January 22, 2008, from http://www.unicef-icdc.org

U.S. Department of Health & Human Services. (1984). *Highlights from the National Survey on Drug Abuse.* DHHS Pub. No. (ADM) 83-1277. Washington, DC: Author.

Ventura, S. J., Moscher, W., Curtin, S., Abma, J., & Henshaw, S. (2001). Trends in pregnancy rates for the United States, 1976–1997: An update. *National Vital Statistics Reports, 49*(4), 1–10.

Vincent, M. L., Berne, L. A., Lammers, J. W., & Strack, R. (1999). Pregnancy prevention, sexuality education, and coping with opposing views. *Journal of Health Education, 30*(3), 142–149.

Vincent, M. L., Clearie, A. F., & Schlucter, M. D. (1987). Reducing adolescent pregnancy through school and community-based education. *Journal of the American Medical Association, 257,* 3382–3386.

Wall Street Journal. (1992, February 20). Schools teach the virtues of virginity, B1.

Weed, S. E., & Olsen, J. A. (1990). Evaluation report of the Sex Respect program: Results for the 1989–1990 school year. Salt Lake City: Institute for Research and Evaluation, 19–25.

Weinstock, H., Berman, S., & Cates, W. (2004). Sexually transmitted diseases among American youth: Incidence and prevalence estimates, 2000. *Perspectives on Sexual and Reproductive Health, 36*(1), 6–10.

Zelnik, M., & Kim, Y. J. (1982). Sex education and its association with teenage sexual activity, pregnancy and contraceptive use. *Family Planning Perspectives, 14,* 117–126.

Zola, I. K. (1993). Self, identity and the naming question: Reflections on the language of disability. *Social Science and Medicine, 36*(2), 167–173.

Resources

Entry-Level and Advanced 1 Health Educator Competencies Addressed in This Appendix

Responsibility VI: Serve as a Health Education Resource Person
Competency A: Use health-related information resources.
Competency B: Respond to requests for health information.
Competency C: Select resource materials for dissemination.
Competency D: Establish consultative relationships.

Responsibility VII: Communicate and Advocate for Health and Health Education
Competency B: Apply a variety of communication methods and techniques.

Note: The competencies listed here are considered both entry-level and Advanced 1 competencies by the National Commission for Health Education Credentialing, Inc. They are taken from *A Framework for the Development of Competency-Based Curricula for Entry Level Health Educators* by the National Task Force on the Preparation and Practice of Health Educators, Inc., 1985; and *A Competency-Based Framework for Health Educators—The Competencies Update Project (CUP)*, 2006.

KEY ISSUES

Entry-level health educator competencies

Advanced 1 health educator competencies

Advanced 2 health educator competencies

Code of ethics for the health profession

Professional organizations

Additional readings

Method Selection in Health Education

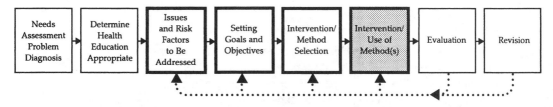

Heavy-bordered boxes indicate subjects addressed in this text; shaded boxes indicate subject(s) of current chapter.

Entry-Level Health Educator Competencies

Area I: **Assess Individual and Community Needs for Health Education**
Competency A: Access existing health-related data.
Competency B: Collect health-related data.
Competency C: Distinguish between behaviors that foster or hinder well-being.
Competency D: Determine factors that influence learning.
Competency E: Identify factors that foster or hinder the process of health education.
Competency F: Infer needs for health education from obtained data.

Area II: **Plan Health Education Strategies, Interventions, and Programs**
Competency A: Involve people and organizations in program planning.
Competency B: Incorporate data analysis and principles of community organization.
Competency C: Formulate appropriate and measurable program objectives.
Competency D: Develop a logical scope and sequence plan for health education practice.
Competency E: Design strategies, interventions, and programs consistent with specified objectives.
Competency F: Select appropriate strategies to meet objectives.
Competency G: Assess factors that affect implementation.

Area III: **Implement Health Education Strategies, Interventions, and Programs**
Competency A: Initiate a plan of action.
Competency B: Demonstrate a variety of skills in delivering strategies, interventions, and programs.
Competency C: Use a variety of methods to implement strategies, interventions, and programs.
Competency D: Conduct training programs.

Area IV: **Conduct Evaluation and Research Related to Health Education**
Competency A: Develop plans for evaluation and research.
Competency B: Review research and evaluation procedures.
Competency C: Design data collection instruments.
Competency D: Carry out evaluation and research plans.
Competency E: Interpret results from evaluation and research.
Competency F: Infer implications from findings for future health-related activities.

Area V: **Administer Health Education Strategies, Interventions, and Programs**
Competency A: Exercise organizational leadership.
Competency B: Secure fiscal resources.
Competency C: Manage human resources.
Competency D: Obtain acceptance and support for programs.

Area VI: **Serve as a Health Education Resource Person**
Competency A: Use health-related information resources.
Competency B: Respond to requests for health information.
Competency C: Select resource materials for dissemination.
Competency D: Establish consultative relationships.

Advanced 1 Health Educator Competencies

Area I: **Assess Individual and Community Needs for Health Education**
Competency A: See Entry level.
Competency B: See Entry level.
Competency C: Distinguish between behaviors that foster or hinder well-being.
Competency D: Determine factors that influence learning.
Competency E: Identify factors that foster or hinder the process of health education.
Competency F: Infer needs for health education from obtained data.

Area II: **Plan Health Education Strategies, Interventions, and Programs**
Competency A: Involve people and organizations in program planning.
Competency B: Incorporate data analysis and principles of community organization.
Competency C: Formulate appropriate and measurable program objectives.
Competency D: Develop a logical scope and sequence plan for health education practice.
Competency E: Design strategies, interventions, and programs consistent with specified objectives.
Competency F: Select appropriate strategies to meet objectives.
Competency G: Assess factors that affect implementation.

Area III: **Implement Health Education Strategies, Interventions, and Programs**
Competency A: Initiate a plan of action.
Competency B: Demonstrate a variety of skills in delivering strategies, interventions, and programs.
Competency C: Use a variety of methods to implement strategies, interventions, and programs.
Competency D: Conduct training programs.

Area IV: **Conduct Evaluation and Research Related to Health Education**
Competency A: Develop plans for evaluation and research.
Competency B: Review research and evaluation procedures.
Competency C: See Entry level.
Competency D: Carry out evaluation and research plans.
Competency E: Interpret results from evaluation and research.
Competency F: Infer implications from findings for future health-related activities.

Area V: **Administer Health Education Strategies, Interventions, and Programs**
Competency A: Exercise organizational leadership.
Competency B: Secure fiscal resources.
Competency C: Manage human resources.
Competency D: Obtain acceptance and support for programs.

Area VI: **Serve as a Health Education Resource Person**

Area VII: **Communicate and Advocate for Health and Health Education**
Competency A: Analyze and respond to current and future needs in health education.
Competency B: See Entry level.
Competency C: See Entry level.
Competency D: Influence health policy to promote health.

Advanced 2 Health Educator Competencies

Area I: **Assess Individual and Community Needs for Health Education**
Competency A: Access existing health-related data.
Competency B: See Entry and Advanced 1.
Competency C: See Entry and Advanced 1.
Competency D: Determine factors that influence learning.
Competency E: Identify factors that foster or hinder the process of health education.
Competency F: Infer needs for health education from obtained data.

Area II: **Plan Health Education Strategies, Interventions, and Programs**
Competency A: See Entry and Advanced 1.
Competency B: See Entry and Advanced 1.
Competency C: Formulate appropriate and measurable program objectives.
Competency D: Develop a logical scope and sequence plan for health education practice.
Competency E: Design strategies, interventions, and programs consistent with specified objectives.
Competency F: Select appropriate strategies to meet objectives.
Competency G: See Entry and Advanced 1.

Area III: **Implement Health Education Strategies, Interventions, and Programs**
Competency A: See Entry and Advanced 1.
Competency B: Demonstrate a variety of skills in delivering strategies, interventions, and programs.
Competency C: See Entry and Advanced 1.
Competency D: Conduct training programs.

Area IV: **Conduct Evaluation and Research Related to Health Education**
Competency A: Develop plans for evaluation and research.
Competency B: Review research and evaluation procedures.
Competency C: See Entry and Advanced 1.
Competency D: Carry out evaluation and research plans.
Competency E: Interpret results from evaluation and research.
Competency F: Infer implications from findings for future health-related activities.

Area V: **Administer Health Education Strategies, Interventions, and Programs**
Competency A: Exercise organizational leadership.
Competency B: Secure fiscal resources.
Competency C: See Entry and Advanced 1.
Competency D: Obtain acceptance and support for programs.

Area VI: **Serve as a Health Education Resource Person**
Competency A: See Entry and Advanced 1.
Competency B: See Entry and Advanced 1.
Competency C: See Entry and Advanced 1.
Competency D: Establish consultative relationships.

Area VII: **Communicate and Advocate for Health and Health Education**
Competency A: Analyze and respond to current and future needs in health education.
Competency B: See Entry and Advanced 1.

Competency C: Promote the health education profession individually and collectively.
Competency D: Influence health policy to promote health.

Code of Ethics for the Health Education Profession

Preamble

The Health Education profession is dedicated to excellence in the practice of promoting individual, family, organizational, and community health. Guided by common ideals, Health Educators are responsible for upholding the integrity and ethics of the profession as they face the daily challenges of making decisions. By acknowledging the value of diversity in society and embracing a cross-cultural approach, Health Educators support the worth, dignity, potential, and uniqueness of all people.

The Code of Ethics provides a framework of shared values within which Health Education is practiced. The Code of Ethics is grounded in fundamental ethical principles that underlie all health care services: respect for autonomy, promotion of social justice, active promotion of good, and avoidance of harm. The responsibility of each health educator is to aspire to the highest possible standards of conduct and to encourage the ethical behavior of all those with whom they work.

Regardless of job title, professional affiliation, work setting, or population served, Health Educators abide by these guidelines when making professional decisions.

Article I: Responsibility to the Public

A Health Educator's ultimate responsibility is to educate people for the purpose of promoting, maintaining, and improving individual, family, and community health. When a conflict of issues arises among individuals, groups, organizations, agencies, or institutions, health educators must consider all issues and give priority to those that promote wellness and quality of living through principles of self-determination and freedom of choice for the individual.

Section 1: Health Educators support the right of individuals to make informed decisions regarding health, as long as such decisions pose no threat to the health of others.

Section 2: Health Educators encourage actions and social policies that support and facilitate the best balance of benefits over harm for all affected parties.

Section 3: Health Educators accurately communicate the potential benefits and consequences of the services and programs with which they are associated.

Section 4: Health Educators accept the responsibility to act on issues that can adversely affect the health of individuals, families, and communities.

Section 5: Health Educators are truthful about their qualifications and the limitations of their expertise and provide services consistent with their competencies.

Section 6: Health Educators protect the privacy and dignity of individuals.

Section 7: Health Educators actively involve individuals, groups, and communities in the entire educational process so that all aspects of the process are clearly understood by those who may be affected.

Section 8: Health Educators respect and acknowledge the rights of others to hold diverse values, attitudes, and opinions.

Section 9: Health Educators provide services equitably to all people.

Article II: Responsibility to the Profession

Health Educators are responsible for their professional behavior, for the reputation of their profession, and for promoting ethical conduct among their colleagues.

Section 1: Health Educators maintain, improve, and expand their professional competence through continued study and education; membership, participation, and leadership in professional organizations; and involvement in issues related to the health of the public.

Section 2: Health Educators model and encourage nondiscriminatory standards of behavior in their interactions with others.

Section 3: Health Educators encourage and accept responsible critical discourse to protect and enhance the profession.

Section 4: Health Educators contribute to the development of the profession by sharing the processes and outcomes of their work.

Section 5: Health Educators are aware of possible professional conflicts of interest, exercise integrity in conflict situations, and do not manipulate or violate the rights of others.

Section 6: Health Educators give appropriate recognition to others for their professional contributions and achievements.

Article III: Responsibility to Employers

Health Educators recognize the boundaries of their professional competence and are accountable for their professional activities and actions.

Section 1: Health Educators accurately represent their qualifications and the qualifications of others whom they recommend.

Section 2: Health Educators use appropriate standards, theories, and guidelines as criteria when carrying out their professional responsibilities.

Section 3: Health Educators accurately represent potential service and program outcomes to employers.

Section 4: Health Educators anticipate and disclose competing commitments, conflicts of interest, and endorsement of products.

Section 5: Health Educators openly communicate to employers expectations of job-related assignments that conflict with their professional ethics.

Section 6: Health Educators maintain competence in their areas of professional practice.

Article IV: Responsibility in the Delivery of Health Education

Health Educators promote integrity in the delivery of health education. They respect the rights, dignity, confidentiality, and worth of all people by adapting strategies and methods to the needs of diverse populations and communities.

Section 1: Health Educators are sensitive to social and cultural diversity and are in accord with the law, when planning and implementing programs.

Section 2: Health Educators are informed of the latest advances in theory, research, and practice, and use strategies and methods that are grounded in and contribute to development of professional standards, theories, guidelines, statistics, and experience.

Section 3: Health Educators are committed to rigorous evaluation of both program effectiveness and the methods used to achieve results.

Section 4: Health Educators empower individuals to adopt healthy lifestyles through informed choice rather than by coercion or intimidation.

Section 5: Health Educators communicate the potential outcomes of proposed services, strategies, and pending decisions to all individuals who will be affected.

Article V: Responsibility in Research and Evaluation

Health Educators contribute to the health of the population and to the profession through research and evaluation activities. When planning and conducting research or evaluation, health educators do so in accordance with federal and state laws and regulations, organizational and institutional policies, and professional standards.

Section 1: Health Educators support principles and practices of research and evaluation that do no harm to individuals, groups, society, or the environment.

Section 2: Health Educators ensure that participation in research is voluntary and is based upon the informed consent of the participants.

Section 3: Health Educators respect the privacy, rights, and dignity of research participants, and honor commitments made to those participants.

Section 4: Health Educators treat all information obtained from participants as confidential unless otherwise required by law.

Section 5: Health Educators take credit, including authorship, only for work they have actually performed and give credit to the contributions of others.

Section 6: Health Educators who serve as research or evaluation consultants discuss their results only with those to whom they are providing service, unless maintaining such confidentiality would jeopardize the health or safety of others.

Section 7: Health Educators report the results of their research and evaluation objectively, accurately, and in a timely fashion.

Article VI: Responsibility in Professional Preparation

Those involved in the preparation and training of Health Educators have an obligation to accord learners the same respect and treatment given other groups by providing quality education that benefits the profession and the public.

Section 1: Health Educators select students for professional preparation programs based upon equal opportunity for all, and the individual's academic performance, abilities, and potential contribution to the profession and the public's health.

Section 2: Health Educators strive to make the educational environment and culture conducive to the health of all involved, and free from sexual harassment and all forms of discrimination.

Section 3: Health Educators involved in professional preparation and professional development engage in careful preparation; present material that is accurate, up-to-date, and timely; provide reasonable and timely feedback; state clear and reasonable expectations; and conduct fair assessments and evaluations of learners.

Section 4: Health Educators provide objective and accurate counseling to learners about career opportunities, development, and advancement, and assist learners to secure professional employment.

Section 5: Health Educators provide adequate supervision and meaningful opportunities for the professional development of learners.

(Adopted by the Coalition of National Health Education Organizations, November 1999.)

The American Public Health Association, Public Health Leadership Society, has developed a "Principles of Ethical Practices of Public Health," which is available at the APHA website: http://www.apha.org/NR/rdonlyres/1CED3CEA-287E-4185-9CBD-BD405FC60856/0/ethics brochure.pdf

They also have a new journal, *Public Health Ethics*, that started in 2009.

Professional Organizations

Organization	Publication	Address	Abbreviation	Approximate Membership
American Alliance for Health, Physical Education, Recreation and Dance	Umbrella organization includes AAHE	1900 Association Dr. Reston, VA 22091 (703) 476-3404 membshp@aahperd.org http://www.aahperd.org	AAHPERD	23,000
American Association for Health Education	*Journal of Health Education*	1900 Association Dr. Reston, VA 22091 (703) 476-3437 aahe@aahperd.org http://www.aahperd.org	AAHE	10,000
American College Health Association	*Journal of American College Health*	P.O. Box 28937 Baltimore, MD 21240 (410) 859-1500 acha@access.digex.net http://www.acha.org	ACHA	3,000
American Public Health Association	*American Journal of Public Health* Umbrella organizations include PHES and SHES	800 I St. NW Washington, DC 20005 (202) 777-2742 comments@msmail.apha.org http://www.apha.org	APHA	50,000
APHA–Public Health Education Section	Newsletter	800 I St. NW Washington, DC 20005 (202) 777-2742	PHES	
APHA–School Health Education and Services Section	Newsletter	800 I St. NW Washington, DC 20005	SHES	
American School Health Association	*Journal of School Health*	7263 Route 43 P.O. Box 708 Kent, OH 44240 (330) 678-1601 asha@ashaweb.org http://www.ashaweb.org	ASHA	2,000
Eta Sigma Gamma	*The Gamman*	2000 University Ave. Ball State University Muncie, IN 47306 (800) 715-2559 ESG@etasigmagamma.org http://www.etasigmagamma .org		3,000

Organization	Publication	Address	Abbreviation	Approximate Membership
National Commission for Health Education Credentialing, Inc.	Newsletter	1514 Alta Drive Suite 303 Whitehall, PA 18052-5642 (888) 624-3248 http://www.nchec.org	The Commission	Membership through examination
Society for Public Health Education	*Health Education Quarterly*	10 G Street, NE Suite 605 Washington, DC 20002-4242 (202) 408-9804 info@sophe.org http://www.sophe.org	SOPHE	4,000

Glossary

Entry-Level and Advanced 1 Health Educator Competencies Addressed in This Glossary

Area VI: Serve as a Health Education Resource Person
Competency A: Use health-related information resources.
Competency B: Respond to requests for health information.
Competency C: Select resource materials for dissemination.
Competency D: Establish consultative relationships.

> Note: The competencies listed above are considered both entry-level and Advanced 1 competencies by the National Commission for Health Education Credentialing, Inc. They are taken from *A Framework for the Development of Competency-Based Curricula for Entry Level Health Educators* by the National Task Force on the Preparation and Practice of Health Educators, Inc., 1985; and *A Competency-Based Framework for Health Educators— The Competencies Update Project (CUP)*, 2006.

Method Selection in Health Education

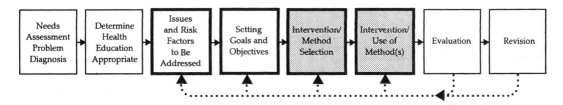

Heavy-bordered boxes indicate subjects addressed in this text; shaded boxes indicate subject(s) of current chapter.

American Sign Language The native language of most culturally deaf Americans, this is a visually based language that bears little relationship to English, particularly in grammar and syntax.

Attention deficit disorder (ADD) A condition characterized by hyperactivity, the inability to concentrate, and impulsive or inappropriate behavior.

Behavioral capability Individual possesses the knowledge and skill to perform a behavior.

Blindisms Movements, often of the head and upper body of a blind individual, thought to result from a deprivation of visual stimulation.

Block plan Used by educators to describe the organizing of educational activities into "blocks" of time. They are presented as sequential "blocks" with only minimal description. The details are found in the methods section of a unit plan.

Case study Practical inquiry that investigates a phenomenon within its real-life context.

CD-ROM Compact disk read-only memory.

Certified Health Education Specialist (CHES) An individual who is credentialed as a result of demonstrating competency based on criteria established by the National Commission for Health Education Credentialing, Inc. (NCHEC) (1990 Joint Committee on Health Education Terminology).

Community health education The application of a variety of methods that result in the education and mobilization of community members in actions for resolving health issues and problems that affect the community. These methods include, but are not limited to group process, mass media, communication, community organization, organization development, strategic planning, skills training, legislation, policy making, and advocacy (1990 Joint Committee on Health Education Terminology).

Community health educator A practitioner professionally prepared in the field of community/public health education who demonstrates competence in the planning, implementation, and evaluation of a broad range of health-promoting or health-enhancing programs for community groups (1990 Joint Committee on Health Education Terminology).

Comprehensive school health program The development, delivery, and evaluation of a planned curriculum, preschool through grade 12, with goals, objectives, content sequence, and specific classroom lessons. It includes, but is not limited to, the following major content areas:
Community health
Consumer health
Environmental health
Family life
Mental and emotional health
Injury prevention and safety
Nutrition
Personal health
Prevention and control of disease
Substance use and abuse
(1990 Joint Committee on Health Education Terminology)

Concepts General principles that make up constructs.

Construct A representation of a concept within a theoretical framework (Green & Kreuter, 2005).

Contact time The time spent with a target group as part of a health education intervention.

Cooperative learning Broad category of learning experiences that center on learning from fellow participants.

Cultural competency An attempt to optimize the likelihood that individuals from all cultures, ethnicities, and races will receive appropriate and sensitive health care.

Curriculum A planned set of lessons or courses designed to lead to competence in an area of study.

Deaf A hearing impairment so severe that an individual is impaired in processing linguistic information through hearing (*Federal Register*, 1977).

Deaf-blindness An impairment caused by a combination of hearing and visual impediments.

Debates Organized discussions of differing points of view.

Demographics Information such as ages, ethnicity, gender, and other characteristics that describe a population and may impact objectives and method selection.

Development delay Occurs when children ages 4–9 experience a disability related to the growth process in one or more of the following areas of maturity: physical, cognitive, communication, social, or emotional.

Diffusion The process of making innovations/methods available and understandable to practicing health educators.

Disability A total or partial behavioral, mental, physical, or sensorial loss of functioning (Mandell & Fiscus, 1981).

Distance learning Includes opportunities to connect learners separated by place or time from the instructor with educational resources.

DVD Digitized video disc or digital versatile disc.

Dyslexia A learning disability that impairs the ability to accurately process information from a variety of sources, including visual notation, speech, written language, and writing systems.

Emotional disability Impairments that adversely affect the educational performance at a significant level over extended periods of time.

Exceptional A label usually associated with an individual whose performance is atypical and often deviates from what is expected. The performance could be superior or inferior to what is expected (Mandell & Fiscus, 1981).

Expectancy As applied to social learning theory, the value an individual places on a particular outcome.

Facilitator The leader or teacher of a method or strategy.

Failure cycle Common among children with learning disabilities. A child fails to master a skill and consequently avoids the activity, guaranteeing that he or she will never achieve competency.

Family life Also known as family living, human sexuality, or sex education. Scope and depth of information can vary in the extreme, according to the specific situation.

Fidelity The degree to which a lesson, program, or curriculum is implemented according to the original intention of the developers.

Field trip Expedition taken by a group of people to a place away from their normal educational environment.

Flame A message written to irritate the recipient.

Gatekeepers Used to describe the key leaders in a community who either get things done, allow things to get done, or prevent action.

Goal A broad statement of direction used to present the overall intent of a program or course. Unlike an objective, it does not need to be stated in measurable terms.

Guided imagery A mental journey led by a guide or leader in person or on tape. Often used in stress management and in seeking behavior change.

Handicap Environmental restrictions placed on a person's life as a result of a disability or exceptionality (Mandell & Fiscus, 1981).

Hard of hearing A hearing impairment, either permanent or fluctuating, that adversely affects an individual's educational performance (*Federal Register*, 1977).

Health advising A process of informing and assisting individuals or groups in making decisions and solving problems related to health (1990 Joint Committee on Health Education Terminology).

Health education (1) A discipline dedicated to the improvement of the health status of individuals and the community. (2) The process of favorably and voluntarily influencing the health behavior of others.

Health education administrator A professional health educator who has the authority and responsibility for the management and coordination of all health education policies, activities, and resources within a particular setting or circumstance (1990 Joint Committee on Health Education Terminology).

Health education coordinator A professional health educator who is responsible for the management and coordination of all health education policies, activities, and resources within a particular setting or circumstance (1990 Joint Committee on Health Education Terminology).

Health education field The multidisciplinary practice concerned with designing, implementing, and evaluating educational programs that enable individuals, families, groups, organizations, and communities to play active roles in achieving, protecting, and sustaining health (1990 Joint Committee on Health Education Terminology).

Health education process The continuum of learning that enables people, as individuals and as members of social structures, to voluntarily make decisions, modify behaviors, and change social conditions in ways that are health enhancing.

Health education program A planned combination of activities developed with the involvement of specific populations and based on a needs assessment, sound principles of educa-

tion, and periodic evaluation using a clear set of goals and objectives (1990 Joint Committee on Health Education Terminology).

Health educator A practitioner professionally prepared in the field of health education who demonstrates competence in both theory and practice, and who accepts responsibility to advance the aims of the health education profession (1990 Joint Committee on Health Education Terminology).

Health information The content of communications based on data derived from systematic and scientific methods as they relate to health issues, policies, programs, services, and other aspects of individual and public health, which can be used for informing various populations and for planning health education activities (1990 Joint Committee on Health Education Terminology).

Health literacy The degree to which individuals have the capacity to obtain, process, and understand basic health information and services needed to make appropriate health decisions

Health promotion and disease prevention The aggregate of all purposeful activities designed to improve personal and public health through a combination of strategies, including the competent implementation of behavioral change strategies, health education, health protection measures, risk factor detection, health enhancement, and health maintenance (1990 Joint Committee on Health Education Terminology).

Healthy lifestyle A set of health-enhancing behaviors shaped by internal consistent values, attitudes, and beliefs and external social and cultural forces (1990 Joint Committee on Health Education Terminology).

Hearing impairment Limitations in the ability to interpret sound, which are not included under the definition of deafness, that adversely affect educational performance.

Hispanic A classification of national background. A Hispanic person may be from any ethnic group.

Impairment Refers to an abnormality in the function of the organs or systems.

Implementation The carrying out of or operationalizing of a plan of action.

Innovation An educational tool or method perceived as being new to potential users.

Intervention The total overall strategy to achieve objectives.

Learning disabled Deficits in the brain's ability to process information, which adversely affects educational performance.

Lesson/presentation plan The organized plan for a presentation.

Locus of control Expectations of reinforcement. The sense of whether or not a person feels in control of their life. Often characterized as external—under the control of outside forces—or internal—under the individual's personal control.

Long-range goals The very broad outcome intentions for the unit. These are optimal behaviors the educator hopes to achieve; they need not be easily measurable.

Mass media Media capable of reaching large audiences. Television and national magazines are examples.

Mental retardation Includes significantly subaverage general intellectual functioning existing concurrently with deficits in adaptive behavior and manifesting during the developmental period, which adversely affects educational performance.

Method One component of the intervention such as an educational game or a health fair. We use the term interchangeably with strategy.

Model Combination of a number of theories to assist health educators understand their specific challenges in a given setting or context (Glanz, Rimer, & Lewis, 2002).

Multiple disabilities Include concomitant impairments (such as mental retardation-blindness and mental retardation-orthopedic impairment), the combination of which causes such severe educational needs that cannot be accommodated in special education programs solely for one on the impairments. Multiple disabilities do not included deaf-blindness.

Needs assessment Formal and informal strategies to determine the needs of the target population.

Normative belief *See* Subjective norm.

Objective A precise statement of intended outcome; it must be stated in measurable terms.

Official health agency A publicly supported government organization mandated by public law and/or regulation for the protection and improvement of the health of the public.

Orthopedic impairment Includes a severe orthopedic impairment that adversely affects a child's educational performance.

Other health impairment Limited strength, vitality, or alertness, including a heightened alertness to environmental stimuli, that results in limited alertness with respect to the educational environment and adversely affects a child's educational performance.

Panel Several people who are invited to speak together on a topic. They may be selected due to expertise, political reasons, or as representatives.

Pedagogy The art and science of teaching.

Peer education Tutoring provided by a person of similar status to the person being tutored.

Performance indicator Quantifiable or qualitative activities that function to measure the accomplishment of the stated objective.

Postlingual deafness Deafness that occurs after spoken language has been developed.

Postsecondary health education program A planned set of health education policies, procedures, activities, and services that are directed to students, faculty, and/or staff of colleges, universities, and other higher education institutions. This includes, but is not limited to:

General health courses for students

Employee and student health promotion activities

Health services

Professional preparation of health educators and other professionals

Self-help groups

Student life

(1990 Joint Committee on Health Education Terminology)

Prelingual deafness Deafness that occurs before spoken language skills have been developed.

Private health agency A profit or nonprofit organization devoted to providing primary, secondary, and/or tertiary health services, which may include health education (1990 Joint Committee on Health Education Terminology).

Problem–solution technique A discussion technique in which a scenario is provided with discussion items of possible contributing factors. It is deliberately set up to cause disagreement and related discussion.

Process objective Mechanism to assess the quality of the implementation of a method.

Public doman Materials considered "public or intellectual property" because they are not owned or controlled by anyone.

Role play Consciously acting out behavior changes to represent an assigned role.

School health education One component of the comprehensive school health program, which includes the development, delivery, and evaluation of a planned instructional program and other activities for students preschool through grade 12, for parents, and for school staff. It is designed to influence positively the health knowledge, attitudes, and skills of individuals (1990 Joint Committee on Health Education Terminology).

School health educator A practitioner who is professionally prepared in the field of school health education; meets state teaching requirements; and has demonstrated competence in the development, delivery, and evaluation of curricula for students and adults in the school setting that enhance health knowledge, attitudes, and problem-solving skills (1990 Joint Committee on Health Education Terminology).

School health services That part of the school health program provided by physicians, nurses, dentists, health educators, other allied health personnel, social workers, teachers, and others to appraise, protect, and promote the health of students and school personnel. These services are designed to ensure access to and appropriate use of primary healthcare services, prevent and control communicable disease, provide emergency care for injury or sudden illness, promote and provide optimum sanitary conditions in a safe school facility and environment, and provide concurrent learning opportunities that are conducive to the maintenance and promotion of individual and community health (1990 Joint Committee on Health Education Terminology).

Self-appraisal A tool that allows individuals to identify strengths and weaknesses through personal assessment.

Self-contained objective Statement that designates the specific behaviors the target audience must demonstrate to indicate learning has occurred. Self-contained objectives are also called behavioral objectives.

Self-efficacy Belief or expectation by an individual that he or she can carry out the desired behavior.

Service learning Offering or requiring hours of service for students either for academic credit or as part of some other requirement such as a general graduation requirement.

Sex educator An individual who teaches about human sexuality. Although professional certification can be obtained through AASECT (American Association of Sex Educators, Counselors and Therapists), many individuals may have little or no training.

Simulation A contrived experience used to expose someone to a certain prescribed set of circumstances based on a model. It has the appearance of some real-life phenomenon.

Social cognitive theory Social learning theory.

Specific learning disability Disorder in one or more of the basic psychological processes involved in understanding or in using language (spoken or written) that may manifest itself in the imperfect ability to listen, think, speak, read, write, spell, or to do mathematical calculations, including conditions such as perceptual disabilities, brain injury, minimal brain dysfunction, dyslexia, and developmental aphasia.

Speech language impairment A communication disorder, such as stuttering, impaired articulation, a language or a voice impairment, that adversely affects educational performance.

Strategy One component of the intervention such as an educational game or a health fair. We use the term interchangeably with method.

Subjective norm The norm or social standard set by the common practice of a group. Example: bell bottom pants become the most common pants in school due to the establishment of a subjective norm. Sometimes referred to as normative belief.

Target population The population for whom we are targeting our health education intervention.

Theory (health) The presentation of a system to explain and predict health behaviors given identified variables.

Transfer learning The ability of an individual to apply learning in one context to another context that shares similar characteristics.

Traumatic brain injury An acquired injury to the brain caused by an external physical force resulting in total or partial functional disability or psychosocial impairment, or both, that advrsely affects educational performance.

Two-committee system A system designed to minimize complaint and maximize community involvement when developing materials and programs that might be viewed as controversial.

Unit plan An orderly self-contained collection of activities designed to meet a set of given objectives.

URL Uniform resource locator, an Internet site address.

Value clarification As the name implies, a method designed to help people clarify how they feel about issues and how they reach decisions.

Visual impairment including blindness Impairments in vision that—even with correction—adversely affect educational performance.

Visually impaired Individuals who have defective or impaired vision. Definitions of impairment or blindness can be either legally or educationally based (Meyen, 1978).

Voluntary health organization A nonprofit association supported by contributions dedicated to conducting research and providing education and/or services related to particular health problems or concerns (1990 Joint Committee on Health Education Terminology).

REFERENCES

Federal Register (Part IV). (1977). Washington, DC: Department of Health, Education, and Welfare, 163, 42.

Green, L., & Kreuter, M. (2005). *Health Program Planning: An Ecological Approach* (4th ed.). New York: McGraw-Hill.

Glanz, K., Rimer, B. K., & Lewis, F. M. (Eds.). (2002). *Health Behavior and Health Education* (3rd ed.). San Francisco, CA: Jossey-Bass.

Mandell, C. J., & Fiscus, E. (1981). *Understanding Exceptional People*. St. Paul, MN: West.

Meyen, E. L. (1978). *Exceptional Children and Youth*. Denver: Love.

Report of the 1990 Joint Committee on Health Education Terminology. (1991). *Journal of Health Education, 22*(2).

Index

A

ABCD&E formula, objectives, 32–34
abstinence education, 367–372
abstracts, citation for, 231
abstract thinking, 337
access to health care, 295
accreditation, 6
accuracy, Internet resources, 228
action, taking, 60
action alert, citation for, 231
ADD (attention deficit disorder), 338–339
ADHD (attention deficit hyperactivity disorder), 338–339
Addiction Research Foundation (ARF), 255
administrative assessment, 52
adult learners, 72–73
advance organizers, 338
advertising, Internet resources, 228–229
advisory committee, 392
affective domain, 34–35
African Americans. *See* minority groups
age, 17–18
AIDS, 300–303, 361–362, 377, 392–393
Ajzen, Icek, 50, 60
alcohol abuse programs, 152–153, 359, 363
American Alliance for Health, Physical Education,

Recreation and Dance (AAHPERD), 4, 408
American Association for Health and Physical Education, 4, 408
American Association for Health Education, 4
American Association of Health Education (AAHE), 243
American Association of School Physicians, 4
American Association of Sex Educators, Counselors, and Therapists (AASECT), 381–382
American College Health Association, 408
American Family Life Act, 379
American Psychological Association (APA), *Publication Manual*, 230–231
American Public Health Association, 4, 408
American School Health Association, 4
American Sign Language (ASL), 343
"An Analysis Checklist for Audiovisuals," 256
anxiety, 64
appropriateness, 77
artistic expressions, 234
Asians. *See* minority groups
assumptions, avoiding, 390–391
attention, deaf audience, 351

Photo Credits

Chapter 1
1-1 Courtesy of Thomas Hanna, School Health Educator; 1-2 Courtesy of Thomas Hanna, School Health Educator

Chapter 2
Page 19 © Monkey Business Images/Dreamstime .com; 2-3 Courtesy of Thomas Hanna, School Health Educator; 2-4 Courtesy of Thomas Hanna, School Health Educator; 2-5 Courtesy of Thomas Hanna, School Health Educator; **page 28** © Dusan Jankovic/ShutterStock, Inc.; 2-7 Courtesy of Thomas Hanna, School Health Educator; **page 43** © Dmitriy Shironosov/Dreamstime.com

Chapter 3
3-6 Courtesy of Thomas Hanna, School Health Educator; **page 73** © Monkey Business Images/ShutterStock, Inc.; 3-8 Courtesy of Thomas Hanna, School Health Educator; **page 76** © Monkey Business Images/ Dreamstime .com; **page 80** © Photos.com

Chapter 4
Page 102 © Avava/ShutterStock, Inc.; **page 109** © Lisa F. Young/ShutterStock, Inc.; 4-2 Courtesy of Thomas Hanna, School Health Educator; **page 113** © Monkey Business Images/ Dreamstime.com; **page 117** © Donna McWilliam/ AP Photos; **page 119** © Photodisc; **page 120** Courtesy of Thomas Hanna, School Health Educator; **page 128** © Rob Marmion/ShutterStock, Inc.; **page 136** © Natallia Khlapushyna/Dreamstime.com; **page 145** © Pryzmat/ Dreamstime.com; **page 152** © Yuri Arcurs/ShutterStock, Inc.; **page 157** © originalpunkt/ ShutterStock, Inc.; 4-21 Courtesy of Thomas Hanna, School Health Educator

Chapter 5
Page 187 © Dmitriy Shironosov/ShutterStock, Inc.; 5-1 Courtesy of Thomas Hanna, School Health Educator; **page 192** Courtesy of Thomas Hanna, School Health Educator; **page 202** Courtesy of Chief Mass Communication Specialist Don Bray/U.S. Navy

Chapter 6
Page 225 Courtesy of Federal Trade Commission; **page 230** Courtesy of CDC; **page 236** © Lee Morris/ShutterStock, Inc.; 6-3 Courtesy of Thomas Hanna, School Health Educator

Chapter 7
Page 254 © Jason Stitt/Dreamstime.com; **page 266** © Eky Chan/ShutterStock, Inc.; **page 268** Courtesy of SMART Technologies ULC; **page 270** Courtesy of SMART Technologies ULC; **page 274** Courtesy of Thomas Hanna, School Health Educator

Chapter 8
Page 289 © Christopher Futcher/ShutterStock, Inc.; **page 295** © Monkey Business Images/Dreamstime.com; **page 297** © Monkey Business Images/ ShutterStock, Inc.; **page 299** © Anette Romanenko/Dreamstime.com; **page 301** © Jonathan Nourok/PhotoEdit, Inc.; **page 304** © Mike_kiev/Dreamstime .com; 8-6 Courtesy of Thomas Hanna, School Health Educator; **page 314** © Greg Gibson/AP Photos

Chapter 9
Page 325 © Marcin Okupniak/Dreamstime.com; **page 332** © Rick's Photography/ShutterStock, Inc.; **page 336** © PhotoCreate/ShutterStock, Inc.; 9.3-A Courtesy of Thomas Hanna, School Health Educator; **page 344** © David Young-Wolff/PhotoEdit Inc.

Chapter 10
Page 365 © Kathy Wynn/Dreamstime.com; **page 367** Courtesy of Thomas Hanna, School Health Educator; **page 368** © Rogelio V. Solis/AP Photos; **page 371** © Patrick Breig/ ShutterStock, Inc.; **page 374** © Michael Newman/PhotoEdit, Inc.; 10-4 Courtesy of Thomas Hanna, School Health Educator

Unless otherwise indicated, all photographs and illustrations are under copyright of Jones and Bartlett Publishers, LLC, or have been provided by the authors.